Diseases of the Nose, Throat and Ear

I. SIMSON HALL MB, ChB, FRCPEd, FRCSEd

Consulting Surgeon, the Royal Infirmary, Edinburgh (Department for Diseases of Nose, Throat and Ear)
Lecturer Emeritus in Diseases of Nose, Throat and Ear, University of Edinburgh

BERNARD H. COLMAN MA, BSc, ChM, FRCSEd

Senior Surgeon, Department of Otolaryngology, The Radcliffe Infirmary, Oxford
Clinical Lecturer in Otolaryngology, University of Oxford

Diseases of the Nose, Throat and Ear

A Handbook for Students and Practitioners

I. SIMSON HALL
BERNARD H. COLMAN

ELEVENTH EDITION

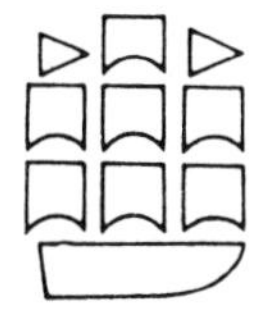

CHURCHILL LIVINGSTONE
Edinburgh London and New York 1975

Churchill Livingstone
Medical Division of Longman Group Limited

Distributed in the United States of America by Longman Inc., 19 West 44th Street, New York N.Y. 10036 and by associated companies, branches and representative throughout the world.

First Edition	1937
Second Edition	1941
Third Edition	1944
Reprinted	1946
Fourth Edition	1948
Reprinted	1949
Fifth Edition	1952
Sixth Edition	1956
Seventh Edition	1959
Reprinted	1962
Eighth Edition	1967
Ninth Edition	1969
Reprinted	1971
Tenth Edition	1973
Eleventh Edition	1975
Reprinted	1977

ISBN 0 443 01313 6

Library of Congress Cataloging in Publication Data
Hall, Ion Simson.
Diseases of the nose, throat and ear.
Includes index.
1. Otolaryngology. I. Colman, Bernard Harold, joint author. II. Title. [DNLM: 1. Otorhinolaryngologic diseases. WV100 H176d]
RF46.H2 1975 616.2 1 75-13874

Printed in Singapore by
Huntsmen Offset Printing Pte Ltd

Preface to the Eleventh Edition

The necessity for another Edition has given the Authors the chance to revise the text and to reflect in it such changes as have taken place since the publication of the 10th Edition.

Descriptions of some diseases, now rarely seen here, have been retained as they are still comparatively common in some countries in which this book is used.

The format has been changed and it is hoped that the new style will render the book more convenient to handle.

The Authors wish to thank the publishers for their continued co-operation in these most difficult times. They would also like to thank Mr Floyd and his Staff in the Department of Medical Illustration of the Radcliffe Infirmary, Oxford, for assistance with the illustrations.

I. SIMSON HALL
BERNARD H. COLMAN

EDINBURGH 1975

Preface to the First Edition

The experience of some years in general practice convinces me that a sufficient knowledge of diseases of the Nose, Throat and Ear is an essential part of the equipment of a medical practitioner. The work of later years, in a busy outpatient department and amongst students, has emphasized that view.

This volume is the result of that conviction and, being designed to meet the needs of the busy practitioner and the student, it is strictly limited in its aim. No attempt is made to describe in elaborate detail diseases of the Nose, Throat and Ear which the student and practitioner, for lack of training, might fail to recognize. For the same reason there must be obvious omissions, but that is balanced by a fuller discussion of the commoner complaints.

In many instances operations are merely mentioned, but particular stress has been laid upon minor technical procedures. Such guidance as it gives is based upon lectures delivered to graduates and students in the course of ordinary teaching in which I am engaged in the Royal Infirmary, Edinburgh, and in certain circumstances, for the sake of emphasis, the direct style is retained.

A short anatomical description precedes each section. This is designed to recall the main features of the part under discussion, and the student is expected to refer to larger works where fuller description is desired.

My thanks are due to the sympathy and opportunity afforded me at all times by my recent chief, Mr Lithgow, and I gratefully acknowledge my debt to Dr A. Brownlie Smith, who has read the manuscript and offered much helpful criticism. The illustrations have been taken from material supplied by the author and from specimens in the Museum of the Royal College of Surgeons of Edinburgh.

EDINBURGH
March, 1937

I. SIMSON HALL

Contents

SECTION III THE PHARYNX

SECTION IV THE LARYNX

SECTION V ENDOSCOPY

SECTION VI THE EAR

INTRODUCTION

Examination Equipment

The equipment required for diagnosis in this speciality is simple. A source of light and a means of projecting that light to the object under examination are all that are needed. It is important that the light should be projected in such a way as to cause no interference with vision.

Illuminants. Usually the light is reflected by means of a mirror on to the part under examination. Daylight may be used, lamps of various kinds or even candles where necessity arises. Naturally, at the present day electricity forms the chief and favourite source of light. Where a universal supply is not available, electricity can be carried in storage or battery form, to supply a head-light worn on the forehead. It is essential that this light can be focussed.

The mirror usually takes the form of a concave 'forehead mirror'. It is a circular mirror of approximately 4 inches in diameter, with a hole in the centre. The mirror is of a definite focal length, the optimum being 8 inches. The hole in the mirror is important. It should be sufficiently large to render minute adjustment unnecessary, and the distance from the outer edge of the mirror to the edge of the hole in the centre of the mirror should not be greater than the distance between the wearer's eyes. The principle is that the examiner looks along the beam of light, the line of sight being parallel to the rays. In this way a very small spot of light can be focussed into deep and narrow cavities.

One of the chief reasons for difficulty in these examinations is that parts of the nose and ear can be seen by one eye only at a time. Stereoscopic vision, upon which we depend for our appreciation of depth, is impossible, and considerable practice is required before the same facility is acquired with one eye only.

To aid examination certain simple instruments are required (Fig. 1). As a rule a *speculum* is used for examining the nose. One of the simplest forms of these is Thudichum's speculum. This consists of a U-shaped spring with nasal plates at the ends. *Tongue depressors* are many and various. One of the simplest is known as Lack's spatula. *Ear specula* may be plain funnels of polished metal, and are to be had in varying sizes, so that the difference in size between a child's external auditory meatus and that of an adult can be met by the appropriate speculum (Fig. 1). Magnification of the drum is now common practice, either by fitting a lens to the speculum or by using an operating microscope or otoscope. Aspiration is sometimes employed as an aid to diagnosis, and a speculum can be fitted with a window so that the speculum may be

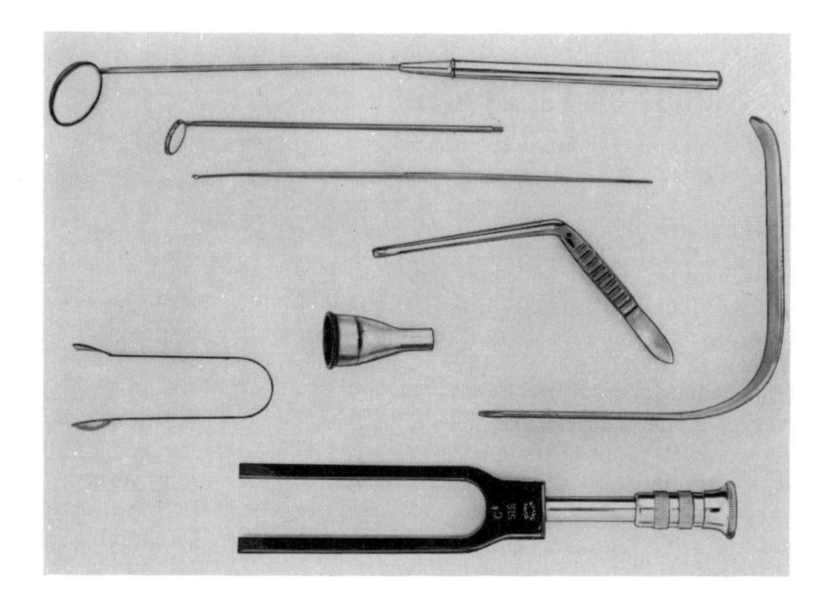

Fig. 1. Instruments used in examination. The basic needs are simple consisting of specula for nose and ear (several sizes), tongue depressor, wax curette, angled forceps, nasopharyngeal and laryngeal mirrors and a tuning fork (preferably 512 c.p.s.).

made air-tight in the external meatus. A rubber bulb can then be attached to the speculum so that suction or pressure may be applied to the drum. Estimation of mobility of the membrane can be a valuable aid to diagnosis of middle ear changes.

INDIRECT EXAMINATION

In cavities, such as the laryngopharynx, pharynx and nasopharynx, examination is carried out by the projection of light by means of a small mirror. Mirrors are of various sizes, from a very small one of approximately one-third of an inch in diameter up to large ones of 2 inches or more in diameter. These mirrors are used to direct the light into the nasopharynx, behind the soft palate, and also to throw the light downwards on to the larynx in what is known as *indirect laryngoscopy*.

ELECTRICAL AIDS TO DIAGNOSIS

Description of the instruments used for diagnosis would be incomplete without reference to the electrically illuminated instruments which have been invented with the object of rendering the examiner independent of outside sources of illumination. The object of these is to provide in one small portable outfit a reliable means of arriving at a diagnosis under all circumstances.

For the practitioner who may be called upon to carry out these examinations at any time, such outfits are of great value on his rounds and owing to their compactness can find a place in his bag. The great disadvantage of these instruments, however, is that they are often of fixed focus so that in certain circumstances, notably in the case of the ear, accuracy of observation is seriously reduced. In general practice a forehead light fed from a battery carried in the pocket is undoubtedly convenient and allows both hands to be free to examine the ear, nose and throat. Electric auriscopes have done much to simplify examination of the ear and although frequently used have definite limitations. Electrically illuminated spatulae and other devices are less satisfactory.

METHODS OF USE OF INSTRUMENTS

Position of patient and examiner. The patient is seated in a chair, and the source of light is placed above and behind the patient's left shoulder. The examiner sits in front of the patient, or at his left side. Should the examiner be left-handed and prefer to use the mirror over the left eye, then the light and the examiner must be on the patient's right. A rotating chair is a valuable aid when examining elderly patients as they find it difficult to turn in a fixed chair for examination of both ears. It is simpler, therefore, to rotate the chair than to have the examiner change his position (Fig. 2).

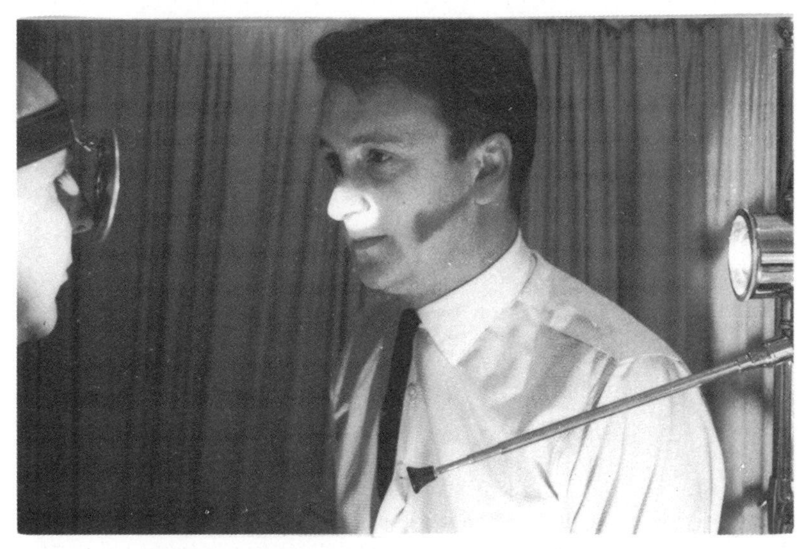

Fig. 2. Positioning is important. The patient sits squarely facing the examiner and leans slightly forwards whilst the beam is focussed. The lamp is near to his left shoulder.

Focussing the light. Before commencing the examination of the patient, it is essential that practice is obtained in focussing the light. The examiner closes his eyes to avoid being dazzled by the lamp which he adjusts until it shines directly into his own eyes. He next brings his head mirror down over his right eye and opens his eyes. The examiner should be looking directly through the hole in the mirror with the right eye and round its edge with his left eye. The light will generally be reflected on to a fairly small area of the patient's face and by varying the position of the patient slightly (usually by bringing him a little forward) the beam will be brought to focus on the part to be examined. This gives bright illumination and by slightly tipping the head mirror the light can be brought exactly to the part required.

It will readily be appreciated that in examining a nose which has a depth of possibly 3 inches or more, it is necessary for the examiner to

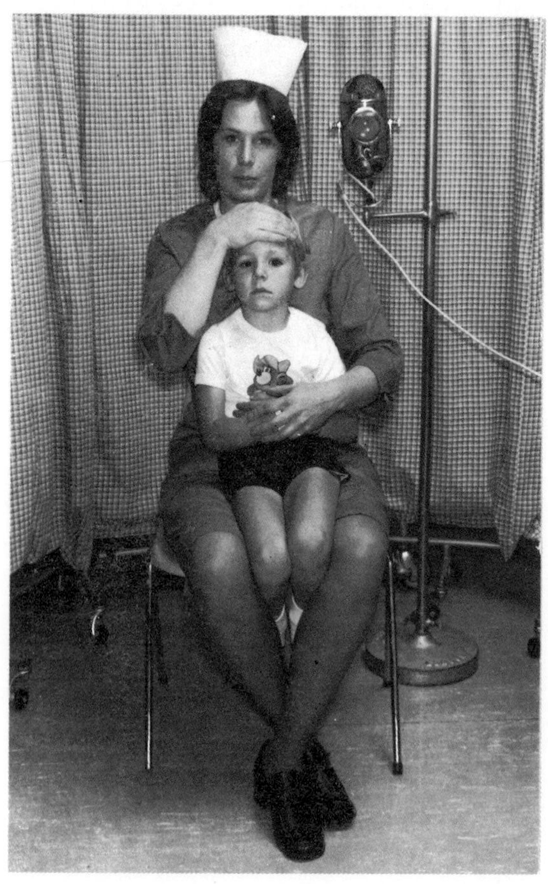

Fig. 3. Control of the fractious child. By this method the child is firmly but gently held.

move either his head or the patient's head as the examination proceeds from the outer part of the nose to the inner part, in order that his light may be kept correctly focussed. It is the failure to appreciate the fact that the light must be moved so that it may be thrown on to each part in succession which causes a great deal of difficulty in the examination of these cavities.

EXAMINATION OF CHILDREN

The successful examination of children requires practice and experience. The confidence of the child in the examiner is essential to success, if the examination is to be carried out without serious disturbance. It will often be found that it is easier and more effective to dispense with the use of instruments, for often the nose of a child can be examined more satisfactorily without the aid of a speculum. The ear can usually be thoroughly examined without an ear speculum and the examiner's finger will sometimes be found to be more sensitive and easily tolerated than the metal spatula. It should be possible for the doctor to examine the average child of three or four years in this way, provided the child is not unusually nervous or refractory.

A useful method of holding the child where resistance is encountered is illustrated (Fig. 3).

SECTION I THE NOSE

1. Anatomy of the Nose

The external nose is a structure composed of bone and cartilage. The bony part is formed mainly by the nasal bone on each side, and the frontal process of the maxillary bone. The cartilaginous portion is formed by several cartilages which support and give shape to the nares. Attached to the cartilages are the muscles for dilating the nares.

The nose is a cavity within the skull having its axis at right angles to the face. It is important to remember this fact in examination of the nose, since it is a common misconception that the nasal axis is parallel to the line of the external nasal structure. The nasal cavity is divided by the nasal septum into two parts which have similar anatomical structure but may be asymmetrical.

The *septum* is a structure composed partly of cartilage and partly of bone. Anteriorly, the septum is formed by the quadrilateral cartilage. Posterior to this is the vertical plate of the ethmoid; while behind that again, the rostrum of the sphenoid bone helps to form the partition. Below, the quadrilateral cartilage articulates with the maxillary spine and with the vomer, while along the lower edge are found two other strips of cartilage which are known as the vomeronasal cartilages.

The *septum* is covered with perichondrium where there is cartilage, with periosteum where there is bone, and outside this with mucous membrane.

On the lateral wall there is a system of ridges known as the *conchae*, or turbinates, each of which overhangs a groove known as a meatus.

The *conchae* or turbinates are three in number – the inferior concha, the middle concha and the superior concha. The inferior concha forms a bone by itself, attached to the lateral wall of the nose. The middle concha and the superior concha are part of the ethmoid bone. The conchae (turbinates) are covered with mucous membrane which is, for the most part, columnar ciliated epithelium (Fig. 4).

Underlying the mucous membrane there is erectile tissue which is found chiefly at the anterior and posterior ends of the inferior conchae, in their lower borders, and at the anterior ends of the middle conchae. The meatus of the nose are of importance since they are the drainage channels of the accessory air sinuses. The appearance of pus in one of the meatus is of diagnostic importance in affections of the nose and accessory air sinuses.

Into the *superior meatus* and spheno-ethmoidal recess drain the posterior group of nasal accessory sinuses. Into the *middle meatus*

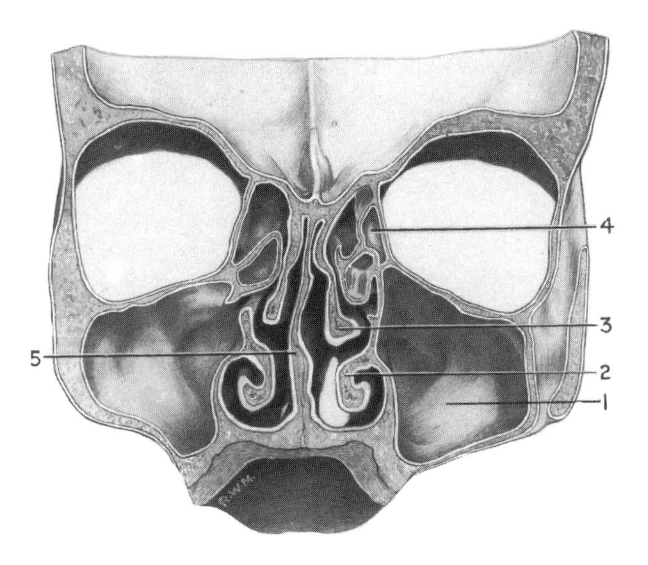

Fig. 4. Section of skull showing nasal cavity. (1) Maxillary air sinus; (2) inferior concha; (4) ethmoidal cells; (5) nasal septum.

drain the anterior group, while into the *inferior meatus* drains the naso-lachrymal duct. It should be noted that while the inferior and middle meatus are open at both ends the superior meatus is closed at the anterior end. This means that pus from the posterior group of sinuses will be seen on posterior rhinoscopy (Fig. 5).

The middle meatus contains several structures of importance. An enlargement is found at the anterior end of the middle meatus, which is part of the ethmoid bone, known as the *uncinate* process. A little farther back can be seen another eminence which is called the *bulla ethmoidalis*, which represents a protrusion into the meatus of one of the air cells of the ethmoidal labyrinth (Fig.6).

In the normal nose these parts can rarely be seen from the front. Between these two enlargements is a groove which is known as the *hiatus semilunaris*, into which the ostium of the maxillary air sinus opens. The hiatus semilunaris, when followed upwards, leads to a narrowing called the *infundibulum*. In many cases the infundibulum continues upwards, becoming the fronto-nasal duct. Owing, however, to the irregularity of the development of the frontal sinus and the anterior ethmoid cells, it is possible that the fronto-nasal duct may open from an anterior ethmoidal cell.

Boundaries of the nasal cavity. Inferiorly the floor of the nasal cavity is formed by the maxilla and by the palatine bones. The roof of the nasal cavity is formed, in front, by the lateral nasal bones. Behind is the

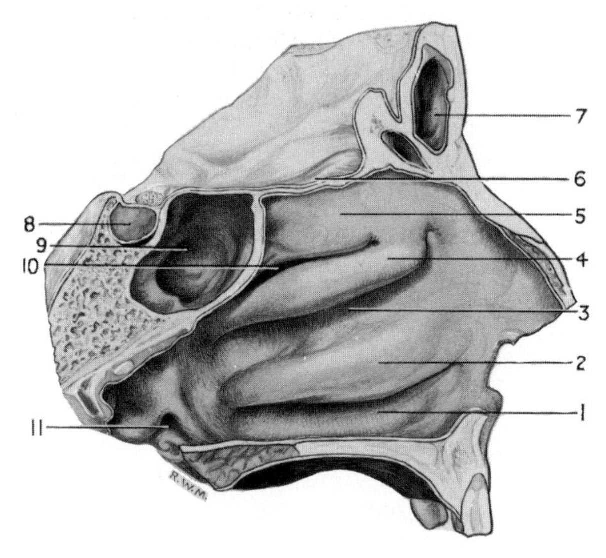

Fig. 5. Lateral wall of nose showing: (1) inferior meatus; (2) inferior concha; (3) middle meatus; (4) middle concha; (5) superior concha; (6) cribriform area; (7) frontal sinus; (8) pituitary fossa; (9) sphenoidal sinus; (10) superior meatus; (11) Eustachian Tube.

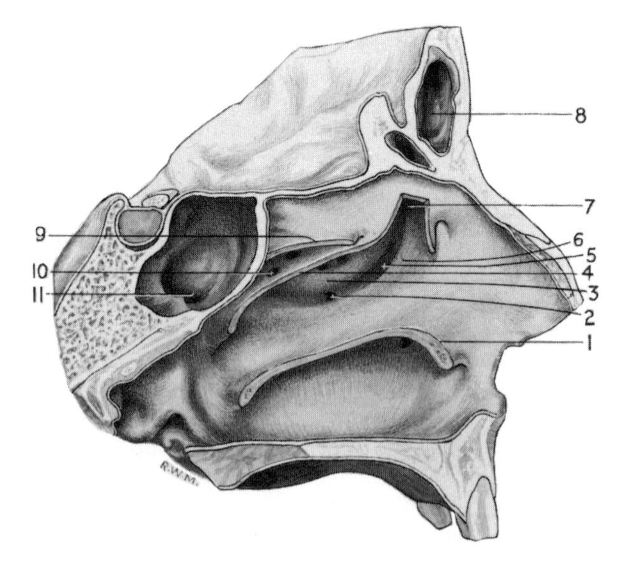

Fig. 6. Lateral wall of nose with middle and superior conchae (turbinates) removed. (1) cut edge of inferior concha; (2) ostium of maxillary air sinus; (3) bulla ethmoidalis; (4) cut edge of middle concha; (5) hiatus semilunaris; (6) uncinate process; (7) infundibulum; (8) frontal sinus; (9) cut edge of superior concha; (10) ostia of ethmoidal cells; (11) sphenoidal sinus.

cribriform plate. This is a bony lamina of the ethmoid bone, which is perforated to permit the passage of the filaments of the olfactory nerves. Posteriorly the sphenoid bone forms part of the roof.

The nerve-supply. The *sensory nerve-supply* is mainly by the sphenopalatine nerves, the fibres of which pass through the sphenopalatine ganglion to join the maxillary nerve. This ganglion is the centre for sensory function in the larger portion of the nose. The anterior and upper part, however, is supplied by the anterior ethmoidal nerves, which are branches from the naso-ciliary branches of the ophthalmic division of the fifth nerve. These find entrance to the nasal cavity at the anterior end of the cribriform plate and finally ramify on the outer surface of the nose as the external nasal nerves. The limitation of the centres of nasal sensation to these points renders block or regional anaesthesia easy and effective.

The *sympathetic supply* to the nose is distributed also from the sphenopalatine ganglion, which it reaches by means of the deep petrosal nerve from the carotid plexus. The *secretomotor* supply is obtained from the geniculate ganglion.

Nerve of special sensation. The olfactory nerves enter the nose through the cribriform plate in the roof and are distributed to the upper part of the nasal septum and the medial wall of the superior concha.

Arterial supply. The upper part of the nasal cavity is supplied by the anterior and posterior ethmoidal arteries which are branches of the ophthalmic artery in the nearby orbit. The ophthalmic arises from the internal carotid artery.

The lower part of the nose is supplied by branches derived from the maxillary artery, the most important being the sphenopalatine arteries and the termination of the greater palatine. Smaller contributions enter from the face.

These internal and external carotid sources anastomose freely in the nose. An aggregation of poorly supported vessels on the anterior part of the septum just behind the skin margin is known as Little's area and is a frequent source of bleeding.

The lymphatic vessels drain posteriorly to the superior deep cervical group.

PHYSIOLOGY OF THE NOSE

The chief functions of the nose are

1. Olfaction.
2. Filtration.
3. Humidification and warming of the air passing to the lungs.

There are other functions, such as vocal resonance, self-cleansing and provision of moisture for protection of the mucous membrane.

The functions depend upon the mucous membrane with its underlying tissues. In certain areas such as the conchae (turbinates) this is a complicated structure of ciliary mucous membrane, glands, blood spaces and connective tissues based upon bone, and is under the control of the autonomic nervous system. In this way the conchae act as a valve-mechanism enlarging or narrowing the air channels and so determining the direction of the air stream. The path of the air column in the nose during inspiration is upwards and backwards towards the middle concha, thence in a curve towards the posterior nares. This can be demonstrated by the inhalation of a small quantity of coloured powder.

In expiration such a definite path is not followed, but there is a more general diffusion of the air column throughout the nose, with an eddy round the middle concha.

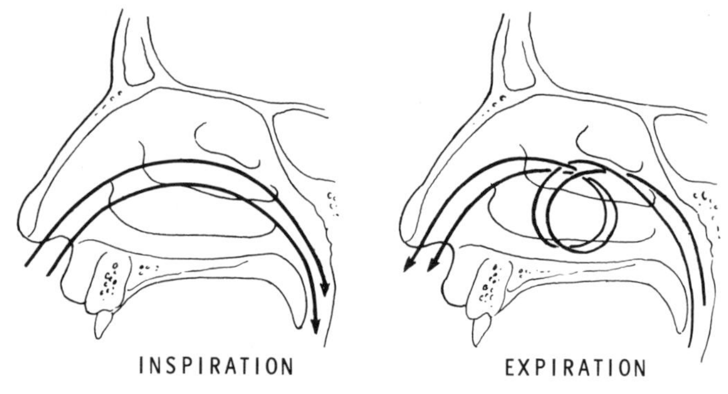

Fig. 7 The direction of air flow in the nasal passage is indicated.

Olfaction as a function may be influenced in various ways. For example obstruction from inflammation or vasomotor changes may prevent air reaching the olfactory area. Sometimes toxic or infective conditions or head injury destroy the nerve endings and the sense of smell.

Filtration is effected by the adhesion to the mucous film of dust, bacteria and other particles. These are removed by ciliary action into the pharynx and swallowed with the secretions.

Humidification. The moistening and warming of the air passing to the lungs is one of the chief functions. Air reaches the lungs at about 30°C and at 75–95 per cent relative humidity. When, during cold weather, the air in a room is heated, the humidity may fall from the optimum 40 per cent to as low as 5 to 10 per cent. To increase this humidity to the level necessary for comfort may cause a severe strain on the nasal mechanism. Unless the mucous membrane is very efficient extreme discomfort may result. Similarly changes in the mucous membrane of the nose caused by disease or trauma may produce symptoms. These are due to the inability of the glands and blood spaces to provide the warmth and moisture demanded by the atmospheric conditions.

Ciliary action is the means by which the mucous membrane cleanses itself and removes unwanted material. By the movement of the cilia which fringe the surface cells, a constant streaming of mucus is produced antero-posteriorly. Any interference with normal action causes unpleasant symptoms. Overaction of the cilia may mean copious nasal secretions and impaired action leads to accumulation of secretion or even to the formation of crusts which cause obstruction by clogging the nose. The post-nasal discharge, so often a cause of complaint, is an expression of the inability of the ciliary mechanism to deal with thickened mucus which slowly finds its way into the pharynx where it accumulates. The conditions necessary for efficient ciliary action are mucus of the correct consistency and adequate aeration. Conditions inimical to ciliary action are excessive drying, inflammation, thick secretions and unsuitable drugs.

Treatment is therefore directed to restoration of the nasal airway where impaired, and the production of conditions favourable to normal ciliary action. Any solutions used should be isotonic and antiseptics are for the most part useless. Salves, oils and snuffs which slow up ciliary action should be avoided. Ephedrine used in saline up to the strength of 2 per cent is a useful drug as it has no ill effects on ciliary action and produces little 'rebound' swelling.

The nose plays an important part in giving resonance to the voice. Malformations of the nasopharynx and obstructions in the nose itself may alter the tone of the voice, making it flat and uninteresting. In the same manner, by interfering with the nasal air column, rigidity or fibrosis of the soft palate may deprive the voice of timbre. For this reason nasal operations upon singers must be approached with great caution and considerable experience is required to judge the probable effects on voice of treatments causing alteration of the nasal structure.

2. The Nose, Examination and Symptoms

Before starting the clinical examination a full and accurate history of the patient's illnesses and social background should be obtained. A frequent source of confusion is the fact that patients mention several complaints in their opening sentence and it is difficult at times to ascertain which is the principal one. Permit patients, however, to give their own story in their own way, although at times it may be necessary to keep them to the point. Avoid leading questions. Get the main complaint clear at once, whatever it may be – nasal discharge, nasal obstruction, dryness of the nose or discomfort. Stick to this symptom and use it as a peg upon which to hang your questions. Ascertain the mode of onset, the duration, the character of the trouble – whether it is sufficiently severe to cause the patient acute discomfort, sleeplessness, etc., or whether it is merely an annoyance. Patients frequently complain that they always have a cold or are never free of colds, a statement which should cause suspicion of a vasomotor basis for the nasal discharge. Find out if the trouble is seasonal – that is, if it comes on at any particular time of the year. It may be found to be dependent on the weather or different atmospheres may have some effect upon the disease. Discover any other symptoms associated with the head, such as headache and giddiness. Never neglect to make careful inquiry about other organs such as the ears, larynx, etc., for the nose is part of a complex mechanism, and laryngeal or bronchial complaints may accompany or follow nasal disease. The general health should always form a subject for inquiry and also the previous medical history, particularly regarding any serious disease. The clue to severe nasal disease is frequently found in some early illness or in some minor complaint upon which the patient will lay no stress unless specifically questioned about it. The family history particularly in regard to nasal disease is of importance. Allergy is important. Respiratory infections in parents or older siblings may produce recurring infections in young patients.

CLINICAL EXAMINATION

Method of holding nasal speculum. Hold the speculum on the point of the forefinger of the left hand, with the blades of the speculum pointing to the examiner. Place the thumb on the hook of the speculum where it crosses the forefinger, and then place the middle finger round the left

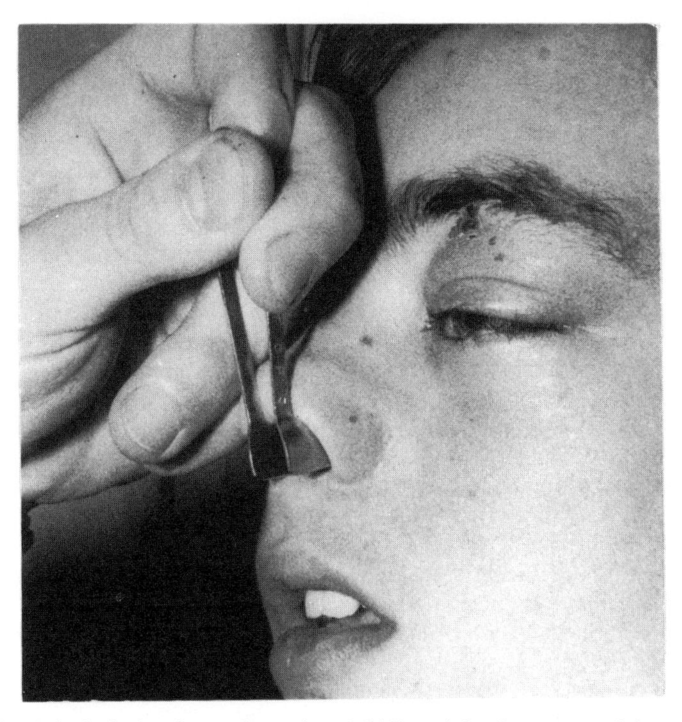

Fig. 8. Method of using the nasal speculum. Middle and ring fingers control the spring, the speculum is introduced obliquely in the plane of the nostril, then lifted into the position shown. Note also the direction of view.

side of the speculum and the ring finger round the right side. The thumb and first finger will then be able to hold the speculum firmly while the other fingers control the spring of the speculum. The hand is then turned away from the examiner so that when the speculum is inserted into the nose the left hand is above the level of the speculum and is well out of the way of interference with the examination. When proceeding to examine the nose remember that the axis of the nose is at right angles to the vertical plane of the face and has nothing to do with the axis of the outer part of the nasal bones as seen upon the face.

How to examine the patient

We will assume that the position described previously has been taken up and that the examiner has focussed his light successfully upon the patient.

The normal nose. The examiner should have a clear idea what he will find in a nose which is healthy. It is quite useless to expect the student to be able to pass judgment on a pathological condition of the nose unless he is sufficiently familiar with the normal. Every opportunity should be taken by the student, and also by the young practitioner who is anxious to enlarge his experience, to examine the normal on every available occasion.

In health the nose should present two approximately equal cavities or passages. These are divided by the septum which is rarely exactly in the mid-line. The septum is vertical and is broader at the base than in the upper part.

Looking towards the lateral side of the nasal cavity there should come into view, near the floor, a smooth rounded projection, which on closer inspection will be seen to be the anterior end of the shelf-like inferior concha, or turbinate. This can then be followed back till it is lost in the shadows of the posterior part of the nose.

If observation is then carried above the inferior concha, a smooth pink mass slightly lighter in colour will be made out. This is the middle concha, or turbinate, of which only the anterior end can be seen. To the medial side of the middle concha a dark crevice appears between it and the septum, which is the olfactory cleft, while to its lateral side in a roomy nose the cleft of the middle meatus will appear.

By tilting the head forward, it may be possible to inspect the inferior meatus below the inferior concha. In many cases, however, where the inferior concha is large, the anterior end may touch the floor of the nose, and render inspection of this part difficult, if not impossible, without previous shrinkage of the concha.

The mucous membrane is smooth and pink and should glisten with a

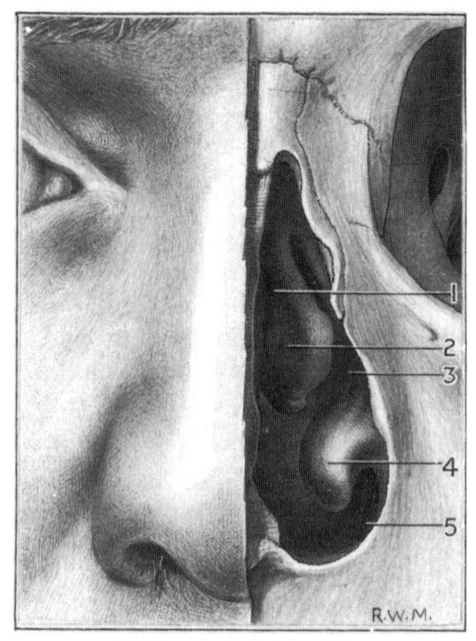

Fig. 9. View of nose on anterior rhinoscopy. (1) Olfactory sulcus; (2) middle concha; (3) middle meatus; (4) inferior concha; (5) inferior meatus.

thin coating of mucus. In health there is little difference in the appearance of the mucous membrane in the various parts of the nose. When the membrane has been subjected to abnormal conditions over a period of time, pathological changes are caused which enable one to differentiate those parts of the mucous membrane having different functions.

Proceeding, then, to carry out an examination of the nose, never neglect the inspection of the outer parts of the nose, and if any external abnormality is observed, find out if there is any cause for this in the past, such as early trauma.

The examiner should always have clearly in mind the order in which he intends to examine the various parts of the nose. The exact order in which these parts are examined is immaterial provided the examiner always follows the same routine. It is only in the practice of routine such as this, that, when more experienced, the examiner can be certain during an examination that nothing has been missed; the following is suggested as a scheme whereby a complete examination may be carried out rapidly.

Examine the *outer parts* of the nose and vestibule.

Look at the *cavities* on each side of the nose; see if they are equal; if they are unequal, ascertain the cause. The cause will probably be septal irregularity.

Examine the *septum* therefore with care. If it is deviated, determine to which side the deviation is greater, whether it is anterior or posterior; whether the deviation is above or below, and whether or not it is seriously obstructing the nose and, if so, which particular portion of the nasal cavity is obstructed.

Then turn the attention to the conchae.

Examine the *inferior conchae* first; determine their size, their colour, and the character of the membrane covering them – whether smooth or rough; if not smooth, where the roughness occurs – its distribution, its extent and character.

Next try to examine the *middle concha*. If it cannot be seen, find out the reason.

The septum may be deviated, the inferior concha may be oedematous. There may be polypi; the light may be badly focussed.

Do not leave this part until a reason can be given for lack of success in the examination.

The conchae are sometimes mistaken for polypi, but unlike the latter are pink, firm, sensitive to gentle probing and immobile. Then look for the uncinate process laterally in front of the middle concha. The superior concha cannot be seen on anterior inspection. The normal mucous membrane should be smooth, pink, slightly moist and glistening.

Examine the nasal secretions; they should be clear and mucoid, neither watery nor sticky. The presence of mucopus or pus should be noted, and its origin decided if possible.

Finally if after this complete inspection the nose appears normal anteriorly, should the complaint be of obstruction, post-nasal disease may be the cause.

The use of cocaine in nasal examination

Cocaine has the property of retracting the mucous membrane to a very marked degree, and in cases where oedema or inflammation renders a view of the interior of the nose impossible, a pledget of wool wrung out of 10 per cent cocaine is placed between the inferior concha and the septum and allowed to remain there for a short time. When removed, it will be found that the concha has retracted to a considerable extent, and the interior of the nose can be inspected. Cocaine may also be applied as a spray when manipulations within the nose are expected. Less toxic synthetic drugs such as xylocaine (lignocaine) may be used, but while they can produce satisfactory anaesthesia they do not cause shrinkage of the mucous membrane. If this is required adrenalin should be added to the spray.

In cases where polypi are suspected the probe is used to touch the portions which are believed to be polypoid. Frequently, if the patient is asked to blow the nose, mistakes in diagnosis will be avoided as mucoid secretion may closely resemble nasal polypi.

In all matters relating to the examination of the nose, the greatest gentleness is essential.

POSTERIOR RHINOSCOPY

Posterior rhinoscopy is probably the most difficult examination procedure. The examiner has to cope with the difficulty of fixing his spot of light upon the very small mirror and then projecting the light with the mirror upon the various structures in the nasopharynx. All this must be carried out without irritating or upsetting the patient and causing 'gagging' or closure of the nasopharynx by the action of the soft palate.

A tongue depressor and a small post-nasal mirror are the instruments required. The mirror is first heated gently to prevent fogging and tested on the hand to avoid burning the patient.

The tongue is depressed and the mirror is then slipped in behind the uvula, the handle of the mirror being usually passed from the left corner of the mouth. The mirror is then rotated gently and the light is made to traverse the nasopharynx.

The mouths of the *Eustachian* tubes are examined.

The upper posterior wall of the nasopharynx is examined for the presence of adenoids. The posterior end of the septum shows as a white pillar and is the chief landmark in orientating the examiner.

The light is then thrown into the *choanae* and the posterior ends of

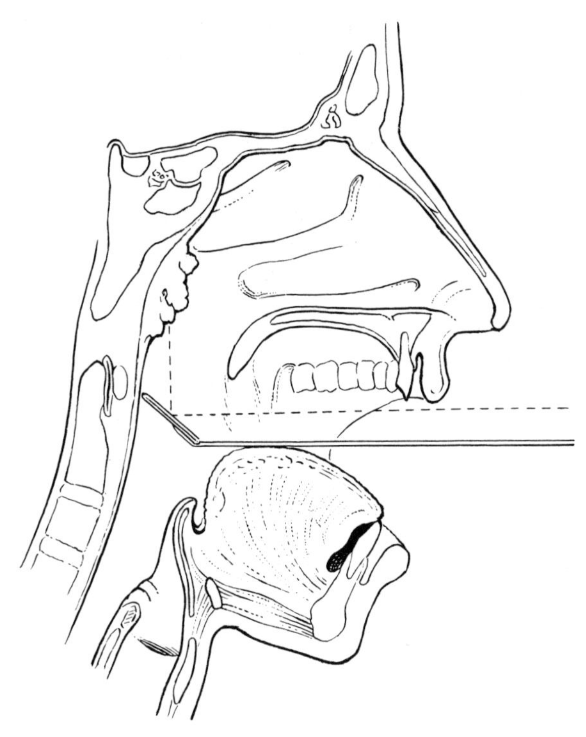

Fig. 10. Posterior rhinoscopy. (Broken line indicates beam of light reflected into the nasopharynx).

the conchae can be examined. The overgrowth of the epithelium, if present, may be noted, and the presence of pus or other secretion in relation to the conchae is observed. If pus is seen the position must be carefully noted; for instance, whether it is above or below the middle concha. The amount of obstruction caused can be judged and the source of the purulent material ascertained by its relation to the various structures.

In cases in which polypi are present, it is sometimes a help to pass a probe along the floor of the nose, and note the position of the polypi in relation to the probe. By such means an opinion may be formed regarding their origin.

From the description this examination sounds comparatively simple, but many difficulties may be encountered.

Difficulties. The chief difficulty which may arise is that the patient may have a sensitive pharynx and may 'gag' easily. This is especially the case with children. Where 'gagging' is considerable an effort should be made to displace the tongue sideways as far as possible. Do not place the spatula in the middle of the tongue and push the tongue down. Try

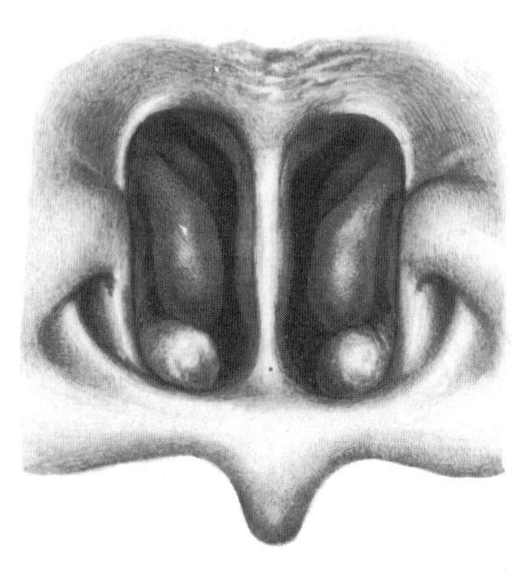

Fig. 11. View on posterior rhinoscopy.

to pass it along one edge and push the tongue across the mouth. Avoid touching the uvula if possible. The patient will frequently tolerate a mirror resting upon the posterior wall of the pharynx, whereas a touch on the uvula or soft palate in passing is sufficient to close the naso-

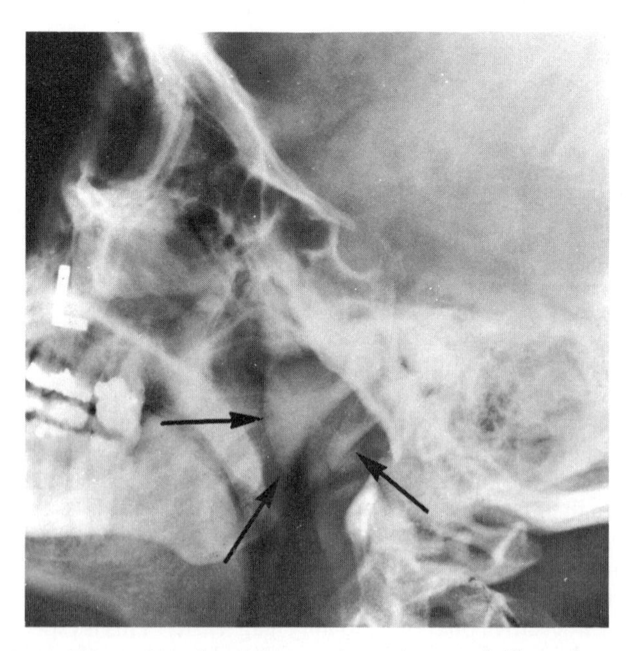

Fig. 12. Lateral X-ray view of nasopharynx. A cyst is arrowed. The patient was quite intolerant of mirror examination. Note how well the soft palate and dorsal surface of tongue can be demonstrated.

pharnyx or even to make the patient sick. The soft palate is often elevated by the patient and one of the chief causes for this is that the patient holds the breath. The patient should be instructed to breathe easily and deeply; if necessary to sniff downwards through the nose.

It may happen that some patients are so sensitive that posterior rhinoscopy is impossible without recourse to other aids. A spray of local anaesthetic may be required and an anaesthetic lozenge is a useful alternative. In some patients, however, inspection of the nose and nasopharynx under general anaesthesia is indicated. Examination of the cavity of the nose can also be aided by the use of the *nasopharyngoscope*, which may best be described as the nasal counterpart of the cystoscope. It is also of use when delicate manipulations in the nasal space demand visual control.

Children. Examination of the nasopharynx with the post-nasal mirror is often impossible in children, but the presence of adenoids, for example, can often be suspected from the history. Nasal obstruction in children in whom the nose looks clear anteriorly is most frequently due to adenoids. A mass can sometimes be palpated through the soft palate, but digital examination of the nasopharynx itself is rarely justified. A lateral X-ray of the nasopharynx may be invaluable. The final step in diagnosis will be examination under anaesthesia if serious doubts persist.

SYMPTOMS OF NASAL DISEASE

Nasal obstruction. One of the chief nasal symptoms encountered is nasal obstruction. This obstruction may be due to a large variety of causes, but there are three main groups:

(1) An anatomical or developmental abnormality in the nose.

In this group are included such conditions as deviations and injuries to the nasal septum, congenital narrowing of the nares or complete atresia of one or both choanae.

(2) The effects of such abnormality causing pathological changes in the mucous membrane.

This group includes such conditions as hypertrophy of the mucous membrane due to repeated rhinitis, the formation of polypi and the accumulation of pathological secretions.

(3) Hypersensitivity of the nervous mechanism of the nasal mucous membrane causing swelling and obstruction.

As in allergic and vasomotor disorders there is an acute swelling of the mucous membrane, with a sudden and excessive outpouring of secretion as well as the temporary obstruction caused by each attack. If these are repeated over a period of time pathological changes are set up such as have already been mentioned.

Nasal discharge. Nasal discharge is another of the chief complaints met with in those suffering from nasal disease. Discharge from the nose may be the result of irritation or repeated acute attacks of inflammation of the mucous membrane of the nose. In acute cases the discharge is thin and watery; it is profuse and is accompanied as a rule by nasal obstruction. In the chronic forms the discharge is thicker than normal and makes its presence felt in the back of the throat. In an acute infection the discharge is the reaction of the mucous membrane to an acute inflammatory condition, and is in some degree a protective measure on the part of the mucous membrane. In the second case the chronic discharge is due to hypertrophy of the elements of the mucous membrane responsible for provision of protecting mucus and is a response to prolonged inflammation. A considerable amount of the discomfort suffered, where this trouble occurs, is due to alteration in the composition of the secretion. The heavier mucoid elements of the secretions are increased in proportion, rendering the nasal discharge thick and sticky. There may be also damage to the ciliary mechanism, either from disease or because it cannot deal effectively with the thickened secretions and expel them readily from the nose. If secretions are not expelled in normal fashion from the nose into the nasopharynx, the patient becomes conscious of the accumulation, and the discomforts of post-nasal discharge ensue.

Pus is occasionally found in the nose and all inflammatory conditions eventually become what is known as 'mucopurulent', the pus cells being those which have been thrown off from the surface of the mucous membrane. Persistent discharge of yellow pus is usually indicative of sinus disease.

In acute nasal allergy excessive watery secretions are produced following exposure to the allergen responsible. Less frequently vasomotor rhinorrhoea is seen. This too is characterized by excessive watery secretions; they are produced continually without exposure to any physical or chemical agents and may not be associated with other symptoms of allergy. An autonomic disturbance is likely.

Pain. Pain is less common as a symptom than obstruction and discharge. A degree of burning irritation is a common accompaniment to acute coryza and it may be severe. Irritation by gases, dust, etc., may also give rise to pain.

More localized symptoms are caused by furuncles or infections of hair follicles at the vestibule. Herpes and eczematous eruptions give rise to varying degrees of discomfort. Small fissures which most frequently form in the roof of the vestibule at the skin margin, and sometimes at the outer and lower corner, may cause distress out of proportion to their apparent importance.

Frequently recurring headaches are often blamed on 'nasal catarrh' and 'sinus trouble', but unless some acute condition is apparent, detailed investigation of nose and sinuses is generally negative.

Sometimes no local cause can be found for pain, in which case a thorough search of the trigeminal nerve distribution is indicated.

Dental pain may be referred to another part and cause confusion. Trigeminal neuralgia and other facial neuralgias and atypical facial pain must be differentiated from pain of local origin.

External deformities. Deformities of the external part of the nose may be developmental or they may be due to trauma or to disease. Cases due to maldevelopment result in abnormalities of the shape of the bones of the nose. The nose may be deviated to one side or the other on account of unequal growth, or it may be narrow and under-developed, owing to insufficient use.

Injury to the nose leads to deformity, such as the sinking of the bridge, or deviation to one side or the other through displacement of the nasal bones. Falling of the bridge of the nose may be the result of a haematoma or an abscess of the septum which has had its origin in injury. The cartilaginous destruction following injury removes the support from the nose with the result that the bridge sinks. The same result may occur after nasal operation in which more support has been taken away than the nose can afford, and a very considerable deformity may result.

Diseases such as syphilis are responsible for some of the most severe nasal deformities. The syphilitic nose is frequently known as the 'saddle-shaped' nose, with a marked sinking of the bridge of the nose and flaring of the nostrils, so that they look forward instead of down. Tuberculosis may affect the soft parts of the nose to such an extent that they may be completely eaten away. Cancer also may be responsible for extensive destruction of the nose and the surrounding parts.

3. Diseases of the External Nose

NASAL INJURY

The common nasal injury encountered is a fracture or mobilizing of the nasal bones, with or without displacement. The injury may be compound or may involve the bony structure only.

If the patient is seen immediately at the time of occurrence (*e.g.* on the football field) before swelling of the soft parts has obscured the deformity, replacement may be attempted, but if not immediately successful the attempt should be abandoned.

When seen some time after the injury, if there has been any laceration of the soft tissues, treatment should be deferred till healing has taken place. In any case, if there is considerable swelling, as usually there is, accurate correction of the deformity will be difficult if not impossible, until the swelling has subsided. The optimum time is ten days after the injury.

Examination usually shows that the chief deformity is a deviation of the nasal structure to one side or the other. Further inspection will show also that one nasal bone has been depressed under the other, so that any attempt at replacement which consists merely of pushing the nose towards the mid-line will be of no value as the depressed bone will prevent any return without excessive force. The first essential is to elevate the depressed nasal bone from within. This can be done with any flat instrument, preferably guarded by rubber tubing. Light pressure only, applied to the side of the nose, is then required to restore the normal contours. The choice of anaesthetic depends upon the extent of the injury and the ability of the surgeon. Simple displacement may be corrected after preparing the nose with a local anaesthetic aided by light general anaesthesia. Where haemorrhage is expected or the injury is extensive, intubation with full protection of the airway is recommended.

The severer forms of injury, and deformity due to disease, belong to the realm of the plastic surgeon, or the maxillo-facial surgeon.

DISEASES OF THE VESTIBULE

Dermatitis

Skin eruptions are frequently seen around the external openings of the nose. The organisms concerned may be staphylococci or streptococci, and when the patient reports for examination the infection will be found to be almost invariably a mixed one. In children there is frequently scab formation and yellow crusting, probably with raw areas where the scabs have been picked off, and the upper lip may be excoriated. These patients may be found to be suffering from chronic nasal discharge, and in planning treatment one of the duties of the examiner is to try to ascertain the underlying cause. Until this has been treated it is of little use to expect satisfactory solution of the condition.

Cleanliness is the first essential. The nose must be cleansed frequently. The crusts should be removed with a little warm olive oil or soap and water, and the part kept covered with an ointment such as sulphur and salicylic acid; or, alternatively, the lesion should be kept lubricated with an ointment such as one of those listed in the Appendix.

Fissures are a frequent complaint, and these will often be found in the upper part of the vestibule. They are generally encountered in adults, the cause of the fissure being a slight, watery nasal discharge which necessitates frequent use of the handkerchief. These fissures often refuse to heal and become very painful and troublesome. They can be treated by frequent application of an ointment containing an antibiotic with a steroid. The use of the ointment should be continued after the fissures are apparently healed.

Boils in the nose

Staphylococcal infection of a hair follicle is not infrequent and results in a boil or furuncle; sometimes several hair follicles may be involved in succession. Pain is often severe because the tightness of the skin over the perichondrium produces a rapid rise in tension.

Infections in this area are always potentially dangerous and should be treated with respect. A spreading thrombophlebitis of the facial vein can involve the cavernous sinus and produce fatal intracranial complications.

The boil should on no account be squeezed, neither should it be incised. In severe cases the patient should be admitted to hospital. Hot fomentations of magnesium sulphate are invaluable; a pledget of wool soaked in magnesium sulphate in glycerine can be inserted between treatments if the lesion is inside the nostril. A systemic antibiotic should be given in full dosage.

During resolution the area should be kept lubricated with a bland ointment and afterwards a search made for a possible focus of infection. This may be in the sinuses or teeth.

To guard against recurrence the patient should be warned against picking or rubbing the nose. Depilation by X-rays is sometimes suggested. Subsequent cleanliness with occasional lubrication of the nasal vestibule should be advised.

Tumours

Warts, rodent ulcers and squamous carcinomas occur in and around the nostrils. Apparently simple warts should always be excised and examined histologically.

4. Diseases of the Septum

Haematoma of the septum

Haematoma is the result of injury, and consists of bleeding between the layers of the septum. The symptoms are those of nasal obstruction, with perhaps a little tenderness over the bridge of the nose if the injury has been fairly severe. Lesser degrees of obstruction may be left alone provided signs of suppuration do not set in. It is essential to avoid infection as this may result in necrosis of cartilage and deformity. If considered advisable, the haematoma may be reduced by lightly cocainizing the anterior part of the septum on one side and aspirating the contents with syringe and needle under strict aseptic conditions.

Abscess of the septum

Abscess formation is a complication of haematoma which should be anticipated. The onset of suppuration is characterized by a rise in temperature, and the occurrence of pain. The nose has a full feeling and may throb. On examination it will be found to be slightly swollen, becoming red and shiny over the bridge and near the tip. There is pain on pressure over the same areas, and this, as well as the swelling, may extend on to the face.

When diagnosed the abscess must be opened and drained. A pledget of wool soaked in 10 per cent cocaine, to which has been added a few drops of adrenalin solution (1/1000), is placed against the mucous membrane of the anterior part of the septum. An incision is then made in the abscess under general anaesthesia in acute cases. When a sufficiently large opening has been made a piece of rubber drain is inserted. There is a tendency to premature closure so care must be taken that the incision remains open for some days. The whole condition may be expected to clear up within a week, although the nasal congestion in all probability will last some days longer.

As a rule no ill effects are experienced, but necrosis of the nasal cartilage may follow, causing a falling of the bridge or other deformity.

Abscess of the septum may also occur in children, without any definite history of injury.

This condition must be regarded seriously, especially in children, as infection passes readily to the orbit or the cavernous sinus through thrombosing veins and may prove fatal. Appropriate antibiotics should be given in all cases.

Septal deviation

The nasal septum may be deviated to one side or to the other, and the deviation may involve chiefly the upper or the lower part of the septum. The origin of the deviation may be developmental or traumatic.

It is possible that the growth of the nasal bones may be unequal. The septum and the lateral nasal bones have, practically speaking, to grow to a single point. When the growth in each bone is not exactly at the same rate, the result is bending of the nasal septum. It may happen in childhood, while the nasal cartilage is in a pliable state, that a blow, unnoticed at the time, forces the septum from the straight path of growth.

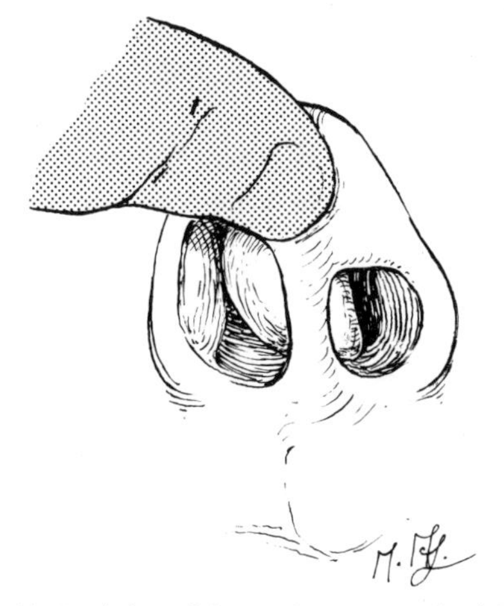

Fig. 13. Deviation of the nasal septum to the right.

Trauma, on the other hand, may cause greater irregularity, especially if it occurs later in life when the nose is formed, the bones have hardened and the cartilaginous or bony septum has been fractured.

Deviations will usually be found to be of two types – cartilaginous and bony.

Bony deviations for the most part cause what are known as 'spurs'. Spurs are outgrowths or ridges encountered in the lower part of the nose; these cause blockage of the part of the meatus which they occupy. Spurs may be anterior or they may be posterior. In an examination of the nose a septum which is seen to be straight anteriorly may possibly present appearances posteriorly which are sufficient to account for nasal obstruction and chronic nasal disease. The cartilaginous deviations, on the other hand, are anterior in position and very frequently involve the upper part of the quadrilateral cartilage.

It will be appreciated that a great variety of septal deformities may be encountered. Any or all of the cartilaginous or bony components of the septum may be bent or angled or dislocated. Not infrequently the quadrilateral cartilage may become dislocated from its groove in the maxillary crest. Occasionally the major part of the deformity is confined to the quadrilateral cartilage, which appears as an ugly swelling in the nostril. The appearance of this is often more embarrassing to the patient than the associated obstruction.

Symptoms. The main symptom is unilateral or bilateral nasal obstruction. In less severe deformities attention may be focussed upon the nose by failure of nasal infections to clear up normally. Headaches are frequently attributed to septal deflection but it rarely causes this symptom. Anosmia is seldom helped by operation on the nasal septum. It is wise to remember that many patients with severe septal deformity are symptom-free and if the condition is found during routine examination its presence should not be mentioned.

Examining for septal deflection

The external appearance of the nose may give a clue to the condition to be found within. On looking into the nasal cavities the septum may be seen to be pressed over to one side so that no view can be obtained into the obstructed side. Usually, in this case, a compensatory hypertrophy of the turbinates will be found on the side opposite to the deviation. This compensatory hypertrophy must be taken into account when planning treatment. Sometimes an 'S'-shaped deformity may be present with an anterior obstruction on one side and a posterior obstruction on the opposite side of the nose.

In all cases a clear view must be obtained of the posterior part of the nasal cavity as bony spurs there may complicate treatment. It may be necessary to insert a pledget of wool moistened in cocaine solution in order to shrink congested mucosa so that the inspection may be completed. The effects on the sinuses are those of obstruction. A severe septal deviation to one side may cause compression or pressure on the

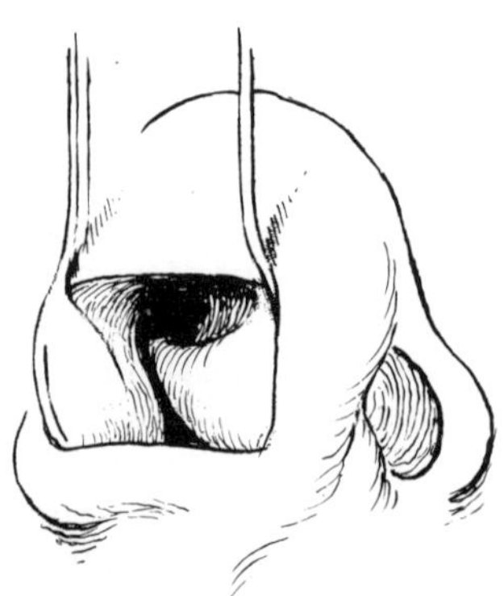

Fig. 14. Bony spur on the right of the nasal septum,

middle concha on the same side, and may cause the ostia of the sinuses to be occluded. This obstruction may be a purely mechanical condition, or it may, in certain instances, be due to the resulting congestion of the mucous membrane, a result which not infrequently follows an abnormal narrowing of the nasal airway.

Septal deviation, therefore, may result in sinus obstruction and infection, and formation of polypi. Relief of such a condition naturally involves not only drainage of the infected sinuses, but correction of the septal deviation. The presence of established infection in an accessory sinus is in general a contra-indication for an operation on the nasal septum, but in certain cases operation may have to be undertaken even in the presence of suppuration. In these operations considerable experience is required on the part of the surgeon if the patient is to obtain relief with safety.

Cure of septal deformity

The operation most frequently performed for correction of the deformity is sub-mucous resection of the septum, but if the injury to the nose has produced a cosmetic deformity this procedure can be combined with a rhinoplasty in order to restore the external appearance of the nose. If desirable the plastic part of the operation can be done at a later date.

Preparation for the operation is the same as for all nasal operations, and is described in the Appendix.

The operation

In addition to preparing the nose with cocaine and adrenalin it is useful to inject Novocain (0.5 per cent) with adrenalin (1 :200,000) into the mucous membrane on each side of the nasal septum. This aids haemosstasis and is helpful even if general anaesthesia is used. An S-shaped incision is then made in the nasal septum upon the side showing the greatest anterior deviation, a quarter of an inch behind the mucocutaneous junction. The mucous membrane is then elevated from the cartilage and from the bone on the side of the incision. The cartilage is incised in the line of the incision and elevation carried out on the opposite side, care being taken not to perforate the mucous membrane. When the mucous membrane has been freed on both sides, first the cartilage and then the bone behind the cartilage are removed with swivel knife and punch forceps. Perforation of the mucous membrane may take place if care is not exercised at the point where the elevation of membrane over a spur is undertaken. The maxillary spine and any bone spurs are then removed with hammer and fish-tail gouge. The removal is continued posteriorly until a clear airway on both sides has been obtained. If the operator is in doubt whether this has been obtained or not, the septal flaps should be replaced and the nose inspected on each side. Only when the airway is perfectly clear is the operation considered satisfactory. When this has been achieved the septal layers are approximated, and packs plentifully lubricated are inserted into each nostril. The object of the pack is to cause close apposition of the flaps of nasal mucous membrane without accumulation of blood clots within the layers. The patient will have greater comfort if the gauze pack is enclosed in a rubber finger-stall but in such circumstances the pack must be securely anchored, to avoid any chance of aspiration, by stitching together the gauze of the packs as well as the rubber, at the front of the nose. It is not considered necessary to stitch the incision in the mucous membrane.

After treatment of septal operations. The packs are removed twelve to twenty-four hours after operation. By careless removal the success of the operation can be jeopardised. Two minutes at least should be taken in slowly removing the packs. This will minimize the chance of haemorrhage within the layers of septal mucosa. Formation of a haematoma will considerably prolong convalescence. After the packs are removed the patient should be instructed to lie quietly for half an hour. A medicated steam inhalation is then given and the patient is allowed to move about more freely. During convalescence decongestive drops followed by an inhalation are comforting; an ointment applied to the nostrils prevents crusting. Nose blowing should be forbidden.

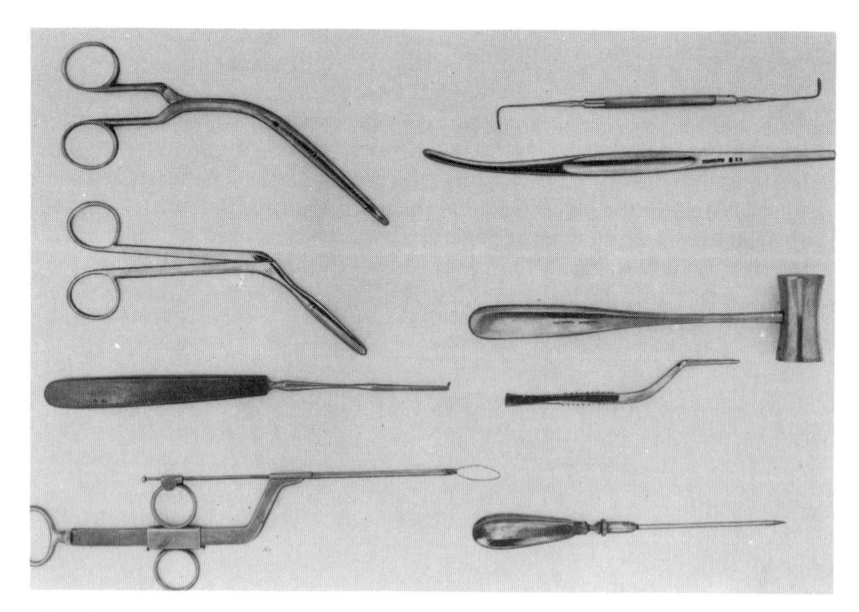

Fig. 15. Instruments commonly used in minor nasal operations. These include Luc forceps and nasal scissors, septal swivel knife, polyp snare, elevators, mallet and gouge, trocar and cannula for antral proof puncture.

Complications of the recovery period

Haematoma. Should a haematoma form between the layers of the septum it will usually be found wisest to leave this alone. If there is any evidence of infection, the incision should be reopened and the haematoma drained. The nose may take three weeks or longer to return to normal and it is well to warn the patient that this is likely to be the case.

Perforation may not make itself evident for some time after the operation. If it is not causing symptoms nothing need be said to the patient. Where it is responsible for nasal discomfort, attempts may be made to close it by swinging a flap of mucous membrane over the gap. Such operations, however, are of great technical difficulty, and as a rule are not successful.

Falling of the bridge. This is due to a too extensive removal of cartilage from the upper part of the nose. When this occurs the nose should be allowed to heal completely and then the deformity is corrected by the implantation of a cartilage graft to support the sunken part of the bridge.

Flapping septum. Following a very complete removal of the septum the membranous curtain which is left may fall to one side or the other of the nose, obstructing each in turn.

The creation of a linear scar by careful application of the electrocautery generally tightens up the septum sufficiently. If unsuccessful a perforation can be made posteriorly.

Meningitis. This, happily, is a rare complication, but may occur where a septal operation is undertaken in presence of an active infection. For this reason, where a patient suffers from a cold or a sinusitis of an acute nature, operation should be postponed.

PERFORATION OF THE SEPTUM

Perforation of the septum by diseases such as tuberculosis or syphilis, while once common, is rarely seen today. It may complicate injury or a sub-mucous resection operation, and it is a recognised industrial hazard, notably amongst chrome workers. In the majority of patients no such factors are operative and the condition appears to arise from a small abrasion of the septum. The traumatic ulcer thus created repeatedly forms a crust, and every time the crust separates the ulcer deepens until cartilage is exposed. Cartilaginous necrosis then occurs and perforation extends through the mucous membrane of the opposite side.

Symptoms may be entirely absent but the patient may be aware of an irritating crust which he separates by rubbing or picking the nose with consequent aggravation of the condition. Slight bleeding may occur when the crust separates. Severe epistaxis may result if the long sphenopalatine artery is exposed in the posterior edge of the perforation. In exceptional cases the shape and site of the perforation may cause a whistling sound with each breath.

Various operations have been designed to close septal perforations but recurrence rate is high. If a penetrating ulcer of the septum is recognised it is important to arrest its progress by the frequent liberal use of a bland ointment.

5. Diseases of the Nasal Cavity

ACUTE RHINITIS OR CORYZA (COMMON COLD)

Acute infection of the mucous membrane with engorgement of the blood spaces results in a generalized hyperaemia of the mucous membrane with enlargement of the gland elements and resulting hypersecretion.

Aetiology. Coryza is due to infection by a virus; transmission occurs by means of air-borne droplets. The disease is highly contagious and the onset of symptoms is precipitated by lack of immunity or by lowering of resistance by chill, fatigue or similar cause. Increased activity of the normal pathogenic bacteria of the nose can then cause secondary infections which may lead to various complications.

Symptoms. The earliest signs of infection may be tickling, irritation, sneezing or dryness of the nose. These sensations may not amount to actual pain and may be felt in the nose or in the nasopharynx.

The acute stage. The prodromal stage is followed by copious nasal secretion. Some degree of obstruction may be present, the eyes are watery, temperature is elevated and the patient frequently feels a general malaise. Headache is often pronounced.

Recovery stage. After the early acute stage of profuse secretion the nose becomes more obstructed and the discharge becomes thicker and more purulent. The general symptoms are improved and after a period of hours or days the nasal passages re-open and normal breathing is re-established. The secretions gradually return to normal.

Pathology. In the early acute stage there is an over-activity of all the gland elements in the nose, producing a profuse secretory reaction to the infection. There is a migration of cells through the capillaries into the tissues and there is a desquamation of the surface epithelium which becomes greater as the infection progresses. In the earliest stages ciliary activity is very great and the secretions are rapidly cleared from the nose, but as the condition becomes established and as the destruction of the surface mucous membrane becomes greater, ciliary activity is lessened with the result that the secretions within the nose become thickened and are difficult to expel. This is the obstructed stage of the coryza and the yellowish nature of the secretions is caused by the number of cast-off cells in the secretions. The process of resolution is determined by the repair of the surface of the mucous membrane and with it the re-establishment of ciliary activity and the return to normal function of the nasal mucous membrane.

Treatment of acute rhinitis

As the disease is contagious the patient should be isolated if possible and nursed in an even temperature about 70°F (21°C) with a humidity of 40 to 50 per cent. If the patient can stay in bed, recovery is hastened and spread of infection is less likely.

Steam inhalations, given frequently, help to soothe the mucous membrane and open up the nasal passages. Anti-febrile drugs such as aspirin and phenacetin tend to reduce the temperature, and codein is effective against the headache.

Decongestants are useful in promoting drainage and preventing occlusion of the sinuses. Ephedrine in saline can be used with safety. (Ephedrine $\frac{1}{2}$ per cent to 2 per cent.) Chemotherapy is of value in preventing bacterial complications, such as sinusitis, otitis media or pneumonia, especially in the very young or the elderly.

If attacks are frequent or prolonged an attempt should be made to ascertain the cause which might be adenoids, allergy, vasomotor rhinitis, or sinusitis. Should there be obvious nasal deformity the question of septal correction should be considered.

Prophylactics. Many prophylactics have been recommended to protect patients against nasal infection. The chief of these are vitamin therapy, vaccine therapy, calcium therapy and ultra-violet radiation. At present there is no unanimity of opinion as to whether these methods of treatment give protection against infection, but it is probable that adequate supplies of vitamins help to raise immunity against respiratory infections. Physical fitness, fresh air and exercise all help to prevent the common cold. Ultra-violet radiation has been used by those whose work precludes a reasonable measure of sunlight. Vaccines do not prevent colds though in some cases they shorten the recovery period, but in specific influenzal epidemics a standard vaccine of a known type of virus may give valuable protection. Unfortunately there is no means of discovering which patients will respond to vaccines except by a system of trial and error, but where vaccines are successful they appear to give good results.

Complications

While inflammation remains localized in the nose, disability is slight; it is the involvement of surrounding structures which renders the common cold such an important factor in loss of work.

The most frequent complications are sinusitis, from direct extension of infection, and otitis media due to the blowing of infected secretions into the middle ear through the Eustachian tubes.

Passage downwards may produce laryngitis, tracheobronchitis and pneumonia.

Severer forms of infection. An acute rhinitis may be of such virulence that it is spoken of as being *purulent*. This form of infection is most commonly encountered in the exanthemata, but it may be met with apart from these illnesses. In such cases an attempt should always be made to identify the causal organism and treatment must be planned according to the bacteriological findings.

Treatment should be a more energetic application of that outlined. The nose must be cleansed by mild alkaline douche, twice or thrice daily, and this part of the treatment must not be left to unskilled hands but must be performed by a competent person. After douching, antibiotic solution or some mild antiseptic such as argyrol should be instilled. The strength of the argyrol solution should be 5 to 10 per cent, according to the age of the patient.

The results of this form of infection may be serious to the patient as it may be followed by permanent damage to the mucous membrane, affecting its function later in life.

MEMBRANOUS RHINITIS

Examination of the nose will sometimes reveal the presence of a membrane of a greyish or yellowish colour. The important point in these cases is to decide whether or not the case is one of nasal diphtheria. This is done by taking a swab for bacteriological examination, and it should be taken in all cases in which a membrane is found. Apart from cases of diphtheria, membrane formation occurs in those who are debilitated, or the subjects of malnutrition.

Treatment of non-diphtheritic cases consists in local cleanliness and correction of the deficiency if that can be identified. The membrane may be removed, if possible, and everything should be done to re-establish the nasal airway. (Also nasal diphtheria, p. 53.)

CHRONIC HYPERTROPHIC RHINITIS

Chronic rhinitis includes conditions of widely differing pathological pattern of which the chief are chronic hypertrophic rhinitis, atrophic rhinitis and rhinitis sicca.

Hypertrophic rhinitis may result from incomplete resolution of acute rhinitis due to causes such as obstruction, trauma, allergy, or vasomotor rhinitis. It may be secondary to unsuspected sinusitis, or the prolonged use of drops and sprays. Environmental factors such as dust, fumes or unsuitable climatic conditions which prevent normal function of the mucous membrane are important.

Appearances. In the early stages examination of the nose will reveal swelling and reddening of the mucous membrane. This is most marked in the covering of the inferior conchae and the nasal septum. The surface of the mucous membrane is smooth, and the secretions are sticky and mucopurulent. Strings of mucus can be seen between the septum and the inferior conchae. The airway is poor and, if septal deflection is the origin, inspection of one side may be impossible. When the condition becomes more firmly established all the elements of the mucous membrane become involved. The ciliated epithelium is replaced by stratified or cuboidal epithelium. There is an increase in fibrous tissue and an infiltration with round cells and plasma cells.

From this stage the mucous membrane may pass into one of permanent thickening or hypertrophy in which all components of the mucous membrane are affected. The gland elements are increased and the surface of the mucous membrane takes on a rounded or roughened appearance called 'mulberrying', which is caused by fibrous changes and cell infiltration round the gland ducts.

Symptoms. Nasal obstruction is the outstanding symptom. In the early stages this is intermittent. It is more marked in certain positions, as in the lower nostril when lying on one side, and it is frequently seen in sedentary occupations. The discharge is sticky and there is much hawking and blowing of the nose particularly in the morning. The chronic discharge may set up Eustachian catarrh and cause deafness.

There is frequently headache and a feeling of fullness in the head. Mouth-breathing and snoring result from the obstruction, and in long-standing cases the voice may become nasal. The obstruction is sometimes responsible for the onset of sinus disease.

Unilateral inflammation and discharge suggest the presence of a foreign body or malignant disease and these must be excluded (pp. 45–50).

Treatment. Before treatment can be planned the extent of the disease must be ascertained. A simple method of doing this is to place a pledget of wool soaked in 10 per cent cocaine solution against the inferior concha. After a few minutes, inspection will show some degree of retraction of the mucous membrane. The more advanced the chronic change the less will be the retraction and in advanced hypertrophic conditions the 'mulberried' portions will stand out clearly.

In the earliest stages of the disease exercise in the fresh air, and avoidance of the excessive use of alcohol and tobacco, especially in the form of snuff, is important. Control of environmental factors is essential, both at work and in the home. No nasal drops should be used except possibly ephedrine for a short time. These measures with the administration of an antihistamine are often sufficient to permit recovery of the mucosa. If secretions are excessive and troublesome an isotonic alkaline douche will be helpful in clearing the mucous membrane.

In more established cases reduction of the bulk of the turbinate can be achieved by submucosal diathermy, by electro-cautery, or by injection of sclerosing solutions. For gross hypertrophy surgical treatment is required.

Submucosal diathermy has the advantage that in contrast to surface electro-cautery the coagulation produced by the needle is obtained deep within the substance of the turbinate. It is claimed that mucosal damage and crusting are thereby minimized.

In electro-cautery the red-hot cautery point is usually drawn along the surface of the mucosa over the inferior turbinate in order to make a deep mark in the membrane. Two such cuts are made on the turbinate. On healing the mucous membrane will contract around the scar with a substantial reduction in the bulk of the turbinate, and the air way is improved.

Submucosal injection of sclerosing solutions is useful when facilities for submucosal diathermy or electro-cautery are not available. The injection is made deep within the turbinate with the intention of producing shrinkage without mucosal damage.

Surgical removal of areas of mulberry or fringe formation is advisable. Such formations are removed by scissors and snare. Among the more usual portions which require to be removed are the posterior ends of the inferior turbinates.

Punch forceps are inserted into the nose. A cut is made just in front of the enlarged posterior end and the cold wire snare is slipped round the hypertrophied end. The butt is pressed into the cut, and the mass can be cut with the wire and removed, the snare always being pressed backwards into the nasopharynx to prevent the concha being stripped forwards. Should this occur, more tissue may be removed than is desired.

Other masses can be clipped or snared off. It should be remembered that more can be removed later if necessary, but if too much is removed the result will be years of discomfort for the patient.

ATROPHIC RHINITIS

Atrophy of the nasal mucous membrane may result from a variety of causes and occurs both in the young and in the old. Changes may be slight (rhinitis sicca) or severe, or there may be obstructive crusting with a foetid odour (ozaena).

Aetiology. Any condition which causes drying of the nasal mucous membrane, if prolonged, will give rise to atrophic rhinitis.

For this reason it may be occupational in origin. It sometimes follows nasal operations which result in undue patency of the passages, and a form, frequently symptomless, is encountered in the elderly.

In the absence of any such obvious cause the aetiology is still undecided. Some suppose that it is due to early acute purulent rhinitis, as the condition is not infrequently met with following the exanthemata. Prolonged nasal and sinus suppuration, or sinus infection remaining undiscovered and untreated, has been one of the most popular theories of causation. Endocrine disfunction and deficiency diseases have been considered as possible factors in its production. Success in certain forms of treatment has recently lent support to this theory.

Pathology. There is a change from ciliated to cuboidal or stratified epithelium. Fibrous tissue is increased and infiltration with round cells and plasma cells is marked.

The glands are atrophied, the vessels narrowed and even obliterated. In advanced cases there may be change in the bone of the supporting conchae akin to a rarefying osteitis.

Similar changes may take place in the nasal sinuses, though these changes are frequently obscured by the infective changes produced in the sinus lining by the stagnant secretions.

Symptoms. The early complaints are usually of dryness of the nose and headache, commonly described as a pain behind the eyes. There may be rawness of the nasopharynx and symptoms due to pharyngitis are frequent accompaniments. Obstruction, however, is one of the chief complaints owing to the formation of crusts. These are due to the destruction of the cilia owing to lack of moisture, and the nasal secretions are therefore not expelled but dry in the nose with formation of crusts.

Rhinitis sicca

This term is used to describe the dry condition of the nasal mucosa sometimes seen in the elderly, in those working in hot, dry dusty conditions, and in some industrial occupations. The change is most marked on the anterior part of the septum and the anterior end of the middle turbinate. Crusting is absent or slight.

The dryness produces irritation and discomfort, and sometimes slight bleeding occurs.

Treatment consists of attention to any cause. Decongestant drops must be avoided, limited use of douches or sprays (see Appendix) is useful. Co-existent systemic disease such as anaemia or avitaminosis may require attention; iodides by mouth are sometimes given to try to stimulate mucus secretion.

Ozaena

In this form the odour is present even before the crust formation becomes established. It is encountered mainly in females. The foul smell in ozaena may be so severe as to render association with the patient impossible, though she herself being totally anosmic is unaware of the odour. This disorder is fortunately becoming less frequent in most countries, being apparently associated with poor living conditions and nutrition.

The aetiology is uncertain but systemic diseases such as syphilis and tuberculosis must be excluded.

Appearances. On examining the nose the nasal passages are seen to be wide. The inferior conchae are flattened and may be difficult to distinguish upon the lateral walls of the nose. The mucous membrane is usually dark in colour; it may be dry, and may even be shiny in appearance. Crusting is common as the atrophy of the mucous membrane makes it impossible for the nasal secretions to be expelled from the nose in the normal way. The crusts are yellow as a rule but may be dark and of a greenish colour, and may fill the nasal cavities.

Examination of the nasopharynx may show crusting, and there is usually glazing of the posterior wall, due to an extension of the atrophic condition. In some cases this change may be traced down to the laryngeal cavity.

Treatment. The majority of patients can be kept fairly free of the worst symptoms by strict attention to local cleansing. Syringing is better than douching, and should be done with a Higginson's syringe fitted with an olive tip. Each side of the nose is syringed in turn whilst the patient pants in and out through the mouth to close off the nasopharynx and thus avoids swallowing the fluid. After syringing the patient blows the nose forcibly to expel the crusts.

Treatment initially should be given four times a day and even when the disease is controlled should be given once daily. Crust formation is discouraged by the use of oily sprays or of 2·5 per cent glucose in glycerine.

In some cases of ozaena a spray of oestradiol in arachis oil (0.5 ml of a solution containing 5 mg per ml) used after cleansing has been found of value, 0.25 ml being sprayed into each nostril daily.

Various surgical procedures are available if medical treatment fails. The airways can be narrowed by insertion of strips of bone cartilage, or plastic materials beneath the mucoperichondrium via a sub-labial approach; teflon suspension can be injected submucosally. The parotid duct can be transplanted into the maxillary sinus to combat the dryness of the nose.

In especially troublesome cases of ozaena, temporary closure of one or both nostrils by suitably based skin flaps has been recommended and is said to give good results. After many months the nostrils are re-opened and apparently the formation of foetid crusts does not recur.

Causative systemic disease, *e.g.* syphilis and tuberculosis, will demand appropriate treatment as will associated sinus suppuration.

6. Diseases of the Nasal Cavity *(contd.)*

NASAL ALLERGY

This is a common disorder, most often affecting young adults but also found in children.

The condition arises essentially as an abnormal response to a foreign material, often a protein, which is known as the antigen. The normal response of the body's reticulo-endothelial system defences is the production of a specific antibody. The allergic patient produces in addition abnormal antibodies which become concentrated in certain tissues such as skin and respiratory mucosa. It is thought to be the interaction between fresh incoming antigen and these antibodies in the tissues which elicits release of histamine, with consequent damage to the cell as a result of which characteristic symptoms appear.

The response described can be produced by a wide variety of allergens which fall into the following main groups.

Inhalants

These are the most common and important group in nasal allergy. Such agents are house and animal dusts, moulds, feathers and pollens. Hay fever is the response to grass pollens, hence in Britain it is confined to May, June and July.

Foods and drugs

Fish, eggs, milk, wheat and their products are important in nasal allergy, especially in children. Drugs include aspirin, iodine, antibiotics.

Contactants

Certain antibiotics and plants are the agents.

Bacteria

These are usually staphylococci, pneumococci or streptococci.

A characteristic of the nasal secretion is the large number of eosinophils, especially just after an acute attack, when the mucosa is infiltrated with these cells. Other histological features are oedema and vasodilatation.

Symptoms. In the acute form there is usually prodromal nasal itching. This is soon followed by violent sneezing and profuse watery nasal discharge. Itching and watering of the eyes are not an unusual accompaniment, especially if the allergen is an inhalant. Attacks may continue intermittently for days or last continuously for an hour or more, leaving the patient exhausted.

A seasonal allergy of this type will suggest a pollinosis. Similar perennial attacks are more likely to be dusts of various kinds.

Chronic nasal allergy is not characterized by such dramatic symptoms. Persistent nasal stuffiness with a tendency to excessive mucoid discharge occurs, punctuated by lesser episodes of sneezing and watering. The differentiation from vasomotor rhinitis (*vide infra*) can be difficult. In children symptoms are not usually acute, but a clue may be provided by a history of previous infantile eczema, a tendency to wheezing bronchitis, or a family history of allergy.

Appearances. In the acute attack the pale oedematous mucosa with excessive thin watery mucoid secretion is typical. Between attacks the nose may look normal, though in long-standing cases there may be hypertrophy or fringe formation of the mucosa over the conchae, or polypus formation.

In the chronic form the mucosa is swollen, but its colour is deeper red or even slightly blue, depending on the degree of venous congestion. The mucosa retracts strongly after cocaine application. The secretions are not so profuse.

Diagnosis is in two stages: (1) of the nasal allergy (2) of the allergens.

At each stage a precise history is most important, and in respect of the former will include evidence of other allergic disorders in the patient and allergy in his family. In addition to clinical examination of the patient, the histological study of the nasal mucosa, preferably of the middle concha, and of the secretions for evidence of eosinophilia is valuable. To find the allergen, history is of prime importance. Prick and scratch tests of the skin – with solutions containing various allergens – are useful if skilfully done and interpreted in conjunction with the history.

Treatment. 1. *Abnormalities* in the nose should be dealt with on their own merits if sufficiently severe (*e.g.* a deviated septum, hypertrophic fringe formation). Sinus infection must also be controlled. Great care is necessary, however, as local nasal surgery can cause a severe exacerbation of, or even initiate, bronchial asthma. Such operations are done under steroid cover.

2. *Local treatment* is of limited value and is capable of inflicting additional damage to the nose if improperly used. Vaso-constrictor drops such as $\frac{1}{2}$ per cent ephedrine or similar solutions can be useful for limited periods; the addition of antihistamines to such decongestant drops is of doubtful value. The use of sodium cromoglycate is valuable during attacks. Reduction of the bulk of the conchae by electro-cautery or by submucosal diathermy is often of help; alternatively the injection of sclerosing solutions, such as sodium morrhuate may achieve the

same result. Zinc ionization is now less popular than previously but still worth considering; it acts mainly by diminishing the sensitivity of the mucosa to inhaled allergens and by rendering it less permeable. The use of Cortisone snuff can be helpful; alternatively steroids may be injected into the submucosa of the turbinates. In either case the amount of the drug is so small that systemic effects are avoided.

3. *Avoidance of the allergen* is clearly ideal. It may be possible in the case of feather pillows, woollen blankets, certain foods, plants, cats and dogs, etc., if these can be removed from the house. Not every sufferer from hay pollinosis can take a long cruise during the grass season.

4. *Suppression* of the allergic response can often be obtained by the careful use of antihistamine drugs, especially if they are supplemented by ephedrine and taken in adequate dosage when an attack threatens. Unfortunately many of these drugs are soporific and should be used only in the evening, and never if the patient has to drive a car, unless he is known to be unaffected by the particular drug chosen. Some, however, of the potent antihistamines are stimulating and should be reserved for use in the earlier part of the day: Phenidamine tartrate is an example.

The steroids suppress the allergic response effectively. A single injection intra-muscularly of a long-acting steroid in depot form is especially worthy of consideration in a patient with a seasonal allergy. One such injection may provide protection for the whole pollen season.

The use of steroids by mouth on a long-term basis requires the most careful consideration and indeed is a form of treatment which is seldom justifiable even when a small dose is given. The use of steroids for relatively short periods can produce long-term effects which may prove disastrous in a medical or surgical emergency at some future date. It is wise to reserve this form of treatment for those patients who have some more serious condition, such as intractable asthma.

5. *Specific desensitization* is a most valuable method of treatment if not more than two or three allergens are causing trouble. The exact identification of the allergen is first necessary. Like skin-testing, this technique requires the utmost skill by the physician and great perseverance by the patient, to be successful. Weekly injections of increasing dosage of the allergen are given for several months before the expected exposure; this implies starting early in the year in the case of hay pollinosis. Yearly boosting injections are also needed. Adrenalin must always be ready when injections are given in case of anaphylactic shock.

The introduction of new stock vaccines and of slow-release depot vaccines promises simplified treatment and fewer injections for certain patients.

The nasal application of steroids, used as beclamethasone, and delivered by aerosol, may give great relief in nasal allergy complicated by asthma. Also it may reduce the dependence on systemic steroids.

VASOMOTOR DISORDERS OF THE NOSE

Patients are not infrequently seen with symptoms very suggestive of nasal allergy but in whom the special tests fail to support such a diagnosis.

Symptoms sometimes originate with a severe upper respiratory infection which may result in permanent injury to the delicate autonomic control of the nose.

The main complaint is of nasal stuffiness, perhaps with excessive nose-blowing and post-nasal 'drip'. There is frequently an active response to changes in temperature or humidity and a tendency to bouts of sneezing when waking.

Treatment is on lines similar to those described for allergy but cannot, of course, be specific. In a few patients the watery discharge is so profuse and disabling as to make life a misery. With these patients some surgeons have reported encouraging results from destruction of the Vidian nerve in the pterygoid canal.

NASAL POLYPI

Nasal polypi are greyish masses of pedunculated tissue resembling a bunch of grapes. They are generally multiple, nearly always bilateral and produce nasal blockage by their presence. They are usually visible on anterior rhinoscopy and may even appear at the nostril. Less frequently they may occupy the posterior choanae where they will be seen on mirror examination. Sometimes a large single unilateral polyp fills a posterior choana or the nasopharynx. This variety usually arises from the maxillary antrum and is known as antro-choanal polypus (p. 43).

Aetiology Polypi are the end product of prolonged oedema in the mucosa of the nose and sinuses, especially of the small spaces which constitute the ethmoidal labyrinth. The sub-mucosa around the middle meatus is especially lax and easily waterlogged, which permits swelling of the tissues. The great majority of polyps originate in the region of the middle turbinate and ethmoids, although polyps can grow from any part of the nose or sinuses in gross disease. Similarly in the small cells of the ethmoidal labyrinth the mucous membrane readily swells to occupy all the lumen available, and then projects through the ostia into the nose. Once the mucosa has squeezed its way through the ostia and become constricted at this point the process readily continues to form further polypi.

It has been stated that in at least 75 per cent of nasal polypi, the initial cause of the oedema is allergy and related vasomotor disorder. The main evidence for this lies in the histo-pathology and the close association with other allergic diseases, notably asthma. In spite of this, however, it has to be accepted that once the tendency to polyposis has developed, the patient's allergic state subsequently seems to have little if any relation to it, and recurrence of polypi is often disappointingly high in spite of anti-allergic treatment. It would appear that once firmly established, the mucosal change is irreversible. On the other hand one sees many patients with nasal allergy or chronic congestion of many years' duration who do not develop polyps, so other unknown factors must play a part. In children nasal polyps hardly ever occur except as a manifestation of mucoviscidosis.

Repeated nasal and sinus infection in which resolution and re-aeration are delayed by anatomical deformity, such as a septal deviation may initiate a vicious circle in which polypi become a pronounced feature. Sometimes suppuration precedes polypi, sometimes it follows. Although on many occasions polypi occur without any sign of suppuration whatever, once polypi become obstructive the resultant stagnation of secretion in the sinuses is liable to cause infection and sinusitis then follows.

Histopathology. Nasal polypi consist of swollen mucous membrane, the spaces of which are distended by fluid. The polypus is covered by a thin epithelial layer which may be pavement or ciliated columnar in type. In polypi which have prolapsed towards the nostril the epithelium may become squamous. The substance of the polypus is infiltrated by plasma cells and lymphocytes, and most characteristic of all, large numbers of eosinophils. The blood supply is scanty.

Symptoms. The main complaint is of nasal obstruction, usually bilateral. There is often some discharge, which may be mucoid or purulent. Frankly yellow pus indicates that the polypi are not of superficial origin around the middle concha but are associated with deep-seated sinus disease. Headaches are not unusual, with or without suppuration, but symptoms of allergy are rarely a pronounced feature.

Examination. In advanced cases the external nose may become broadened; the condition is known as 'frog-face'.

On examining the interior of the nose attention should first be directed to the region of the middle concha, though in obvious cases a view of this part will be obscured by the large, grey, polypoid masses. These masses are freely mobile on their pedicles, insensitive to probing and nearly always multiple and bilateral.

In less advanced cases, smaller polypi may closely resemble blobs of mucus but are not cleared by blowing the nose. If doubt remains a probe should be used to palpate the area; the patient will feel discomfort only if the probe touches the nasal mucosa.

The presence and origin of any pus should be noted, also the state of the mucous membrane. The appearances of allergy are often absent.

Posterior rhinoscopy should also be done: the nose can look perfectly normal anteriorly in the presence of a large choanal polypus, the narrow pedicle of which cannot be seen in the middle meatus. The obstruction in antro-choanal polypi is often valvular, *i.e.* present only on expiration. If masses of polypi are seen on posterior rhinoscopy treatment should be planned accordingly.

Treatment. Small polypi occasionally undergo spontaneous regression if the cause is removed. In the vast majority of instances, however, polypi must be removed surgically. The nose is cocainized, and a cold wire snare is passed around each polypus in turn and gradually tightened as high up around the pedicle as possible.

It is important that the pedicle should be avulsed and not cut or torn through, otherwise early recurrence is inevitable. Any small tags remaining can be removed with a broad-bladed forceps. It is wise to re-examine the nose a few days later: small tags not present at the end of the operation may become apparent when the shrinking effect of the cocaine wears off and necessitate further treatment. This can be done in the out-patient department. After-treatment is minimal, decongestant drops, and medicated steam inhalations for a week are comforting.

Simple removal of polypi must be combined with an attempt to control the underlying cause; associated allergy and sinus infection must be energetically treated or recurrence is almost inevitable. Sinus infection may be dealt with by antral wash-outs or by radical antrostomy, whichever is appropriate. A severe septal deformity can also predispose to recurrence and interfere with adequate access for complete clearance of polypi, and so should be corrected.

It is wise to see patients at intervals after polypectomy rather than await a recurrence of actual nasal obstruction; any polypi beginning to re-form can then be dealt with easily and without inconvenience to the patient. Steroids should be avoided in cases of recurrent polypi unless demanded by some underlying allergic condition.

In the case of persistent early recurrence, if extensive sinus disease is diagnosed then an attempt should be made to remove the polypus-producing area. This may be achieved by means of an intranasal ethmoidectomy. In skilled hands this can be a completely excisive operation, but the surgeon is inevitably working near the orbit and dura, and disasters have occurred. There is thus an increasing tendency in favour of an external ethmoidectomy, in which the danger areas can be seen. The scar around the inner canthus soon becomes invisible.

An alternative, if a radical antrostomy is needed and has not already been done, is to perform a combined clearance of antrum and ethmoid together. This can be carried out from above via an incision approximately along the infra-orbital margin (Patterson) or through the canine fossa (transantral ethmoidectomy).

ANTRO-CHOANAL POLYPUS

As already mentioned, this presents as a valvular obstruction generally in adolescents and young adults. Inspiration is relatively free but impaction of the polyp in the posterior choana on expiration produces almost total blockage. Anteriorly the nose may look normal, yet posteriorly the nasopharynx can be almost filled by the single smooth polyp (Fig. 16).

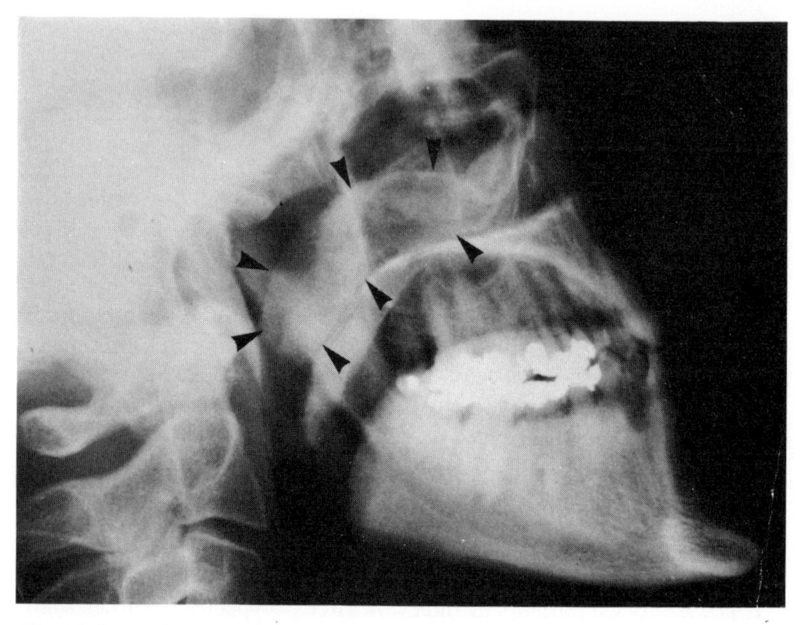

Fig. 16. Antro-choanal polyp. – A clue to the diagnosis sometimes arises from the fact that inspiration may still be possible, but expiration becomes totally blocked as the polyp impacts in the posterior choana.

The condition is occasionally bilateral. The precise cause is unknown.

There is generally no associated evidence of active allergy or infection, though radiologically the sinus is opaque due to the thickened mucosa, which in prolapsing through the abnormally wide ostium has formed the choanal part of the polypus. Careful removal of the polyp by grasping its pedicle and avulsing as much antral mucosa as possible is followed by cure in some patients.

In those which recur the antrum must be opened through the canine fossa and diseased mucosa removed as necessary.

7. Diseases of the Nasal Cavity *(contd.)*

FOREIGN BODIES

Foreign bodies are often found in the noses of children. They consist, for the most part, of pebbles, peas, pieces of indiarubber and other small objects which are handled by the child. The place of impaction is usually the lower part of the nose. The symptoms are those of unilateral obstruction and discharge. In a child a unilateral purulent discharge is pathognomonic. Removal of the foreign body by means of fine nasal forceps or hook is, as a rule, simple, though not infrequently it necessitates the use of general anaesthesia. In these cases great care must be taken in searching for the foreign body, as it is surprisingly easy to push it into the pharynx, from whence there is some danger of its being inhaled. This may happen to the inexperienced as the foreign body becomes covered by mucus and is difficult to identify. To prevent this accident it is wise to place one finger in the nasopharynx when searching for the foreign body if it is deeply embedded in the nasal cavity.

In adults, foreign bodies usually take the form of rhinoliths, which sometimes are calcium deposits on pieces of gauze or other substances which have been used to plug the nose in a case of haemorrhage. If these foreign bodies have been in the nose for a considerable time, a degree of atrophy of the mucous membrane will be observed when they are removed. A douche should be given for a short period after removal of the foreign body, and then the nose should be allowed to recuperate. As a rule there is little discomfort following this condition, even where there is quite a marked degree of atrophy.

HAEMORRHAGE FROM THE NOSE (EPISTAXIS)

The blood supply of the nose is described on p. 9.

As a rule bleeding in young and middle-aged patients is commonly from an anterior site low down and is unassociated with systemic disease. In older patients bleeding is often from an inaccessible site high up or far back (*i.e.* ethmoidal) and frequently associated with systemic disorder, but in both groups, especially if bleeding recurs in spite of adequate local treatment, search must always be made for a particular cause. The actual attack may be initiated by minimal trauma such as rubbing or nose-blowing.

Systemic causes. These include hypertension (in which epistaxis may provide a safety-valve), arteriosclerosis, cardiovascular, renal and blood diseases. Hereditary telangiectasia usually shows first as epistaxis.

Local disorders. These include the presence of prominent unsupported vessels especially in Little's area, ulcerations, tumours and trauma. Pressure change from high altitude may provoke bleeding.

Treatment of an attack

1. In the younger patient: the nose is blown to expel loose clot, the nostrils are then firmly pinched between finger and thumb continuously for ten minutes. A cottonwool pledget soaked in 10 per cent cocaine with an equal amount of 1/1000 adrenalin and squeezed out can with advantage be inserted into the nose and retained during this time whilst the patient breathes gently through the mouth. Very often the bleeding will have stopped as a result of direct pressure (if from Little's area) or from the vasoconstrictor action of the cocaine-adrenalin (if further back). A search is then made in the clean dry nose for the responsible vessel. This is frequently identified without difficulty and can be cauterized. If it cannot be cauterized and if bleeding continues a pack or a nasal balloon may be needed (p. 48.)

2. In the elderly: the nose is dealt with as before. Preliminary sedation with morphine is often helpful, also the patient should keep the mouth open and be forbidden to swallow. This closes off the nasopharynx, and encourages the formation of a firm clot. After ten minutes the nose is inspected and any bleeding vessel is cauterized, but in many elderly

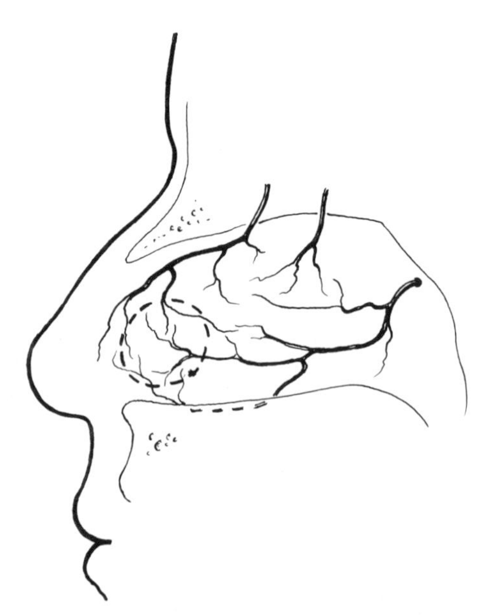

Fig. 17. Anastomosis of vessels on Little's area.

patients the site is ethmoidal and inaccessible. If bleeding is uncontrolled or recurs the patient should be confined to bed, the nose packed, and attention directed to any causative factors. The pack can generally be removed after one day and the patient gradually mobilized again. Sometimes re-packing is necessary for another day. Occasionally even a well-inserted pack fails to control severe bleeding and a post-nasal pack is necessary. Severe blood loss in all patients should be made good, but in the elderly care must be taken not to overload the circulation.

Frequently repeated bleeding in old patients, which demands packing, rapidly reduces the patient to a seriously exhausted condition. This is unnecessary and should be avoided by ligation of the appropriate artery if control by non-operative means is unsuccessful.

If bleeding is from the upper part of the nose the ethmoidal arteries are ligated in the orbit. This is a minor procedure which can be carried out under local anaesthesia. Bleeding from the lower part of the nose may call for ligation of the external carotid or the maxillary artery. The latter procedure requires a transantral approach and a general anaesthetic.

Patient seen between attacks

A search should always be made for a prominent or weakened vessel which should be cauterized. This is often impossible in the elderly. Attention is paid to causative factors and if disabling attacks continue ligation of the ethmoid or maxillary arteries should be considered as an interval procedure.

Methods of cauterization

If the bleeding vessel can be identified the nose is cocainized and the area coagulated by the electric cautery; care must be taken to avoid touching the region otherwise the crust is pulled off and bleeding continues.

Alternatively the area can be cauterized by chemical means and for children this is less frightening. The cocainized area is touched with a wool-dressed probe which has been very lightly dipped into trichloracetic acid. This penetrates, tends to run and can cause deep burns. It should therefore be used with the utmost care and preferably only by an expert. Excess is neutralized by gentian violet. If these means are not available a bead can be made from chromic acid, but again this demands care in use. A chemical cautery should not be used on both sides of the nose on the same occasion, for this may cause perforation of the septum. After cautery the nose is kept lubricated for one week.

Methods of packing

The nose is anaesthetized by inserting a strip of ribbon gauze wrung out of 5 per cent cocaine and leaving it in the nose for 10 minutes. If gauze ribbon (about 1 metre) is used for packing it should be well lubricated with liquid paraffin to which a small amount of iodoform paste has been added. Adrenalin packs are to be avoided. The first part of the ribbon is inserted double along the floor of the nose, the remainder of the pack being built up lengthwise on this until every part of the nasal cavity is firmly filled. In the majority of cases this controls the bleeding. If suitable inflatable bags are available they can be used instead and there is much to be said in their favour. They are more convenient, equally effective, less uncomfortable and less damaging to the nasal mucosa if properly used.

A well-inserted anterior pack seldom fails to control bleeding, but sometimes it is insufficient and a post-nasal plug or a balloon must be inserted. (Fig. 18). These balloons may be single or double and apart from saving the patient a great deal of discomfort, are much less traumatic to nasal mucosa than packing.

Insertion of a post-nasal pack is painful to the patient and unpleasant to the surgeon if not done under general anaesthesia, but circumstances may permit of cocainization only. This should include the soft palate as well as the nose. The pack is prepared from gauze and is of such size as to fit firmly into the naso-pharynx (about 5 cm × 2.5 cm).

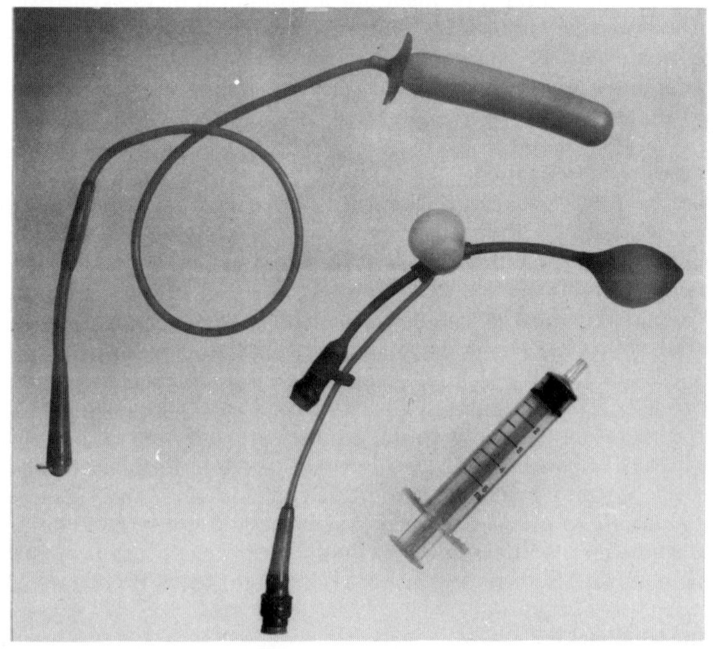

Fig. 18. Epistaxis balloons.—The ordinary and the double balloons are illustrated. The latter occludes both the posterior and the anterior nares. Air is injected to obtain gentle pressure by means of a 5 ml. syringe.

A strong tape is tied round its middle and it is soaked in liquid paraffin and iodoform. The end of the tape is picked up from the patient's pharynx by an instrument passed backwards through the nose. The tape is then drawn forwards through the nose.

Traction on the tape above and the help of a guiding finger below enable the pack to be positioned firmly in the nasopharynx. The tape is anchored to the side of the face and the nose packed anteriorly as before. When post-nasal pressure is required, a double balloon of the Brighton Wadsworth type (Fig. 18) can be recommended as an alternative to the conventional post-nasal gauze pack.

If properly inserted, anterior packing together with a posterior pack will control any haemorrhage.

Chemotherapy is essential for all patients with a post-nasal pack and for patients retaining an anterior pack or balloon longer than one day.

CHOANAL ATRESIA

This is a developmental defect in which there is failure of one or both nares to canalize. Suffocation may occur before the child learns to breathe with the mouth. Severe feeding difficulties also occur. When one posterior naris is blocked, all the secretions from the nose and sinuses are forced to come through the anterior naris. The obstruction may be composed of membrane or of bone.

Treatment. Problems of feeding and breathing may arise in bilateral cases, often demand urgent attention soon after birth. Breathing can be helped on a first-aid basis by inserting an ordinary anaesthetic airway or similar tube, which is then kept in place by adhesive tape until skilled surgical help is available. Operative treatment is difficult, but the obstruction, which may only be membranous, should be pierced and a sufficiently large opening maintained.

Keeping the hole open by in-dwelling tubes and later by frequent dilatation may succeed. More usually it is necessary to remove the atretic plate and prevent stenosis by making suitable muco-periosteal flaps. The approach can be either transpalatine or transnasal, using microsurgical techniques and an operating microscope.

In unilateral cases treatment is not urgent and operation can be delayed until the child is older and the structures are larger. In older patients the obstruction is usually removed by the transpalatine approach.

NEW GROWTHS IN THE NOSE

Benign tumours

Warts, *i.e.* squamous papillomata, occur in the skin of the vestibule and must always be regarded with suspicion. Excision sometimes shows the lesion to be a squamous carcinoma. The so-called bleeding septal polyp is usually an infective granuloma, occasionally it may be a true fibroangioma or some rarer lesion and accordingly such polyps should always be examined histologically after removal. Angiomata occur in the ethmoids and though histologically benign are always serious. Transitional cell papilloma is often diffuse when first seen and has a great tendency to recur unless treated by adequate excision. It can become malignant.

Malignant tumours

These are commonly squamous cell carcinomata, but any type of lesion can occur, including adeno-carcinomata, malignant melanomata and sarcomata.

The most common site in the nose for these lesions is the ethmoidal region, but the nose and sinuses are one area as far as these diseases are concerned and one is seldom treating a purely nasal condition. The real point of origin is rarely determined.

Irritation of the nasal passages by the dust of certain hard woods has been shown to cause nasal cancer amongst woodworkers.

Symptoms. The chief symptom of new growth in the nose is unilateral obstruction. There may be haemorrhage or a purulent and sanguineous discharge. Also broadening of the nasal bones may occur as the growth increases in bulk. Headache is a late complaint.

Treatment. The treatment of these diseases of the nose depends upon their site, their size and their character. Benign growths can be removed by excision or diathermy with all precautions for histological verification.

Treatment of malignant tumours can seldom be considered separately from treatment of the sinuses and is generally a combination of irradiation and surgery, the approach being either sub-labial or via a lateral rhinotomy.

The planning of treatment should be an exercise in collaboration between surgeon and radiotherapist. Opinions differ as to whether radiation should be used to reduce the tumour before surgery is attempted or should follow surgical excision. Some surgeons prefer radiotherapy before surgery and intra-cavitary radium after. Results are encouraging and are likely to improve with the introduction of the newer cytotoxic drugs. These are given intra-arterially, the alkylating agents and the antimetabolites being those most commonly used. So far they have been used mainly for palliative purposes, especially for relief of pain. Certain drugs may have their main use prior to radiotherapy and subsequent radical surgery.

SYPHILIS

Syphilis of the nose may be encountered in its primary, secondary, tertiary or congenital forms.

Primary nasal syphilis

This is exceedingly rare, but when seen causes swelling and reddening on the affected side of the nose, simulating a boil or dermatitis, and unless the examiner is alive to the possibility, the presence of syphilis may easily be overlooked.

Secondary syphilis

This is most frequently seen in infants as the condition known as 'snuffles'. This develops within the first few weeks of life, and is accompanied by crusting and fissuring of the anterior nares. Secondary syphilis may occur, however, in adults, and mucous patches and shallow ulcerations are found, as on other mucous membranes. The symptoms caused by these changes are those of obstruction and offensive discharge.

Tertiary syphilis

This stage commences with gumma formation. When seen it is usually of nodular character and if it affects the septum the swelling is bilateral. There may be some swelling and tenderness of the nose. Chronic nasal discharge occurs when the gumma breaks down, and when the nose is examined the appearance is of a swelling which is in reality the indurated edge of an ulcer. Extensive destruction of the nasal structures may follow, with foul crusting in the nose. The bridge of the nose is the part most commonly affected, but the whole nasal structure may be destroyed.

Congenital syphilis

In the congenital disease the lesions are those of secondary or tertiary syphilis, snuffles being the most common manifestation in infancy.

Diagnosis. Although nasal syphilis is now rare in the United Kingdom, cases still occur and can cause confusion. Diagnosis is aided by clinical awareness, bacteriological methods in early cases, serological tests and biopsy in later ones. Tuberculosis, tumours, ozaena and certain ulcerations of doubtful origin must be differentiated. As some tropical diseases such as yaws may closely resemble syphilis, enquiry about travel abroad should be made in all doubtful cases. It is emphasized that syphilis may co-exist with some other disease.

Treatment. This consists of local cleanliness, combined with management of the general disease along conventional lines. Deformity may later require plastic surgery.

RHINOSPORIDIOSIS

This disease is caused by a yeast-like organism – the *Rhinosporidium seeberi*. It is encountered in India, in South America and other tropical countries.

Clinical features. It appears usually as nasal polypi, but may affect the mucous membrane of the cheek, the uvula and other parts. Spread in the body is haematogenous and the liver, spleen and skin may be affected in this way. The mode of dissemination of the disease is undetermined.

Treatment. This is wide removal of the polypoid masses by cutting diathermy snare; histological examination should be carried out always, owing to the similarity of the disease to carcinoma. Antimony has been used with some success.

RHINOSCLEROMA

The causative factor is the *Klebsiella rhinoscleromata* (of Von Frisch). Distribution of the disease is world wide, but in Europe it is found chiefly in Poland, Hungary and the Ukraine, though it has been reported in Switzerland and in Italy. The condition appears to be associated with lack of hygiene.

Clinical features. Any part of the upper respiratory system may be the site of the painless chronic inflammatory masses which are limited to the mucous membrane. These consist of plasma cell infiltrations, exceedingly dense, and containing the characteristic foam cells. Increasing sclerosis is a feature and neighbouring glands tend to become affected.

Diagnosis. The identification of the typical foam cells by histological examination is conclusive. The complement fixation test is invariably positive.

Treatment. Rhinoscleroma is specific. Antibiotics should be used. The local deformities can be dealt with by plastic surgery.

TUBERCULOSIS OF THE NOSE(LUPUS)

Tuberculosis of the nose is found chiefly in the anterior part of the nasal cavity. It may on occasions spread into the nose from the skin, but the usual site is the mucous membrane of the inferior concha and the anterior part of the septum, a short distance behind the muco-cutaneous junction. From these sites it may spread round the nasal cavity. It may involve the soft parts of the nose and the cartilages and cause severe ulceration and destruction. The bone is rarely attacked.

Pathology. The histo-pathology is similar to that of tuberculosis in other sites. The nasal lesion varies from a comparatively acute ulcerative form to a fibrotic type of slow progress, usually called lupoid, or simply lupus. Between the comparatively acute lesions and the fibrotic, many different degrees of activity are encountered.

The usual clinical variety of tuberculosis in the nose is the subacute form in which sessile warty vegetations may fill the nares. They bleed readily and cause discharge and obstruction. Ulceration is frequently present and on the septum can progress to perforation.

In lupus the disease is fibrotic in type and of slow progress. The 'apple jelly' nodules which characterize the skin condition can be demonstrated if the nose is swabbed with cocaine and adrenalin solution.

Diagnosis. This is chiefly by exclusion. The blood Wassermann reaction should be taken to exclude syphilitic infection, not only to make a differential diagnosis, but because syphilis is sometimes co-existent. The chest should be examined, as tuberculosis of the chest may be present. The diagnosis finally rests with the microscope, and a portion of tissue should be removed in all cases which are suspicious. This can be done by cocainizing a small part of the mucous membrane and removing a portion of the tissue with punch forceps or scalpel.

Treatment. Streptomycin is the drug of choice combined with P.A.S. as used in the treatment of tuberculosis elsewhere in the body. If possible the customary tuberculosis regime should be instituted until the disease is under control, but during later treatments patients may continue their occupations since further treatment can be an out-patient measure.

Against lupus, calciferol alone may be adequate as the tendency to healing is high. Diathermy now has a less important part to play but can be used to destroy nodules which are slow to heal. Where diathermy is not available a galvanocautery point may be used instead.

Treatment of tuberculosis and lupus is prolonged, and the patient must continue attendance for a considerable time after apparent cure, as there may be recurrence after a lapse of some years.

DIPHTHERIA OF THE NOSE

This is encountered most frequently in children. It is characterized by nasal obstruction and discharge which is sometimes bloodstained and which may excoriate the upper lip. In the majority of cases seen in nasal clinics the patient is not severely ill and the condition is liable to be overlooked. Inspection of the nasal cavity may reveal a greyish white membrane covering the inferior concha and the adjacent parts. This bleeds when removed. In every case in which there is any doubt, or in which a membrane is seen in the nose, a swab should be taken for bacteriological examination.

PROGRESSIVE ULCERATIVE GRANULOMA

Also known as lethal mid-line granuloma this rare and dangerous disease is of unknown etiology. It possesses features of inflammatory and neoplastic diseases but is characteristic of neither. It may be an auto-immune disorder.

The granuloma begins as a locally destructive ulceration in the nose or sinuses. If not controlled, and if the patient survives long enough, it becomes associated with granulomata and necrotizing arteritis throughout the body and ends fatally. The diffuse form involves lungs and kidneys especially and is known as Wegener's granulomatosis.

No treatment is specific. Steroids are valuable, as is radiotherapy. The latter is given in small dosage over a prolonged period. Cytotoxic drugs are reported to be of use. Antibiotics help control secondary infection.

SECTION II NASAL ACCESSORY SINUSES

8. Anatomy

The nasal accessory sinuses are air spaces which are developed in the bones of the skull and have communication with the nasal cavity. They are divided into two groups – the anterior group and the posterior group. The anterior group comprises the frontal air sinus, the maxillary air sinus and the anterior ethmoidal air cells. The posterior group comprises the posterior ethmoidal air cells and the sphenoidal sinus. This grouping of the sinuses is arranged more from the point of view of drainage than from actual anatomical distribution. The sinuses vary so widely in their positions during development that the distinction between 'anterior' and 'posterior' might be completely misleading. The anterior group of sinuses drains into the middle meatus, and the posterior group drains into the superior meatus and the spheno-ethmoidal recess (Figs. 4–6).

THE MAXILLARY AIR SINUS

At birth this sinus is represented by a small space on the lateral wall of the nose, high up in the middle meatus, and communicates with the nasal cavity. As growth proceeds the space enlarges by a process of pneumatization of the maxillary bone. There is a double process at work. In the young child the second dentition lies in the upper part of the maxillary bone, a very short distance below the orbit, and the descent of the dentition is brought about by the laying down of new bone. This bone, as it is laid down, becomes pneumatized, forming the maxillary air sinus. Development proceeds downwards and forwards until at the age of, approximately, nine years, the floor of the maxillary air sinus is on the same level as the floor of the nose. This manner of growth, its direction and approximate extent at any particular age, is of importance in carrying out the operation of proof-puncture upon children, for allowance must be made for the probable position of the sinus at any particular stage in its development. From this time development proceeds until the antrum is finally completed by the descent of the third molar tooth. This takes place between the twenty-third and twenty-fifth years.

The fully developed maxillary air sinus should extend from the first premolar to the third molar tooth. The sinus reaches up to the floor of the orbit and thus occupies practically the whole body of the maxillary bone. Its medial boundary is the lateral nasal wall with the attachment

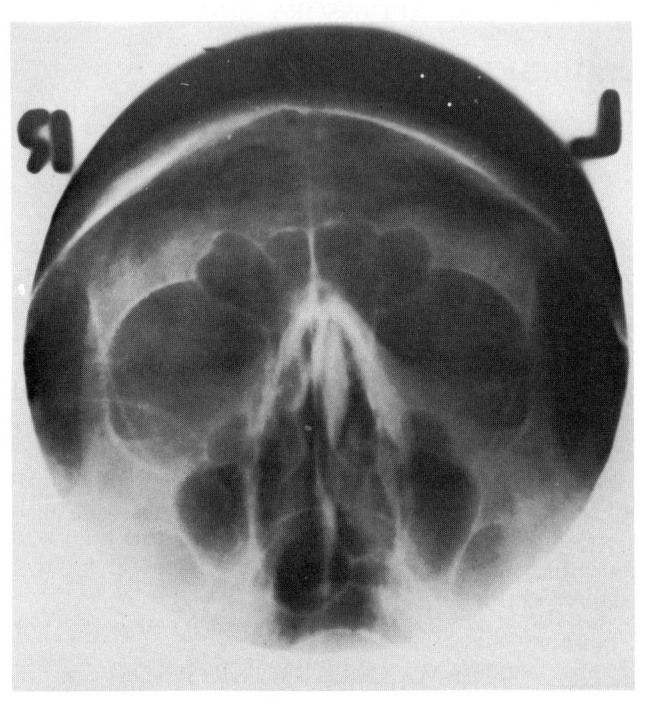

Fig. 19. Postero-anterior view of normal nasal sinuses. View for maxillary sinuses.

of the inferior concha, while the upper posterior part of the medial wall frequently shows a bony dehiscence which is closed by membrane. This is known as the membranous part of the middle meatus, and the ostium lies in this part of the wall. In addition to the normal ostium there is sometimes a small accessory ostium below and in front of it. It is important to remember that the infra-orbital nerve traverses the roof of the maxillary air sinus and appears at the infra-orbital foramen in the upper part of the anterior maxillary wall.

In the floor of the sinus runs the superior alveolar nerve, and the roots of the teeth not infrequently project into the maxillary air sinus. They may be covered with only a thin plate of bone, in which case the reason for infection of the maxillary air sinus in apical tooth abscess becomes obvious. Extraction of such a poorly covered tooth can result in an abnormal communication between mouth and antrum. This is known as oro-antral fistula. In the upper wall of the antrum anteriorly is a hollow bounded medially by the canine ridge. This depression is known as the canine fossa, and within the bone of the anterior wall run twigs from the infra-orbital nerve to the teeth of the upper jaw.

The hard palate forms a large portion of the floor of the maxillary air sinus. The pterygoid fossa with the sphenopalatine fissure at its inner or

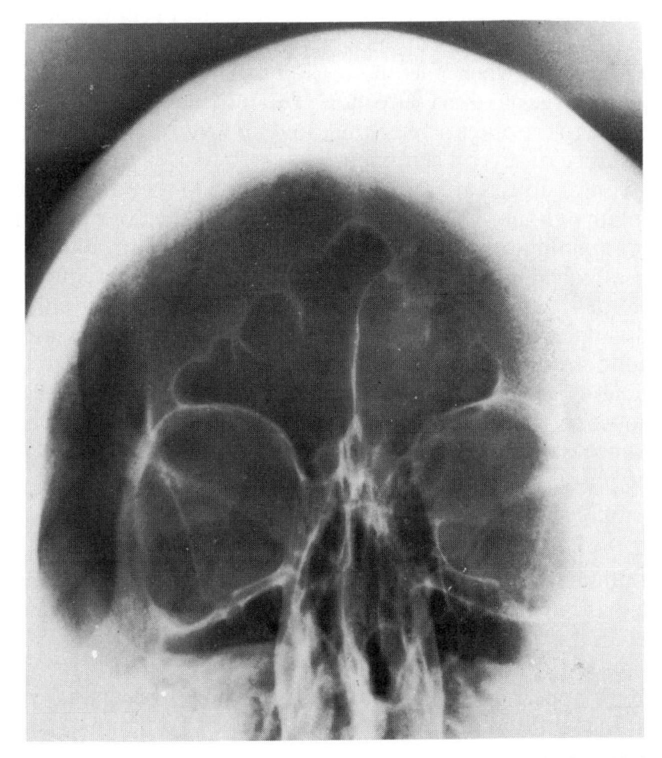

Fig. 20. Postero-anterior view of nasal sinuses to show frontal and ethmoid sinuses.

medial end is posterior. The maxillary air sinus may consist of one whole cavity or it may be divided by septa into two or more cavities which may or may not communicate with one another. The shape of the maxillary air sinus varies with different types of facies. In persons with projecting face bones it will be found that the anterior and medial angle of the sinus is narrow with the nasal wall bulging into the sinus, so that it is not unknown when opening through the anterior wall of the maxilla to open through into the nasal cavity, missing the sinus altogether. This point must be remembered in carrying out operations upon the sinus.

The maxillary air sinus is lined by ciliated columnar epithelium. It is richly provided with glands, which are situated chiefly around the ostium.

THE FRONTAL SINUS

The frontal sinus occupies the space in the frontal bones between the inner and the outer tables. The sinus is not present at birth, but becomes the frontal sinus about the age of five when the air cells extend above the level of the supra-orbital ridge. The frontal sinus is developed from a recess in the anterior part of the nose. One or both sinuses may remain rudimentary, but when pneumatization extends into the frontal bone proper it enlarges in every direction. The fully developed frontal sinus may extend to the outer orbital angle and upwards into the frontal bone for a distance of several centimetres.

The frontal sinuses are rarely symmetrical, and they are separated by a thin plate of bone. The roof of the orbit forms the floor of the frontal sinus, containing towards the inner angle the supra-orbital nerve and having attached to it, more medially, the trochlea of the superior oblique muscle. The frontal sinus is lined with columnar epithelium. The cilia of the frontal sinus, according to some authorities, are generally found around the opening of the fronto-nasal duct. Between the frontal sinus and the orbit are frequently found narrow cells which are known as the orbito-ethmoidal cells, and these may or may not communicate with the frontal sinus. They may have their own openings into the nose.

THE ETHMOIDAL CELLS

The ethmoidal air cells, although divided into two groups, must be regarded as one from the point of view of development and treatment. To explain this division of the ethmoidal cells properly, it is necessary to go back to their development. In the primary nasal cartilage, grooves and ridges appear on the lateral wall, the ridges becoming conchae, and in the embryonic nose may number five ethmo-conchae. As development proceeds adhesions form on these ridges, parts of the grooves being cut off and thereby forming cells. Eventually one of these ethmo-conchae becomes more prominent than the others and forms the middle concha. This appears to be a more or less arbitrary process, and therefore all cells above this ridge become posterior ethmoid, while all those below it become anterior ethmoid, drainage being respectively above and below the middle concha, so that an anterior ethmoidal cell might quite well be behind, anatomically speaking, a posterior ethmoidal cell. In contrast to the other sinuses the ethmoids consist of very many small air cells without regular disposition, symmetry or fixed number. They lie in the upper part of the lateral wall of the nose. Laterally is the orbital periosteum. Below is part of the maxillary air sinus and above the cells meet at an apex, though in the anterior part the frontal sinus might be said to bear a superior relationship. The lining of these cells is similar to that of the other sinuses, drainage, as before, being effected by ciliary mucous membrane.

THE SPHENOIDAL SINUS

The sphenoidal sinus occupies the body of the sphenoid bone. At birth the sphenoidal sinus is seen as a small depression at the posterior end

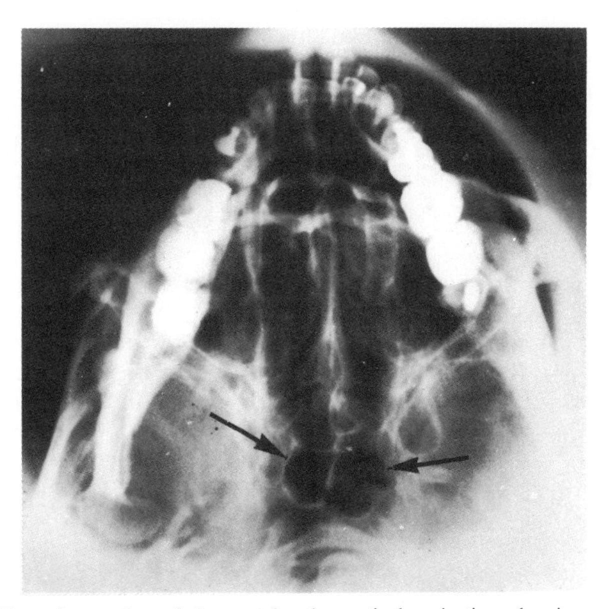

Fig. 21. View of normal nasal sinuses taken by vertical projection, showing sphenoidal sinuses.

of the nasal cartilage. As development proceeds the depression deepens and in effect the posterior end of the nasal cartilage becomes constricted, the point of constriction becoming the ostium of the sphenoidal sinus. At the age of nine to twelve years the sphenoidal sinus does not encroach upon the sphenoidal bone, and is still confined to cartilage; but after this period pneumatization of the sphenoidal bone begins, and may extend down into the pterygoid process of the sphenoid. The sphenoidal sinuses are capable of wide variation in shape and position. They may be of unequal size and one may be almost on top of the other.

Abnormal pneumatization accounts for certain unusual complications of sphenoidal sinusitis. In most skulls pneumatization extends inferiorly below the pituitary fossa which bulges into the sinus. The transphenoidal route to the pituitary takes advantage of this, so that the sphenoidal sinus now provides the usual means of access for hypophysectomy. At the outer part of the roof the Gasserian ganglion may form a superior relationship, while at the outer anterior angle, where the roof and the lateral wall meet, the optic foramen, containing the optic nerve, is in close apposition to the sphenoidal sinus. The lateral wall is in contact with the cavernous sinus, with the nerves and vascular structures which it contains. In the floor there is one important structure, the Vidian nerve or the nerve of the pterygoid canal. As a rule this nerve is in the substance of the bone, but it may be lightly covered on the floor of the sinus and may even be carried in a bony arch across it.

The ostium of the sphenoidal sinus is, as has already been pointed out, high up on the anterior wall. The lining of the sphenoidal sinus is similar to that of the other sinuses and the nasal cavity.

It will be seen that the accessory sinuses form a system into which the nasal lining is continued unbroken, and which, therefore, must share in some degree in all the pathological changes which infection is likely to produce in the nasal cavity.

9. Sinusitis

Sinusitis means an inflammation of the lining membrane of the sinuses.

Aetiology. Most frequently it is an extension from a nasal infection, but any condition within the nose which interferes with drainage and aeration of a sinus renders that sinus liable to infection. When infection is established the blockage of the natural drainage channels renders spontaneous recovery more difficult.

Any condition which tends to narrow the nasal passage, especially in the region of the middle meatus, pre-disposes to sinusitis, through the tendency to obstruct the drainage of the sinuses. Such causes are deflection of the septum, foreign bodies and new growths. Excessive vasomotor changes associated with extreme temperature variations or with improper air conditioning resulting in excessive humidity or dryness appear to predispose to sinus infection.

Infection of the roots of the teeth may be the cause of maxillary sinusitis, particularly in those cases in which the roots project through the floor into the sinus cavity. Infection sometimes takes place when part of the floor gives way in the extraction of teeth from the upper jaw.

Excessive blowing of the nose during an acute infection may determine the onset by driving infected material into the sinus. Nasal douching for the same reason should not be carried out during the early stages of inflammation. Some instances of infection have been recorded in which the sudden inrush of infected material was caused by diving or underwater swimming.

Pathology. The mucous membrane passes through all the usual stages of infection. There is an outpouring of secretion which rapidly becomes purulent. At first there is increased ciliary activity; later, as infection becomes established, ciliary action becomes ineffective and there may even be destruction of the cilia. Thickening of the membrane of the sinuses occurs to such an extent that the membrane may become polypoid, and in very acute cases the whole of the space of the sinus may be filled with oedematous mucous membrane, the cavity being obliterated. In cases of long-standing suppuration the mucous membrane may be similar to granulation tissue, and organisms are found in submucous tissues and may even be found in the bone. Fibrous tissue formation may be marked and new bone is sometimes laid down.

Occasionally all the sinuses on one side or on both sides may be affected. The condition is then spoken of as pansinusitis.

DIAGNOSIS OF SINUSITIS

Certain symptoms of sinusitis are common to all sinuses – such symptoms as headache or pain, usually referable to a particular sinus, general disturbance with elevation of temperature and pulse rate. There may or may not be nasal discharge, depending upon whether the ostium of the sinus is patent or occluded. There is usually tenderness over the affected sinus. One sinus alone may be infected, but it is more frequent in the acute forms for the whole group of sinuses to share in the inflammation.

When the sinusitis follows a nasal infection the earliest symptoms are usually those of the causal condition. When this does not exist or has passed unnoticed, in severe cases the onset may be characterized by a rigor, with elevation of pulse and temperature.

In the examination of the sinuses the position and time of the headache is of importance and the points of maximum tenderness are valuable guides.

Nasal inspection is of the greatest importance and the presence of pus and its origin should be ascertained if possible.

Studies by X-rays should be made in all cases of suspected sinusitis,

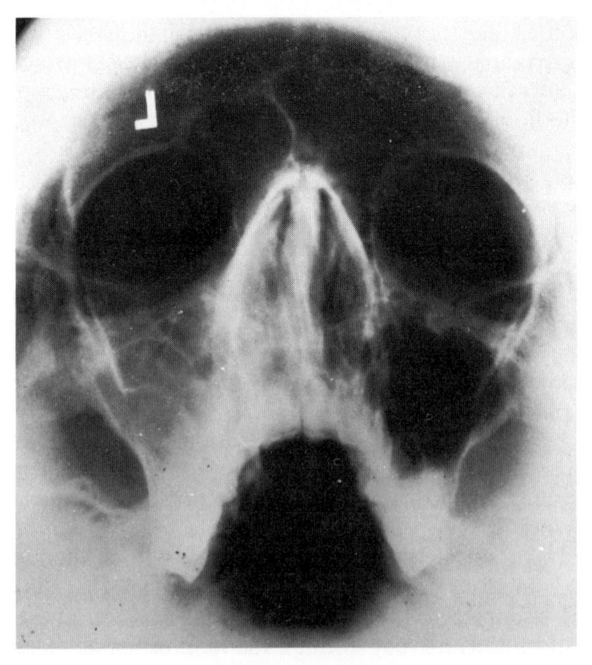

Fig. 22. Unilateral maxillary sinusitis. Note the opacity of the homolateral nasal cavity due to associated mucosal swelling. The other sinuses are clear, the frontals being well developed.

or if these are not available, transillumination can be carried out. Finally, cannulation or puncture of certain sinuses may be done and the contents examined bacteriologically.

Points of tenderness. *Frontal sinusitis* pain and tenderness are greatest over the floor of the sinus; tapping over the frontal region may be painful.

Ethmoidal headache is deep-seated behind the eyes; tenderness is felt at the sides of the nose just below the inner canthus.

Maxillary sinusitis causes pain localized to the upper teeth and to the canine fossa; pressure over the fossa and behind the maxilla may reveal tenderness.

Sphenoidal headache is described as being in the centre of the skull; it may seem far back, as if in the temple, and may spread down the back of the neck, the sides of the neck and behind the ears.

Nasal signs. In the majority of cases of acute sinusitis changes will be found within the nasal cavity. The mucous membrane will be reddened and oedematous according to the location of the infection. If the sinusitis occurs in the course of an acute rhinitis, the nose will be congested throughout and will give very little information as to the individual sinus affected. In the case of individual sinuses in the anterior group the middle concha is usually to be seen reddened, swollen and glistening. The uncinate process will also be prominent. The middle meatus will be closed, or a trickle of pus will be seen coming from it. In the posterior group of sinuses the appearance of the mucous membrane will be confined to the upper and posterior part of the nose and pus will be seen above the posterior end of the middle concha or coming down from the spheno-ethmoidal recess, but if seen anteriorly it appears in the olfactory sulcus.

MAXILLARY SINUSITIS

Acute stage. The maxillary sinus, owing to its large size, gives acute symptoms less often than the other sinuses. When infected, however, neuralgic pains in the upper teeth may be the first sign. There is a beating sensation in the cheek and a feeling of fullness below the eye on the side affected, while frequently a spot of tenderness can be indicated just lateral to the alae nasi. Tenderness may be found on pressure behind the maxilla on the edge of the pterygoid fossa.

Examination of the nose may reveal the presence of pus in the middle meatus. In the early stages probably there will be some discharge from the nose. This may completely dry up as the mucous membrane in the sinus swells and occludes the ostium. A point is reached, however, in which the tension rises inside the sinus, and a certain amount of purulent fluid is forced out through the ostium. At this stage there is extremely severe pain, and after a little discharge the pain may subside. This condition of affairs may continue for some days until the infection

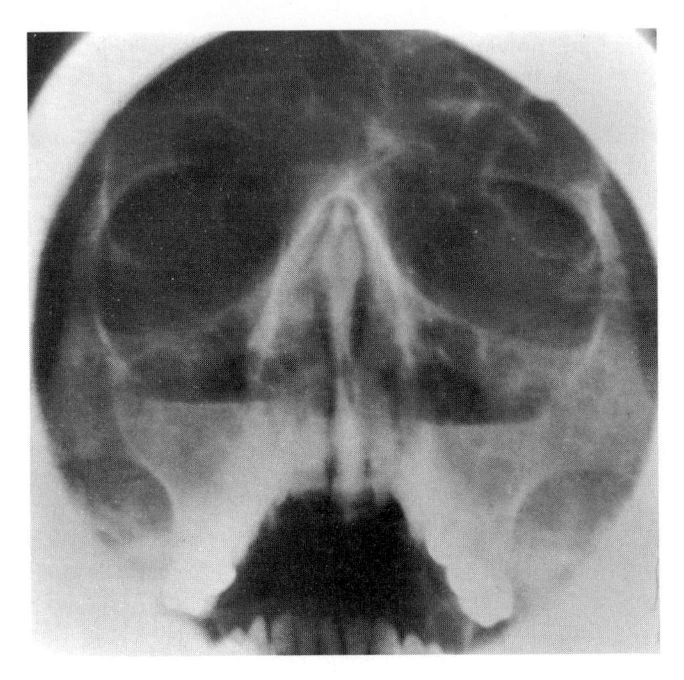

Fig. 23. Fluid levels in maxillary antra. A second view with the head tilted sideways is confirmatory.

finally begins to recover, when drainage is re-established from the ostium and there is a copious flow of pus from the infected sinus. If complete resolution takes place it may be expected within two or three weeks.

Chronic stage. On the other hand, resolution may be incomplete, and the damage to the mucous membrane may be such that ciliary activity is seriously impaired and the mucous membrane takes on a polypoid and thickened character. This condition may progress until the sinus is filled with polypi and pus, which is discharged at frequent intervals into the nose. The patient may come to seek advice regarding purulent nasal discharge, but, on the other hand, symptoms are varied and the complaint may be of frequent colds, or the tardy resolution of colds. An unpleasant taste or a bad smell in the nose may have drawn the patient's attention to the condition, or general poor health and appetite may require investigation. The discharge is frequently foul, and where the origin of the disease lies in a dental infection the discharge is extremely foetid.

As the condition settles into the chronic state, pain and tenderness disappear. It is a very rare complaint in chronic maxillary sinusitis for the patient to have any pain which is actually referable to the sinus itself. In fact, if the patient is sent to the hospital out-patient department for chronic pain in the face, a diagnosis of chronic sinusitis is rarely made.

Diagnosis of maxillary sinusitis

The chief points in the diagnosis of maxillary sinusitis will be evident from the foregoing. But as the maxillary sinusitis is frequently only one item in the clinical picture, further investigation is required to determine the extent of the infection. It often happens that patients are seen whose symptoms include some, if not all, of the symptoms of maxillary sinusitis, but in such indefinite form that further accurate knowledge is necessary before a diagnosis can be arrived at. Other investigations have therefore to be carried out.

Transillumination. In view of the wide availability of X-rays this method of diagnosis of sinus infection is now largely abandoned.

X-rays. A complete radiological study of the sinuses is our most reliable guide to the condition obtaining in the sinuses. Good radiological films, carried out stereoscopically for preference, will show even slight departures from normal in the contour of the linings of the sinuses. They will show clearly the presence of fluid and its extent, and one can visualize the actual condition to be found on opening the maxillary air sinuses. Different positions are devised for the proper demonstration of the various sinuses, and those used will vary with the preference of the specialist concerned. The most important point in the diagnosis of films of the sinuses is that the surgeon should be familiar with the type of view taken and that he should be sufficiently familiar with the fallacies which are likely to occur. This ability can be gained by experience alone, combined with accurate clinical observation.

Diagnostic puncture (proof puncture). Investigation of the maxillary air sinus can be carried out either by puncture through the inferior meatus or by cannulation through the ostium. Either method may be used, but in general the route through the inferior meatus is the more usual, especially where there is obstruction to the middle meatus by deviated septum or other condition. There is also less trauma to the natural drainage channels, and in inflamed conditions of the sinuses this is an important consideration.

Proof puncture is a diagnostic procedure to demonstrate the contents of the maxillary sinuses when X-rays have shown an opacity. Aspirated pus is sent for bacteriological examination; opaque media can be inserted to show changes in outline in more detail and give some idea of the emptying time. When combined with antral lavage, proof puncture is important in treatment of infection. The method is described on page 76.

ETHMOIDAL SUPPURATION

Infection of one group of the ethmoid cells alone rarely occurs without infection of other sinuses. The pathology of ethmoidal suppuration is similar to that of other sinuses. The location, however, of the ethmoid cells and their surroundings give them certain characteristic symptoms in the acute stages.

Acute ethmoidal suppuration

Acute ethmoidal suppuration, if drainage should be inadequate, will quickly find a way of extension of the inflammation through the thin plates of bone which surround it. One of the chief directions in which the ethmoidal suppuration can extend is outward into the orbital cavity, and an acute ethmoidal suppuration may frequently be diagnosed by the appearance of a thickening and swelling at the inner part of the orbit. The swelling in the orbit will be tender to the touch. It may consist of little more than a thickening of the periosteum of the walls, but in more advanced cases it may be tense and fluctuating, while the oedema may cause complete closure of the eyes by swelling of the lids. At this stage there is a collection of pus under the periosteum of the orbit. Failing treatment, the pus may break through the skin and form a discharging sinus in the corner of the orbit.

This condition in the early stages must be differentiated from acute orbital abscess resulting from skin infections, boils on the face, trauma and dacryocystitis. The onset is acute, the patient is ill. It is essential in these cases that a careful history should be obtained, and an examination will usually enable a diagnosis to be made. (Also 'Acute Orbital Abscess', p. 94.)

Chronic ethmoiditis

Chronic infection of the ethmoid is characterized in most cases by the formation of polypi. A necrosis of the ethmoid may occur without the polypi being formed and cells may be filled with pus. In most cases the linings of the ethmoid cells project through the ostia or the openings of the cells and thus help to form the masses of nasal polypi which have been described.

To aid diagnosis a careful radiological study should be made wherever possible. (For treatment, p. 80.)

FRONTAL SINUSITIS

Acute frontal sinusitis frequently accompanies or is accompanied by acute ethmoidal suppuration. The earliest sign of frontal sinus inflammatory change is known as a 'vacuum frontal headache'. This is generally supposed to be due to a blockage of the fronto-nasal duct by oedema in the nose. Absorption of the air in the sinus results, which again gives rise to hyperaemia and so causes headache of vascular type. The relief of the vacuum by readmission of air should result in these cases in cessation of the pain.

The infective form of sinusitis is the result of a nasal infection. It is a complication of influenza and may be seen in the exanthemata which are accompanied by nasal discharge, particularly in scarlet fever.

Symptoms. A distinctive symptom of frontal sinus infection is pain above the eye. The pain has frequently a definite periodicity, coming on about 10 a.m., and lasting to 4 or 5 p.m. It is of a dull, boring character, or it may come in acute spasms, being accompanied by a certain degree of photophobia and inability to use the eyes. The pain on using the eyes is due in some measure to the pull of the trochlea upon the inflamed frontal sinus floor. Infection may be so acute as to cause oedema and puffiness over the brow, and the upper eyelid may become swollen. Tenderness is frequently extreme, and the slightest pressure over the floor of the frontal sinus or over the orbital ridge may give the patient intense pain. The tenderness extends over the whole area of the frontal sinus.

Transillumination

This may be of value occasionally for outlining a frontal sinus, but now is little used.

X-ray examination

This is of greater importance in the case of the frontal sinus than perhaps of any other sinus. The reason for this is the extreme variability of the sinus in size, position, or, indeed, presence. Symptoms which would confidently be referred to a frontal sinus are frequently found to be due to the ethmoid, or the maxillary sinus when the frontal sinus is rudimentary. Treatment of an operative nature undertaken under these circumstances might be followed by disastrous results. The views favoured by different surgeons and radiologists vary greatly, but it is important that both sinuses are included to enable a comparison to be made between them. A lateral view is always useful to show the depth of the sinus.

As the condition advances the bone becomes involved, and as the inflamed mucous membrane prevents adequate drainage through the ordinary channels, perforation of the bone may occur.

Penetration posteriorly produces various intracranial complications. More frequently perforation occurs through the floor into the upper part of the orbit and in most cases takes place in the inner third. The condition thus closely resembles that of an acute ethmoiditis, previously described, in that the upper lid is swollen and the eye possibly closed, and a slight fluctuating swelling can be felt filling up the inner angle of the orbit. Sometimes the perforation of the bone occurs near the middle of the orbital roof and in such cases the abscess may spread upwards over the frontal bone. Perforation of the soft tissues may take place, and the sinus may drain through the opening above the inner canthus and the condition settle down. Sometimes complete resolution takes place and the sinus returns to normal. On the other hand, chronic infection may develop as in the case of the maxillary sinus, and the mucous membrane lining the frontal sinus may become polypoid. This leads to a condition of chronic frontal sinusitis which is very intractable and, owing to the very long and tortuous drainage channel, is difficult to cure.

The nasal signs are similar to those of chronic ethmoiditis and pus can usually be seen coming from the middle meatus under an oedematous and inflamed middle concha. Provided that no obstruction takes place, apart from slight nasal discharge, it is characteristic of chronic frontal sinusitis that it should give the patient a minimum of trouble, and perforation into the orbit may take place in cases in which the patient is unaware that any real suppurative condition exists.

SPHENOIDAL SINUS SUPPURATION

Acute sphenoiditis is a disease which is in many cases difficult to diagnose. It is usually encountered as part of a generalized sinus infection. It is frequently discovered as the result of failure of more conservative measures to clear up a sinusitis.

Diagnosis. The chief indications are severe deep-seated headache and by the appearance of pus in the spheno-ethmoidal recess. X-ray examination should never be neglected in cases of suspected sphenoidal infection, and diagnosis may be further confirmed by proof puncture of the sinus by the method described in the section on the technique of proof puncture. Suppuration of the sphenoidal sinus, however, is more frequently encountered as part of a chronic suppurative condition in the posterior sinuses, and in these cases the mucous membrane lining may become polypoid and may project from the sinus in the form of polypus.

Occasionally empyema of the sinus occurs. Sphenoidal infection has been blamed for many conditions, such as neuralgic pains about the head, eye disorders and mental instability. Sinus infection may exist, but there is little acceptable evidence that it is an aetiological factor. In retrobulbar neuritis any connection is very doubtful.

10. Sinusitis—Treatment and Complications

Principles of treatment

The principles underlying health in the accessory sinuses are the same as those in the nose. Ciliary activity is important in that, if secretions stagnate owing to its absence, infection takes place and surgical drainage eventually becomes necessary. To prevent loss of ciliary activity renders it essential that the ostia of the nasal accessory sinuses should be kept patent. In planning treatment of accessory sinus infection, two main objects are kept in view, the stimulation of ciliary activity and the provision of adequate drainage through the normal channels. Also, just as aeration plays an important part in nasal health, adequate aeration of the sinuses becomes of the utmost importance.

TREATMENT OF ACUTE SINUSITIS

In the acute stages treatment should be directed primarily towards restoring the patency of the ostia of the sinuses and so promoting drainage and relieving pain. Nasal congestion is the condition responsible to a great extent for prevention of drainage, and agents which will tend to shrink the mucous membrane of the nose and keep it in this condition should be employed.

Medical treatment enables most cases of acute sinusitis to resolve satisfactorily. The patient should be confined to bed in a warm but adequately ventilated room. To promote sinus drainage nasal decongestive drops or sprays should be used frequently (Fig. 26), followed by an inhalation. Ephedrine (1 to 2 per cent in normal saline) or Tuamine is best in that both have a prolonged shrinking effect, are followed by little or no rebound congestion, and do not interfere with ciliary action. Other applications (*e.g.* cocaine and adrenalin) often paralyse the cilia and this cancels out the benefit arising from their decongestant action. Menthol or Friar's Balsam are recommended for use as inhalations. Both are soothing and give a feeling of clearness, but the effect of these drugs is minimal and the essential factor in the treatment is the steam itself.

To relieve pain and headache analgesics are given in adequate dosage. Local heat is also comforting. Short-wave diathermy, however, is contraindicated in the acute stage. Douching during the acute stage of sinusitis is likewise to be avoided.

Sulphonamides or antibiotics are necessary in the more virulent

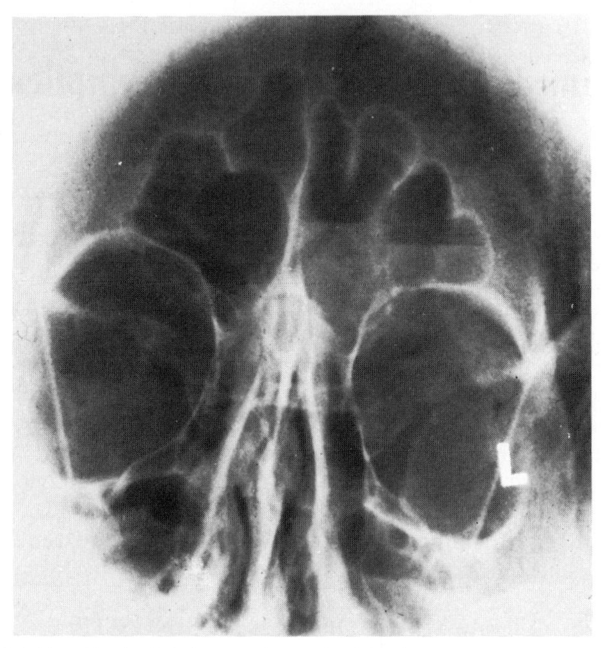

Fig. 24. Fluid level in the left frontal sinus. Fluid level will tilt with movement of the patient's head.

infections and must be given systemically in full dosage. Many infections respond to sulphonamides or penicillin, but chemotherapy should be controlled by bacteriological studies of the organisms and their sensitivities.

Surgical treatment is occasionally needed in acute sinusitis. It is reserved for those patients in whom improvement is not being obtained, especially if pain or headache is severe. It is imperative to remember that for the acutely inflamed sinus, operative treatment should be the minimum necessary to relieve tension and promote drainage. It is not to be undertaken without continuing effective chemotherapy.

Surgical drainage is most frequently necessary in the case of the *maxillary sinus*, and as the approach is through a thin layer of non-diploetic bone there is not the same anxiety as in the case of the frontal sinus. Proof puncture through the inferior meatus is preferable to attempted cannulation of an already swollen ostium. The method of proof puncture is described in page 76. Pus usually washes through without difficulty, but sometimes insertion of a second cannula is necessary to obtain a free return. A sample is taken for bacteriological examination. Ephedrine in saline can be left in the sinus to assist continuous drainage by maintaining the patency of the ostium. It is dangerous to expel fluid by injecting air; fatal air embolism can occur.

Once drainage has recommenced it usually continues, but lavage can be repeated especially if pain returns. Introduction of indwelling catheters or provision of an intra-nasal antrostomy are seldom indicated in acute infection.

In the case of acute infection in the frontal, ethmoid or sphenoid sinus which is not responding to conservative treatment the possibility of an associated maxillary sinus infection should not be overlooked. This is very often present and is the key to the whole problem: antral wash-out may be necessary before the other sinus infections will resolve.

Acute frontal sinusitis also sometimes demands surgical relief. Attempts to open up the fronto-nasal duct by intra-nasal procedures are to be avoided. Instead, via a small incision just below the medial end of the eyebrow, an opening is made in the floor of the sinus. A swab is taken for bacteriological study. Two plastic tubes are sutured firmly into position and the wound closed around them. The one tube serves for the injection of a decongestant such as ephedrine in saline, the second tube serves for drainage and should not be removed until the fronto-nasal duct has regained its normal patency as demonstrated by the free passage of fluid into the nose. It is essential not to overlook the associated maxillary sinusitis which is nearly always present. In *acute ethmoiditis* surgery is very rarely necessary except in those patients who develop an acute ethmoidal abscess or orbital involvement. This demands prompt external drainage and is described under complications of sinusitis. Intra-nasal procedures such as removal of the anterior end of the turbinate and opening of the anterior ethmoidal cells are still occasionally recommended. The necessity of treating an associated maxillary sinus infection by lavage is again emphasized.

In *acute sphenoidal sinusitis* surgical interference is hardly ever necessary; a co-existent maxillary sinusitis may again need proof puncture and lavage. If symptoms persist which are attributed to continuing infection in the sphenoid, cannulation or proof puncture is to be considered. This may be sufficient to allow the ostium to re-open. Some ephedrine in saline is left in the sinus to encourage continued drainage and promote resolution.

TREATMENT OF CHRONIC SINUS SUPPURATION

When suppuration in the various sinuses has become chronic, treatment has to be continued along lines which take into consideration the condition present in the sinuses. For instance, if there are polypi which have their origin in a chronic inflammatory condition of the sinuses, the removal of the polypi must form part of the treatment. Should the determining cause be septal deviation, the deflection of the septum may require correction. For the proper understanding of chronic sinus suppuration efficient X-ray films are of very great assistance in planning treatment. If the thickening of the mucous membrane does not suggest a very advanced condition of polypus formation, and does not show a fluid level of pus, conservative treatment is worth considering.

Proper cleansing of the nose by douching and by frequent instillation of drops of ephedrine in saline (1 to 2 per cent) may be sufficient to cause the chronic inflammatory condition of the membrane to subside and enable the resulting aeration of the sinuses to clear up the chronic infection.

Repeated washing of the sinus either by the ostium or by puncture through the inferior meatus may hasten recovery by clearing out the infected material. This gives the mucous membrane of the sinuses a chance to return to normal, and for the cilia to recover and perform their usual function. Absence of fairly rapid improvement in the character of the washings, however, generally indicates that repeated lavage will not be successful and more radical treatment is required.

Displacement treatment with $\frac{1}{2}$ per cent ephedrine in normal saline by the method of Proetz is useful where the change in the sinus lining has not progressed too far.

Short-wave diathermy is sometimes helpful in hastening recovery in a sinus which is showing reluctance to clear up.

On the other hand, if infection has been present for a considerable period and X-rays suggest serious disease, then more radical treatment is indicated. The various sinuses are treated by means of their appropriate operations, which will be referred to later.

COMPLICATIONS OF SINUSITIS

These may follow an acute infection or an exacerbation of a long-standing chronic sinusitis. Complications may be multiple.

Orbital cellulitis and abscess

These conditions complicate both ethmoid or frontal sinus infection. Aching around the orbit is followed by swelling of the eyelids and later of the conjunctiva. The movements of the eyeball are progressively limited until the eye is fixed and displaced. Tension on the optic nerve can produce blindness. Lack of rapid improvement or presence of more advanced change denotes abscess formation and urgent external drainage is needed. This can be provided by an incision in the superomedial quadrant of the orbit. By separating between periosteum and bone pus will be reached. A drain is then inserted (see also p. 94).

Meningitis

This is generally due to direct extension but may occur from spreading thrombophlebitis. The principles of diagnosis and treatment are the same as those as described for meningitis of otitic origin (p. 307). The sinus responsible may be the frontal or ethmoid and each demands urgent treatment.

Brain abscess

Abscess occurs mainly from chronic frontal sinus infection. It may be extra-dural or within the frontal lobe and follows erosion of the posterior wall of the sinus. Diagnosis is difficult but abscess should be suspected if headache persists after adequate treatment of the sinus, or if defects develop in memory, behaviour or personality. Treatment consists of repeated aspiration through an appropriately sited exploratory burr-hole. In the case of an extra-dural abscess diagnosed in the course of an operation on the sinus, drainage through the enlarged defect in the posterior wall is likely to suffice.

Osteomyelitis

This is a rare and dangerous extension of frontal sinus disease into the diploetic bone between the inner and outer tables of the skull. Initial spread follows the venous channels as a septic thrombosis. It is not

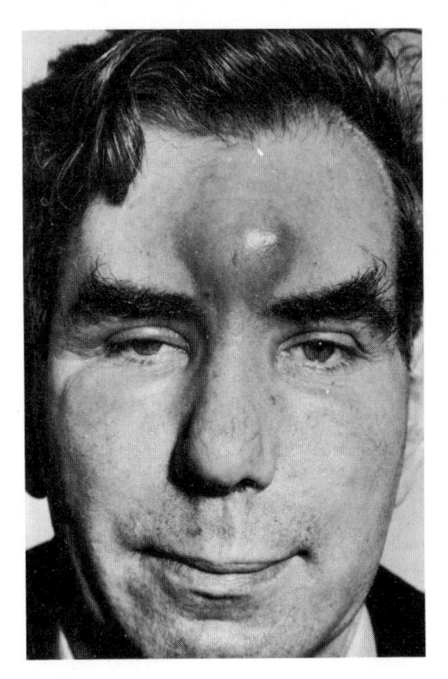

Fig. 25. Osteomyelitis of the frontal bone with abcess formation. It is important to recognise the significance of this type of swelling. The condition is dangerous, although the patient does not seem very ill. In this patient there was a large extra-dural collection of pus.

limited by suture lines. Intracranial complications are frequent and may be multiple.

Initial symptoms are minimal and the patient often seems remarkably well even though there may already be a large extra-dural collection of pus. A limited area of swelling and tenderness above the sinus ('Pott's puffy tumour') is soon followed by another similar area at a distance. X-ray changes are very late. Intensive chemotherapy combined with drainage of the sinus may abort the early case, but if progress is not entirely satisfactory the scalp must be turned down and all diseased bone widely excised. This may expose a large area of dura, but this is not important and the residual deformity can be corrected later. Half-hearted measures carry a high mortality.

Cavernous sinus thrombosis

Occasionally this follows ethmoid infection. The signs resemble orbital abscess, but the second side usually becomes involved, the retinal veins are engorged and the patient is much more ill. The classical picture is now rare because chemotherapy modifies and masks the disease. Accordingly, the complication is often merely suspected. Intensive chemotherapy, and treatment of the cause now give a better prognosis to what formerly was a fatal disease. The role of anti-coagulants is still undecided.

Mucocele is a late complication and is described on page 85.

Cutaneous fistula is occasionally seen. Fistulae are usually situated near the inner canthus or eyebrow, although occasionally they may be on the forehead if they arise from a large frontal sinus. They may develop spontaneously, or occur when a subcutaneous abscess is incised. This may arise from an unrecognized empyema of the underlying sinus or osteo-myelitis of the frontal bone. The treatment is that of the underlying disease.

SINUSITIS IN CHILDREN

Special mention of infection in children is necessary as the frequency is greater than is sometimes recognized.

In addition to the causes mentioned, the presence of infected tonsils and adenoids predisposes to sinusitis; allergy probably plays a large part owing to its frequency in children.

Diagnosis. In young children the ethmoid and the antrum are the sinuses commonly affected. Their development is a governing factor, and so until the age of five frontal sinus infection is not to be expected.

Treatment. A conservative attitude should be adopted. If the predisposing cause such as infected tonsils and adenoids or allergy can be treated the tendency towards spontaneous recovery is great.

In acute sinusitis treatment should be given along the lines already described. Ephedrine in saline or Tuamine sulphate is recommended as

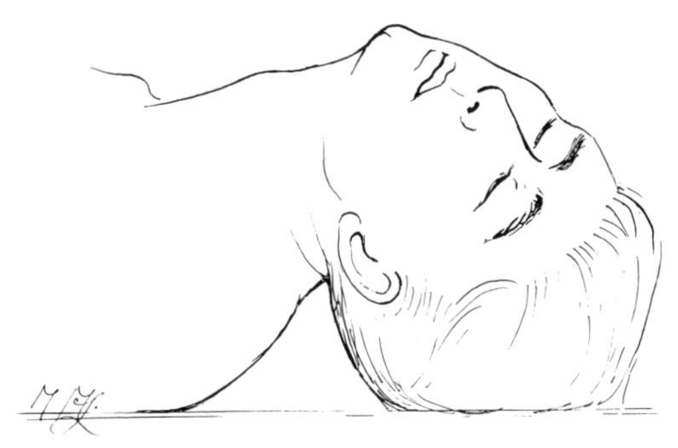

Fig. 26. Position of patient for instillation of nasal drops. The head is turned to one side or the other according to which nostril is being treated.

drops or sprays, with the appropriate antibiotic given systemically if needed.

Operation is seldom indicated but may be necessary for maxillary antrum or ethmoid infection. In the former, lavage may be repeated: as an alternative, an indwelling tube can be inserted through the inferior meatus. This allows for repeated washing-out and instillation of ephedrine. An intra-nasal antrostomy can be done instead. A radical antrostomy should be avoided because in younger children it endangers the second dentition.

External drainage of the ethmoid is sometimes necessary in children, when an abscess is pointing near the inner canthus.

11. Operations for Sinusitis

ANAESTHESIA

Before undertaking any operation on the nose it is advisable to prepare the nose with cocaine and adrenalin (see Appendix). This in many cases will give sufficient anaesthesia to carry out the lesser procedures, but where the operation is likely to be extensive, and particularly where it involves the posterior part of the nose, the packing must be supplemented.

This may be done in a variety of ways.

Good anaesthesia can be obtained by blocking the spheno-palatine ganglion with concentrated cocaine. A finely dressed probe carrying 25 per cent cocaine paste is placed over the spheno-palatine foramen. The cocaine penetrates the mucous membrane and anaesthetizes the ganglion. In addition, a probe is placed in the roof of the nose over the point of emergence of the ethmoidal nerve. For operations on the maxillary sinus an effective regional block can be obtained by injecting around the maxillary nerve as it emerges from the foramen rotundum and lies in the pterygo-palatine fossa.

Most major sinus operations, however, are done under general anaesthesia with endotracheal intubation. Local preparation of the nose is still necessary to promote shrinkage and haemostasis.

THE MAXILLARY SINUS

Proof puncture

The inferior meatus and the lateral wall of the nose under the inferior turbinate are cocainized, either by means of ribbon gauze soaked in cocaine and adrenalin solution and packed into the inferior meatus, or by a dressed probe carrying cocaine and adrenalin placed under the inferior turbinate anteriorly. A Lichtwitz trocar and cannula are used to carry out the puncture (Fig. 27). The trocar is inserted under the anterior end of the inferior concha in an upwards and backwards direction, being made to impinge upon the lateral wall of the nose about one inch behind the anterior end of the concha. The handle of the trocar is carried to the mid-line against the columella, and aim is made for a point just below the outer canthus. The butt of the needle rests in the palm of the hand, while the first or second finger of the hand rests on the canine fossa of the upper jaw and prevents the cannula being forced too far whenever it enters the maxillary air sinus. The trocar is pressed inwards until it impinges upon the posterior wall of the sinus. It is then withdrawn slightly and the trocar is removed, leaving the cannula in place. A record syringe containing 3 to 4 ml of sterile solution, *e.g.* saline is attached to the Lichtwitz cannula (Fig. 27). The plunger of the syringe is then withdrawn to aspirate any fluid contents of the sinus. If nothing appears in the syringe, the saline is then injected and again aspirated so that a wash is obtained of the sinus cavity, or if the pus is too thick to be aspirated in the first place, it will flow into the syringe after dilution with the saline. This sample may be used for bacteriological examination in the laboratory should it be so desired.

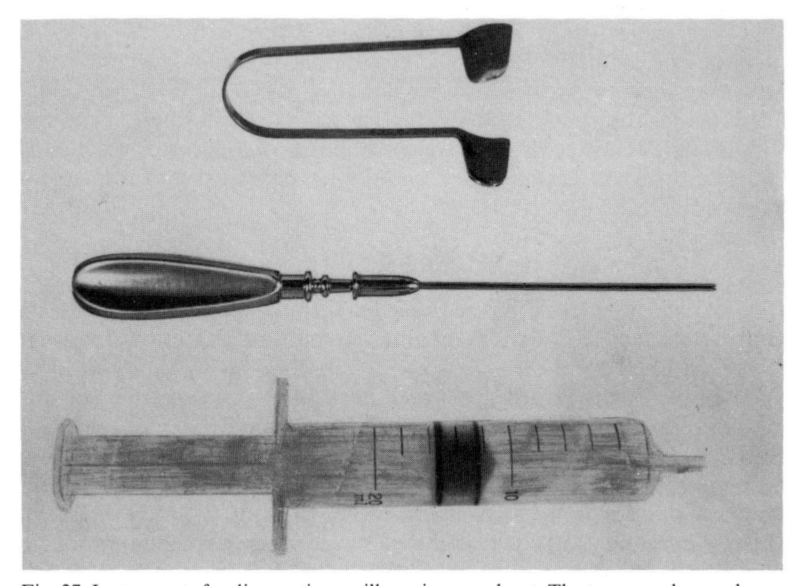

Fig. 27. Instruments for diagnostic maxillary sinus washout. The trocar and cannula are inserted high up beneath the inferior turbinate. The syringe fits directly on to the cannula so that saline can be injected and aspirated to obtain a specimen for bacteriology. Further lavage can be carried out with either the reloaded syringe or with a Higginson's syringe.

Difficulties of proof puncture. Complete anaesthesia of the mucous membrane through which the puncture is being made is desirable. Therefore the patient should be left sufficiently long after packing before the puncture is done. The exact time will vary according to the nature of the case and the amount of packing used. As a general guide at least ten minutes should be allowed, and if an acute inflammation is present twice this period may be insufficient to obtain a painless puncture. The wall of the sinus may be too thick at the point selected. If this is so trial is made a little higher up and farther back. If difficulty is still encountered a slight boring motion may be given to the trocar and this will frequently be sufficient to find a way into the sinus. The sinus may be extremely narrow anteriorly or posteriorly, in which case the trocar may strike the opposite wall before it is properly through the nasal wall. If the cannula is entered too far forward, there is danger of passing the trocar into the tissues of the cheek. An injection made in this position causes a swelling in the face. The consequences of this accident are not serious. If the puncture is made too high up there is a danger of injuring the floor of the orbit. Should it be found difficult to aspirate or to obtain a return of the fluid being used for the puncture, make sure that the patient's head is placed so that the ostium is higher than the point of the cannula. If it is still impossible to obtain a return flow after moving the cannula about, the reason is that the sinus is full of polypoid tissue and no space exists.

It may be useful to insert a second cannula alongside the first. Thick pus may then be washed out even though the ostium is completely blocked. A Higginson's syringe and warm sterile normal saline are employed for lavage. Ephedrine in saline can be left in the sinus. If antibiotics are necessary they should be given systemically under bacteriological control.

ANTROSTOMY

The maxillary antrum may be opened through the nose (intra-nasal antrostomy) or through the canine fossa (radical antrostomy or Caldwell Luc operation).

Intra-nasal antrostomy provides improved drainage and permits efficient lavage of the antrum, although it seldom results in a permanently patent stoma. It is useful in sub-acute sinusitis which is resistant to conservative treatment, especially in children in whom permanent mucosal damage in the sinus is considered unlikely to have developed. Also, the second dentition in children is less vulnerable in this approach.

Radical antrostomy is used in cases of chronic infection or recurring sinusitis in adults, in whom irreversible changes are suspected in the mucosal lining of the antrum. The operation has the great advantage of allowing direct inspection of the cavity and also allows the creation of a stoma which should remain permanently patent. A further advantage of the radical operation lies in the fact that the whole procedure can be carried out with minimal interference within the nasal cavity itself.

Both operations should be done under general anaesthesia supplemented by the local application of cocaine adrenalin. In adult patients local anaesthesia combined with maxillary nerve block provides an alternative.

Intra-nasal antrostomy

As the inferior concha is in many cases close to the floor of the nose the first step in the operation is the displacement of the anterior end of the inferior concha or its removal with punch or wire snare.

This gives access to the lateral nasal wall.

With a trephine or other perforating instrument an opening is made in the wall of the sinus under the inferior concha. This opening should be made as far forward and as low down as possible. It is then enlarged forwards and downwards so that the ridge between the sinus and the nose is as small as possible.

Through this opening the sinus can be washed out.

Radical antrostomy (Caldwell-Luc)

In this operation the maxillary air sinus is opened through the canine fossa. Intratracheal general anaesthesia is preferable and permits packing of the post-nasal space and the pharynx. This prevents blood and secretions finding their way into the trachea.

A haemostatic injection containing adrenalin solution made into the area of the incision is of assistance.

The opening is made with hammer and gouge and then enlarged with punch forceps till a clear view can be obtained of the interior of the sinus. The condition of the mucous membrane then decides whether the sinus lining requires to be stripped in part or in whole.

A counter-opening is made in the nasal wall working from the sinus, and after the bone has been removed the mucous membrane is cut so that it falls into the sinus as a flap and covers the raw bony ridge in the floor. This renders adhesions and premature closure of the opening unlikely. If the inferior concha interferes with the drainage the anterior end can be removed, but this is unnecessary in the great majority of cases.

As a rule no packing is required in the nose, but where there is free bleeding a small pack of ribbon gauze soaked in paraffin can be left in the inferior meatus for a few hours. The mouth wound is closed with three or four interrupted catgut sutures.

AFTER-TREATMENT OF MAXILLARY SINUS OPERATIONS

No packing of nose or sinus is advised under normal circumstances, and if the operation is carefully performed, swelling of the cheek is exceptional. Should it occur, a fomentation of a saturated solution of magnesium sulphate will quickly reduce the swelling and relieve any discomfort which may be present. On the day of operation and for two days following, a fair amount of oozing of blood-stained serum may be expected. The second morning after operation the maxillary sinus is washed out. This is carried out through the nose, by means of a bent cannula and a Higginson's syringe or gravity douche. Boric lotion or saline solution is used, and the intention of the douche is simply a mechanical cleansing of the sinus of accumulated blood clot, and a clearing of obstructing secretions. In cases of marked sepsis, the douche should be repeated daily, but in those cases in which there has been small interference within the sinus continuance of the douche will not be required.

In addition to these measures for cleansing the sinus, steam inhalations should be given thrice daily for some days. This helps to reduce the nasal congestion, and opens up the nasal airway. An oily spray or drops of sterile liquid paraffin will prevent crusting and add considerably to the patient's comfort. The stitches, being of catgut, do not call for removal, and if the incision has been made in the position recommended, the wearing of artificial dentures can be resumed almost immediately after the operation.

OPERATIONS ON THE ETHMOIDS

The ethmoidal labyrinth can be approached intra-nasally, through the maxillary antrum, or through an external incision.

Intra-nasal ethmoidectomy

This operation, if it is to be complete, requires a high degree of skill and carries the risk of damage to important nearby structures, namely the dura, the optic nerve and the contents of the orbit. The tendency therefore is towards the external or transantral approach, both of which permit more precise observation and accuracy.

The nose is well cocainized to promote shrinkage and haemostasis, and the ethmoid is entered with a curette just behind the anterior end of the middle concha, commencing with what are known as the *agger nasi* cells. The curette may be used until the external ethmoidal wall is felt, and the cell walls and the lining of the cells are removed with a pair of punch forceps. Removal is carried backwards until firmer bone is met. Possibly the outer wall of the ethmoid may be removed, in which case the tough, resistant orbital periosteum will be felt. Great gentleness should be used, for this is potentially a dangerous operation in the hands of the inexperienced. The most important point is to keep outside the middle concha.

Trans-antral ethmoidectomy

Antrum and ethmoid are generally both involved in patients with gross or recurrent polyp formation and these sinuses can be satisfactorily dealt with by this approach.

The antrum is opened via the canine fossa as already described in the Caldwell-Luc operation. Using round-ended forceps such as Luc's, entrance is made into the ethmoids through the corner of the antral roof in a posteromedial direction. Complete clearance of the disorganized ethmoid cells and polyps is obtained posteriorly as far as the sphenoid sinus which can be opened if necessary, and superiorly up to the roof of the ethmoids under good visual control. Some difficulty is generally encountered anteriorly where clearance is at an awkward angle and it is necessary to work simultaneously through the nose to free diseased tissue.

No packing is necessary; the incision is sutured as in an ordinary Caldwell-Luc operation.

External ethmoidectomy

A curved incision is made, starting below the inner end of the eyebrow and coming down on to the lateral nasal wall half-way between the nasal bridge and the canthus of the eye.

The structures are divided down to the periosteum and the lachrymal sac is carefully mobilised laterally. Bone is then removed beginning in the region of the lachrymal fossa and the whole of the contents of the ethmoid labyrinth are exenterated under direct vision. Particular care is taken to remove cells lying anteriorly and also in the roof of the ethmoids. All diseased cells posteriorly are likewise cleared and the sphenoid sinus entered. At the end of the operation the wound is repaired by catgut stitches followed by skin sutures. A properly designed incision results in a scar which is often invisible.

An alternative procedure is the Norman Patterson operation, carried out through an incision in the infra-orbital skin crease. This approach gives access to ethmoids and antrum, but it is somewhat limited as the lacrimal duct crosses the operation field.

After care is simple following ethmoid operation. As in the case of the antrum, decongestants and inhalations are helpful. Gentle aspiration of secretions is comforting, but nose-blowing is forbidden as it encourages bruising, swelling and surgical emphysema. A simple lubricant is sometimes necessary to discourage crusting.

OPERATIONS ON THE FRONTAL SINUS

The intra-nasal operation

Because of the technical difficulties, potential dangers and poor results, the intra-nasal operation is nowadays hardly ever indicated. In it search is made for the fronto-nasal duct using a special frontal sinus probe, in certain cases this may be facilitated by removing some of the anterior ethmoid cells although it is wise to retain the middle concha as long as possible to act as a landmark. More efficient drainage and less risk of damage to the inflamed fronto-nasal duct is obtained by trephining the frontal sinus.

Frontal Trephine. This is indicated in patients with frontal sinusitis in whom pain and swelling are not improving in spite of effective chemo-therapy and the use of suitable decongestants. Under local or general anaesthesia a small incision is made in the medial end of the eyebrow. A small circle of bone is removed from the floor of the frontal sinus using either a small hammer and gouge or the drill. The surgeon should take care to enter the sinus fairly far medially where its diameter is greatest. Pus usually appears under pressure and a swab is taken for bacteriological study. Two plastic tubes are sutured in position and the wound is closed around them. One tube is used for injecting $\frac{1}{2}\%$ Ephedrine several times daily, the second tube allows its free return until the fronto-nasal duct regains its normal patency. This is indicated by the appearance of fluid in the nose on gentle lavage. At this stage both tubes can be removed.

External frontal operations

Howarth's name is associated with those operations in which the anterior wall is preserved intact. Through a curved incision beginning in the line of the eyebrow and extending on to the side of the nose the bony floor of the sinus is exposed, the periosteum of the orbit being carefully preserved intact. The sinus is entered through its floor, and then the floor is removed in each direction until the condition of the mucosa can be assessed with accuracy. Polypoidal or irreparably diseased mucosa is removed. The anterior ethmoid cells are cleared, but great care is taken to preserve a continuous strip of mucosa between sinus and nose in the line of the now enlarged fronto-nasal duct. A plastic tube of at least 1 cm diameter is inserted down this channel through the anterior ethmoid region, and the wound is closed. The tube must be retained for about three months. Thiersch grafting with skin has been employed in the past to discourage stenosis but has little effect in doing this or in aiding drainage.

An osteoplastic flap is utilized in the operation developed by Macbeth in which a coronal incision is used and the tissues of the scalp are turned downwards. Excellent access is provided to both fronto-ethmoidal regions and the method is particularly valuable in patients with extensive disease, or with large osteomas, and also in patients who have previously had unsuccessful operations. Meticulous removal of mucosa is necessary; the space obliterates by fibrosis without the need for inserting fat or connective tissue as has been advocated.

Killian's obliterative operation is now less often performed, but still has a use for those patients in whom non-obliterative procedures have failed to control disease. The following brief description is given because it may be an emergency operation carried out by those unaccustomed to major sinus surgery, when access to a special clinic is not possible and it is essential to eradicate frontal sinus infection. The sinus is opened through its anterior wall and this and the floor are removed completely. It is essential that no recesses remain and that all mucosa is meticulously removed. The posterior wall of the sinus is examined and if necessary an extradural abscess can be uncapped, all diseased bone being excised. The soft tissues of forehead and orbit are allowed to fall back and obliterate all dead space. The wound is closed, drainage being provided for two to three days. A pressure dressing aids obliteration by preventing formation of pockets. The frontal contour can be restored at a later date by plastic measures.

OPERATIONS ON THE SPHENOID

Proof puncture of the sphenoid sinus

This may be carried out under local anaesthesia either for bacteriological investigation or to ascertain the presence of pus. The nose is cocainized carefully in the area embracing the middle concha, the cocainization being carried as far as the posterior wall. A proof-puncture trocar and cannula with a blunt-pointed trocar should be used for this investigation. It is passed backwards in the olfactory sulcus just above the lower edge of the middle concha, until it reaches the posterior wall of the nose. It is then turned slowly outwards and search is made for the ostium of the sphenoidal sinus. In some cases it may be necessary to dislocate the middle concha outwards, but this can be done without any real discomfort to the patient. When the sphenoidal sinus has been entered investigation should be carried out with a syringe and inner cannula, as described for the maxillary air sinus. If it is considered desirable to open the sphenoidal sinus, some operators prefer to remove the greater part of the middle concha. This, however, is not necessary except under exceptional circumstances, as in most cases the opening of the sphenoidal sinus is done in conjunction with an operation on the ethmoid cells and the middle concha can be dislocated to one side or the other to allow of further access to the sphenoidal sinus. A blunt probe with a fairly broad point, or some other instrument such as a Heath's nasal forceps, should be used first to localize the ostium of the sphenoidal sinus. When this is found the forceps are passed back until the posterior wall is felt. This is hard and solid and gives a characteristic sensation to the probing instrument. When the sinus has been identified the instrument is changed to the sphenoidal punch forceps, which is passed through the ostium into the sinus. Part of the anterior wall below the ostium is removed in a downward direction with the punch forceps until the anterior wall is level with the floor of the sinus.

After-treatment consists in frequent administration of steam inhalations and the instillation into the nose of some drops of sterile liquid paraffin to act as a lubricant and to prevent crusting.

COMPLICATIONS FOLLOWING OPERATIONS ON THE SINUSES

Haemorrhage

This sometimes occurs after operation on the sinuses. It is rarely of serious significance, but occasionally it may be of major importance. The spheno-palatine artery has been damaged and also the cavernous sinuses during operations on the sphenoidal sinuses. In such circumstances these accidents must be dealt with by packing and by the ligature of the main vessels where possible.

Haemorrhage into the tissues surrounding the sinuses may give cause for concern. Discoloration of the cheek not infrequently follows operation on the ethmoid or maxillary air sinus. This may take the form of the familiar black eye. Haemorrhage into the deeper tissues behind the orbit is a more serious complication, since it may give rise to blindness from pressure on the optic nerve.

Meningitis

This may occur as a complication of either acute or chronic suppuration, or in consequence of operative interference. It may be due to direct extension of the infection from the sinus, or to thrombosis of vessels, leading to the infection of blood spaces within the brain. Thrombosis of the ophthalmic veins may lead to thrombosis of the cavernous sinus and infection of the meninges.

Diagnosis and treatment of meningitis are described on p. 307. When this complication arises from operative injury to the meninges cerebro-spinal fluid rhinorrhoea may occur. Craniotomy will probably be required for repair of the dura.

Optic nerve injury

This is a rare complication of operations on the posterior ethmoids and sphenoid sinuses. It can arise as a consequence of direct surgical injury, but more often it is probably caused by a reactionary oedema or by bleeding. The optic atrophy which occurs is associated with permanent loss of vision.

12. Miscellaneous Diseases affecting the Sinuses

MUCOCELE

Mucocele is the name given to a condition of distension of the air cells by mucoid fluid. The absence of drainage gives rise to a sterile accumulation inside the bony wall of one of the cells and increase of tension enlarges and distends the sinus so that disfigurement and displacement of other structures may be caused. For instance, the orbit may be displaced by mucocele of an orbito-ethmoidal cell (Fig. 28).

Diagnosis. The main complaint is generally that of external swelling of slow onset. Headache or pain occur only if infection supervenes. The swelling gradually displaces the orbital contents and results in diplopia. Initially the swelling is bony hard, but as the bone is thinned this gives place to egg-shell crackling. Occasionally the swelling is seen only inside the nose or a posterior ethmoidal mucocele may cause

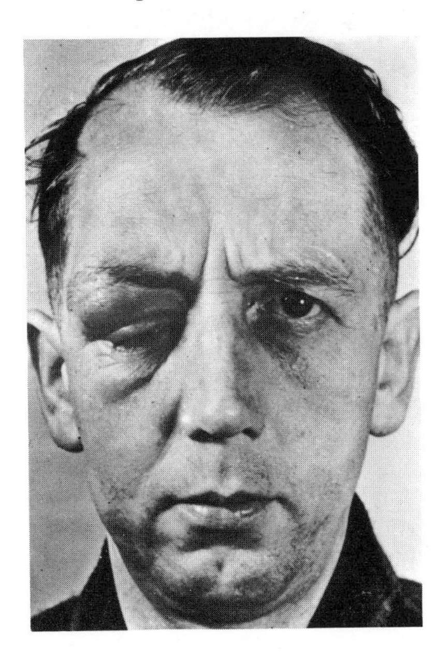

Fig. 28. Mucocele of the frontal sinus. Displacement of the eye was of some duration, the patient's symptoms were those of a superimposed infection. (By courtesy of Mr. Macbeth).

proptosis. X-rays show enlargement of the sinus with rounding of the borders of the bone.

Treatment of a small ethmoidal mucocele can sometimes be carried out intra-nasally, but in most instances an external frontal or ethmoid operation is necessary in order to deal satisfactorily not only with the mucocele but also the sinus in which it lies. If suppuration has occurred treatment is along the lines already indicated for treatment of sinus infection.

CYSTS

Cysts around the upper jaw and sinuses are infrequent but of almost endless variety. Most commonly seen is a retention cyst in the mucosa of the antrum. It is symptomless and shows up as a rounded swelling on X-ray. On proof puncture clear yellow fluid escapes and the cyst collapses.

Cysts of congenital origin occur around the pre-maxilla. Naso-alveolar cysts occur superficially and produce a swelling which obliterates the normal naso-labial fold.

Cysts of bone and cystic tumours such as osteoclastoma and adamantinoma occur but are rare.

Dental cysts may be large and extend widely into the antrum; they occur only around a devitalized tooth, the apex of which is within the cyst.

Dentigerous cysts are a developmental abnormality of a tooth follicle and can be identified by the fact that a tooth is missing from the dentition. On X-ray the deformed unerupted tooth is shown inside the cyst.

Treatment. Cysts may be treated according to their individual requirements. Cysts which involve the alveolus only, should be opened and scraped and then packed to encourage granulation formation. If, on the other hand, the cyst involves the maxillary air sinus, success is more likely to be achieved by removing the cyst lining carefully, throwing the space into continuity with the sinus, and providing for adequate intra-nasal drainage.

Infected cysts

Infected cysts, dental or dentigerous, may simulate acute maxillary sinusitis, or may actually cause it. If the cyst happens to be completely shut off from the sinus by a bony partition there may be no involvement of the sinus; but, on the other hand, it may be difficult or impossible to deal adequately with the cyst without opening the maxillary air sinus.

ORO-ANTRAL FISTULA

Extraction of a molar or premolar tooth can produce a fistula between mouth and antrum. It may be large or small, depending on how much bone adheres to the tooth. A fistula can occur when a tooth has only a very thin covering of bone over its apex or when dental infection has produced absorption of bone. Malignant growths also sometimes erode the alveolus.

Small acute fistulae probably occur not infrequently and close spontaneously if the clot in the dental socket organizes without interference.

Larger fistulae become epithelialized and then are chronic. A foul sinusitis develops and the patient is aware of leakage of pus or air into the mouth. When he drinks leakage of fluid may occur into the nose. Treatment is surgical and generally consists of a radical antrostomy (Caldwell-Luc operation) combined with removal of the epithelialized track and repair of the defect using a plastic flap dependent on the greater palatine artery. Smaller procedures are seldom successful.

TUMOURS OF THE SINUSES

A large number of innocent tumours have been described, such as fibromata, angiomata and osteomata. Angiomata most frequently occur in the ethmoidal region; osteomata in the frontal sinuses.

Papillomata

Transitional cell papillomata of the nose and sinuses are histologically benign, but have a great tendency to recur. They may have multicentric origin and usually involve the antrum, ethmoids and nasal cavity when first seen. They expand the containing bone, but do not infiltrate it. Irradiation is to be avoided. Adequate excision is essential. The risk of malignant change is debatable.

Angiomata

Angiomata of the ethmoid cause obstruction of the nose and profuse haemorrhage, which is repeated and is increasingly difficult to stop. Fortunately they are rare.

The treatment for this form of tumour is unsatisfactory. Injection with sclerosing solutions has given some success. The tumour may first of all be reduced with X-ray treatment, and, when it has shrunk to a smaller bulk, radium may be packed into the nasal cavity to try to obliterate the tumour completely. Cryosurgery may offer a better chance of control.

Osteomata

Osteomata of the frontal sinuses are usually discovered during routine X-ray examination of the sinuses. They may cause headache, but are frequently silent until the sinus becomes infected.

Osteomata are most frequently found in the frontal sinus, but they may be seen also in the ethmoidal region. The common site of attachment is the floor of the frontal sinus near the mid-line, and from this point they may extend in all directions in the sinus. Their bulk may cause a protrusion of the anterior sinus wall, and by pressure erosion it may expose the dura through the posterior sinus wall.

Symptoms may occur when the osteoma causes obstruction, and so produces infection.

Treatment. A small frontal osteoma discovered accidentally may remain under observation. An osteoma likely to block the fronto-nasal duct, and this includes all ethmoidal osteomata and all osteomata of any size, should be removed by the appropriate external frontal or ethmoidal approach. The osteoplastic operation is especially valuable for large fronto-ethmoidal lesions. Whatever route is used great care must be taken to avoid injury to the dura and to ensure that no remnants of the osteoma remain.

CANCER OF THE SINUSES

The great majority of these tumours are squamous-cell carcinomata. Adeno-carcinomata, transitional-cell carcinomata and sarcomata occasionally are seen. Many other growths occur, but all are rare.

The maxillary antrum and the ethmoid are generally both involved when the patient is first examined and it is impossible to say where the growth originated. Frontal and sphenoid are rarely the primary site.

Diagnosis. Reference should be made to nasal tumours (p. 50); these lesions cannot be considered apart and most patients complain of nasal symptoms. Obstruction and blood-stained discharge are common. Occasionally the first symptom is toothache, or loosening of teeth. Less frequently the patient may have a facial swelling, or symptoms arising from orbital involvement.

In the earliest stages the examining finger may feel, in the canine fossa, an elastic sensation which may progress to crackling. In many instances the initial diagnosis is that of chronic sinusitis.

The growth is often visible in the nose as a fleshy polyp. A warning must be given about ordinary looking mucous polyps which are present unilaterally: there is always the possibility that a growth may have caused them.

X-rays and tomograms give valuable information about destruction of bone and the direction of the spread of a growth. Biopsy is an essential step in diagnosis; tissue can generally be obtained from the nose, but if doubt persists the sinus should be opened (Fig. 29–30).

Treatment. There is no unanimity between surgeons and radiologists regarding the best sequence of treatment or its extent. Tumours in the anterior and inferior parts of the maxillary air sinus and some in the ethmoidal region offer a better prognosis than those in the posterior and

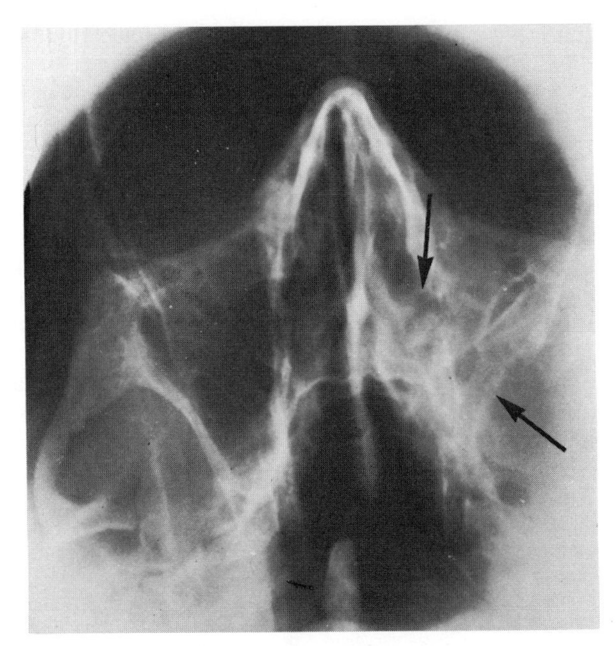

Fig. 29. Malignant disease of the maxillary antrum. The antrum is opaque, arrows indicate erosion.

superior part of the maxillary air sinus. Dissemination into the gland drainage areas is comparatively late, and good results can be expected in those cases in which the growth is small and is dealt with adequately.

Treatment in most cases is a combination of various forms of irradiation and of surgery.

Irradiation may be from a linear accelerator or a cobalt source and generally precedes operation. Intra-cavitary radium may be used after operation, depending upon the histological findings in tissue removed from various sites in the operation cavity, whether or not there has been preliminary external irradiation.

The type and extent of surgical resection will vary according to the nature and size of the tumour. Surgery may take the form of palatal fenestration, a resection en bloc or a lateral rhinotomy. The contents of the orbit require clearance if there is any suspicion of orbital involvement, especially in the case of ethmoidal cancers. This is a difficult decision to make, especially in patients with good eyesight on the diseased side.

Palatal fenestration consists of removal of half of the hard palate together with the alveolus and lateral nasal wall. It provides access for exenteration of the contents of the antrum and ethmoid through an intra-oral approach which can be supplemented if necessary by lateral rhinotomy.

Resection *en bloc* of the maxillary and ethmoidal labyrinth to the level of the cribriform plate is probably preferable for extensive growths, especially those encroaching upon the orbit. The operation is best done through a hemi-facial incision and the soft tissues of the cheek and upper lip are turned laterally. Excellent access to the ethmoids is possible by this approach which is particularly valuable if orbital involvement is suspected.

At the end of both types of operation the cavity is packed and an upper denture is wired firmly into position. This simplifies talking and feeding and adds greatly to the patient's comfort. Lateral rhinotomy may be the operation of choice in tumours confined to the ethmoids and again is easily combined with exenteration of the orbit.

Operations in the nature of an extended Caldwell Luc operation are seldom justifiable except in patients with tumours of borderline malignancy in whom the palate is free from growth, but even in these patients retention of the palate gives very little advantage. It limits the

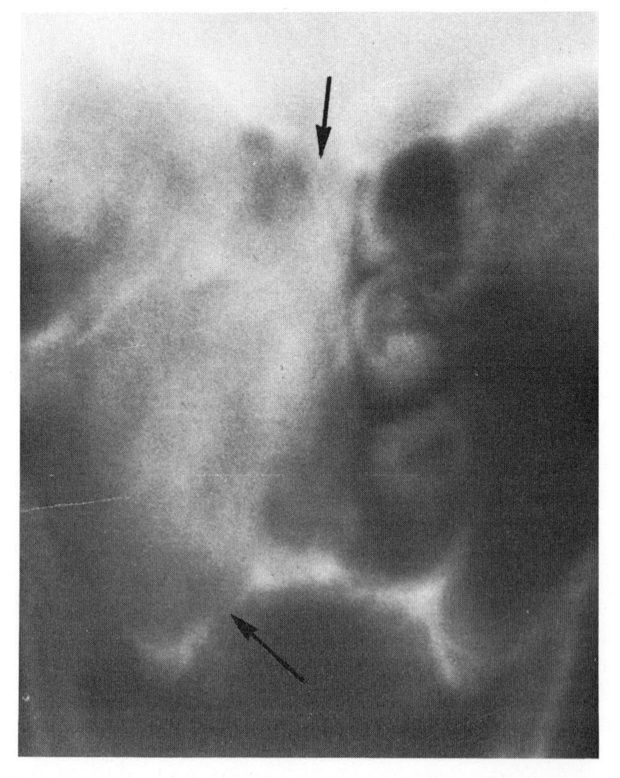

Fig. 30. Tomogram; cancer of antrum and ethmoid. Malignant disease involving the right side of the nose and right maxillary antrum. Arrows indicate erosion. Ordinary films failed to show erosion of palate and cribriform plate. (arrows).

access for surgery and for subsequent observation of the cavity. Its removal gives no great disability providing a well fitted, permanent prosthesis is supplied. Indeed, the special denture is often more comfortable than the type necessary for patients in whom only a small segment of alveolus has been sacrificed. Cervical nodes if enlarged should be included in the preliminary radiation, and where response is inadequate dissection of neck glands should be considered.

Intra-arterial chemotherapy sometimes has a part to play in cancer of the jaw although its precise role remains undecided. Infusion is carried out by a catheter inserted into the external carotid through its superior thyroid or superficial temporal branch. The position of the tip of the catheter is verified by the initial injection of a dye. The main use of this treatment at present seems to be in those patients with incurable disease who are suffering severely from pain.

SINUS BAROTRAUMA

The sinuses, in particular the frontal and maxillary sinuses, may be affected by rapid changes in barometric pressure, as in flying and diving. Also in diving, infected material lying in the nose may be forced into the sinus and give rise to sinusitis.

If there is blockage of the ostium by inflammation or other cause, the lack of rapid equalization of pressure within and without the sinus may cause hyperaemia, exudation, or haemorrhage into the sinus, giving rise to acute pain.

Such conditions appear in radiographs as dullness, therefore cannulation or proof puncture should be avoided as this might introduce infection. If left alone the sinus will clear up in most cases. Search must then be made for the underlying cause of the obstruction.

FRACTURES OF THE SINUSES

These injuries may be slight or very severe, causing haemorrhage and shock.

Diagnosis is made by inspection and palpation, if the local swelling will permit, and above all by careful X-ray studies. The presence of diplopia, dental mal-occlusion, and cerebrospinal fluid leakage must be determined.

Frontal sinus

Fractures of the frontal sinuses are chiefly fissures of the anterior walls, but in severe cases may involve the inner table and the dura. Infection is not common. The patient must be warned against blowing or douching the nose, and chemotherapy or antibiotics should be administered early.

Where the outer wall is displaced it may be elevated if necessary through an opening made in the floor, or the deformity may be corrected at a later date by cartilage or bone implants.

Ethmoid sinus

Serious results may be expected if the fracture extends into the cribriform area with tearing of dura mater. The same warning against douching and blowing the nose must be given, and the advice of a neurosurgeon should be obtained as soon as possible, though small dural tears usually heal spontaneously.

Maxillary fractures

These may involve the middle third of the face in which both maxillae are pushed bodily backwards. Initially very gross swelling obscures the displacement. If this is not quickly recognized and reduced an ugly 'dish-face' deformity occurs.

Zygomatic fractures

Zygomatic fractures result from a blow or kick on the cheek bone and are not uncommon. Generally the zygoma is displaced inwards and downwards towards the antrum. The fracture line passes through the infra-orbital foramen. Consequently a step-like deformity occurs in the rim of the orbit, diplopia and anaesthesia occur, and there is bleeding into the conjunctiva and antrum. Disimpaction and reduction can usually be achieved by passing a strong elevator downwards within the temporalis fascia, deep to the zygoma through an incision within the hair line. If reduction is unstable or if the maxilla is very comminuted the fronto-zygomatic joint may be wired or the antrum opened and packed.

Fractures of the arch are easily recognized; they can be reduced readily and remain stable.

FACIAL PAIN AND HEADACHES

Although patients are not infrequently seen with headache and a self-made diagnosis of 'sinusitis', it is seldom that sinus disease is in fact the cause. Nevertheless it is important that patients with persistent headache or facial pains should receive a careful examination of the teeth, ears, nose and throat, and that certain disorders should be borne in mind. Occasionally malignant disease in the sinuses or naso-pharynx has referred pain as its first symptom.

Referred pain may also occur as a post-herpetic neuralgia. Frontal or occipital headache may complicate cervical osteoarthritis, fibrositis, or 'whiplash' injuries of the neck. Pain from nerve injury may complicate fractures of the nose or occasionally radical antrostomy operations. Other conditions include the following:

Migraine headache

This is an intense paroxysmal hemicranial headache. It is probably due to vasomotor disturbance in the meningeal arteries. Prodromal eye symptoms are common, and there may be gastrointestinal symptoms. Duration, severity and frequency of attacks are variable. Ergot preparations do much to control this disorder.

Anterior ethmoidal neuralgia

This has been blamed upon compression of this nerve at its point of emergence in the roof of the nose. Diagnosis is made by abolition of the pain when the nerve is cocainized by a dressed probe soaked in cocaine (5 per cent) and inserted into that part of the nose.

Facial migraine

This syndrome is easily recognized, although not well known. It goes by a number of names including cluster headaches, histamine headache, spheno-palatine neuralgia and ciliary neuralgia. The patient is usually a youngish man who complains of severe, recurring episodes of pain, centred around the eye. Attacks may last up to two hours and often occur at night. They occur in clusters and then a remission, lasting many months, may occur. The eye and the nose on the homo-lateral side are often congested and watering. Ergot preparations are usually effective.

Trigeminal neuralgia (tic douloureux)

The pain of this form is intense, even intolerable, and spasmodic. It may affect any or all of the branches of the fifth nerve and may radiate widely. The presence of 'trigger' points is characteristic, and the touching of these as in shaving or the movement of the mouth in eating may determine an attack. Spasms can occur frequently but there may be remissions lasting months. The etiology is obscure, but trauma and dental disorders sometimes appear to play a part. Atypical varieties are not uncommon.

In many patients the pain can be controlled by carbamazepine ('Tegretol'), therefore alcohol injection of the appropriate division of the nerve, injection of the ganglion, or section of its sensory root are now less often necessary.

Mandibular malposition (Costen's syndrome)

This consists of pain around and in front of the temporo-mandibular joint in patients without adequate molar support owing to removal of these teeth. Permanent changes in the joint and its cartilage are often present by the time the disorder is diagnosed, but even in these patients provision of an adequate denture is of great help. Tinnitus and deafness have been included in the syndrome, but there is no valid evidence for this.

Atypical facial pains

These are not infrequent and as no physical basis is demonstrated it is easy to label patients as neurotic. A psychological overlay undoubtedly develops in some, but there is probably a basic abnormality which is not properly understood. Many of these patients have already suffered nerve blocks, sinus operations and repeated dental extractions without benefit. Although no specific treatment can be provided it is important to recognize this entity in order to save the patient from unnecessary surgical interventions. Diagnosis is largely by exclusion of those conditions which have already been mentioned. It is also important to remember that multiple sclerosis can produce atypical facial pain; so can brain-stem disease.

ORBITAL ABSCESS AND CELLULITIS

Three forms of this affection may occur.

1. Collateral oedema.
2. Subperiosteal abscess.
3. Orbital cellulitis.

Collateral oedema is due to inflammation and suppuration in neighbouring sinuses. This is usually in the ethmoid or the frontal sinus; the diagnosis and treatment are similar to those in sinusitis and the latter includes the administration of antibiotics. With treatment the condition recovers quickly and without ill effects.

Subperiosteal abscess may result from extension of oedema, but occasionally no sinus infection is diagnosed. There is formation of pus under the orbital periosteum. General symptoms are more marked and limitation of movement of the eyeball is greater in one direction than in the other. The condition responds readily to antibiotics, but there is danger of blindness in the affected eye.

Orbital cellulitis

This is a virulent and dangerous affection which may prove rapidly fatal through its extension to cavernous sinus thrombosis and subsequent meningitis. Blindness is a common sequel and in spite of the greatest vigilance the patient may be overwhelmed by the rapidity of the infection. the cause may be a boil on the face, erysipelas or other infection and there may be high temperature and sickness. Occasionally owing to the overwhelming nature of the infection there are few general signs apart from prostration. There is acute pain in the orbit and early fixation of the eyeball. Oedema is uniform over the eyelid and there is tenderness on pressure over the globe. The condition closely resembles cavernous sinus thrombosis but is distinguished by the presence of pain and tenderness and the absence of papilloedema. As, however, this must be considered a stage in the development of cavernous sinus thrombosis, treatment with antibiotics is of the utmost urgency. It is possible that surgical drainage of the orbit may be effective in preventing the spread of infection and the blindness which is a common sequel (see also p. 72).

ACUTE DENTAL ABSCESS

Acute dental abscess in the upper alveolus frequently causes confusion with sinusitis, as the pus spreads up over the anterior surface of the maxilla. A careful examination, however, which should always include inspection of the teeth, will reveal the true state of affairs. Appropriate dental treatment should then be applied.

TRANS-SPHENOIDAL HYPOPHYSECTOMY

In trans-sphenoidal hypophysectomy, access is obtained via an external ethmoidectomy, or via the nose or by a combination of these routes.

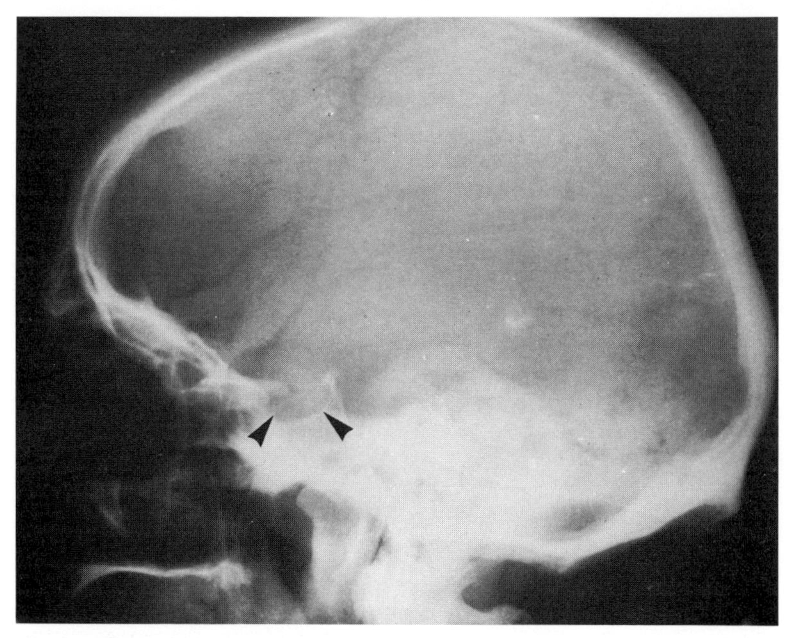

Fig. 31. Lateral view of skull in acromegaly. Note the expansion of the pituitary fossa and compare it to the normal view as shown for example in fig. 12.

Excellent exposure is obtained without the risks of a major intracranial procedure or of optic nerve injury.

The operation is carried out most frequently for uncontrolled breast cancer and is particularly indicated when painful bone metastases are present. There is unfortunately still no practical method by which hormone-dependent tumours can be identified, but subjective relief is obtained in about a third of patients operated upon and objective regression in another third. This improvement occasionally lasts up to three or four years or more, especially in post-menopausal patients.

Replacement therapy is relatively straightforward, and consists essentially of administration of cortisone and of thyroid tablets.

Hypophysectomy by this route also has important applications in the management of prostatic carcinoma and Cushing's syndrome. This is also the route of choice when hypophysectomy is required in acromegaly and basophil adenoma as well as for tumours of the pituitary which are giving rise to pressure symptoms. Suprasellar extension is not necessarily a contraindication for removing pituitary tumours by the trans-sphenoidal route.

SECTION 3 THE PHARYNX

13. Anatomy

The pharynx comprises three parts – the *nasopharynx*, the *oropharynx* or the *pharynx proper*, and the *laryngopharynx*. The boundaries of the nasopharynx are the basisphenoid above to a line at the level of the soft palate below; the oropharynx commences at the level of the soft palate and extends to the level of the tip of the epiglottis; the laryngopharynx commences at the level of the tip of the epiglottis and extends to the level of the cricoid cartilage, or the commencement of the oesophagus.

The pharynx, as a whole, has several features common to every part. The lining mucous membrane is of similar character throughout and is one continuous sheet of stratified squamous epithelium. Inflammation of one part of the pharynx is readily transferred to the other, so that all inflammatory conditions of the pharynx must be considered in their relation to the other parts, and cannot be regarded as individual diseases without effect upon other structures.

The lymphoid tissue of the pharynx forms an important part of its structure and is concerned with many diseases encountered in this area.

NASOPHARYNX

The posterior wall of the nasopharynx arches forward into the roof. The roof is formed by the basisphenoid, and may contain a small embryonic remnant known as *Rathke's* pouch. At the junction of the roof and the posterior wall is situated the aggregation of lymphoid tissue called *adenoids* or the pharyngeal tonsil. In the anterior wall open the choanae, and below them is found the attachment of the soft palate. On the lateral wall there are the openings of the *Eustachian* tubes. Behind these are the eminences known as the Eustachian cushions, behind which again are the hollows called the fossae of *Rosenmuller*. These hollows should be kept in mind in the investigation of the Eustachian tubes.

Oropharynx. Passing down into the oropharynx, the soft palate is seen as a membranous muscular structure arching across the pharynx, and in the centre is the uvula, which in some people may be divided owing to the non-union of the two halves of the palate. The condition is spoken of as a bifid uvula. From the palate stretch down on each side two folds of mucous membrane and muscle to meet the side of the tongue. These are the pillars of the fauces; they are anterior and posterior. Between these pillars are the faucial tonsils, while below the tonsils, in the side of the tongue, are masses of lymphoid tissue which are called the lingual tonsils (Fig. 32).

The dorsum of the tongue can be followed down until it reaches the base of the epiglottis, to which it is attached by the glosso-epiglottic ligament.

On the posterior wall of the oropharynx are many little aggregations of lymphoid tissue which are liable, in certain conditions, to enlarge and become inflamed.

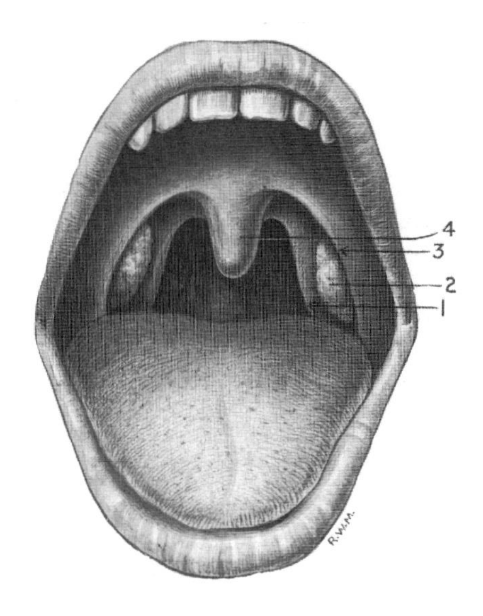

Fig. 32. Normal pharynx showing; (1) posterior pillar; (2) tonsil; (3) anterior pillar; (4) uvula.

The laryngopharynx

This is the part of the pharynx which contains the larynx, and in front of the epiglottis are found two spaces which are known as the *valleculae*. They are divided in the mid-line by the glosso-epiglottic ligament and bounded posteriorly by the pharyngo-epiglottic ligaments. These are folds of mucous membrane which are attached to the posterior part of the base of the epiglottis. Behind these ligaments commence the *pyriform sinuses*—one on each side. The pyriform sinuses are potential spaces which are formed by the bulk of the larynx dividing the lowest part of the pharynx into two. They open to some extent on phonation and to permit of the passage of food.

Muscles of the pharynx

The pharynx is a channel of mucous membrane surrounded by muscular tissues and supported at a distance by bony structures. To fulfil its functions of respiration and deglutition, muscular movement is essential. The chief muscular group is the constrictor group, which is composed of the superior, medial and inferior constrictors. These surround the pharynx in a more or less circular direction. Two other groups are necessary – one to shorten the pharynx as required and the other group to manipulate the soft palate, to ensure that the nasopharynx can be shut off from the mouth to prevent food entering the nose in swallowing, and to open the nasopharynx again for respiration.

The muscles providing vertical movement are chiefly the *stylopharyngeus* muscle and the *palato-pharyngeus* muscle. Those which control the soft palate are, chiefly, the *levator palati*, the *tensor palati* and the *palato-glossus*. There is another small muscle called the *salpingopharyngeus*, whose function it is, together with the *levator palati* and the *tensor palati*, to control the patency of the auditory tube.

The motor nerve supply of the pharynx is from the *accessory nerve* through the pharyngeal plexus.

The blood-supply of the pharynx comes through the ascending palatine and the tonsillar branches of the facial artery, and the ascending pharyngeal artery, and branches from the *internal maxillary artery*. (For methods of examination, p. 104.)

14. Adenoids and Tonsils

ADENOIDS

Adenoid tissue plays an important part in the development of the nasopharynx. In the pre-natal stage adenoids may occupy the posterior wall of the pharynx from the roof of the nasopharynx to the level of the larynx. As term approaches this adenoid tissue comes to occupy the position with which we are accustomed to associate it, that is the uppermost part of the posterior wall of the nasopharynx.

Adenoids are composed of masses of lymphoid tissue which are usually disposed in vertical ridges of three or more. The adenoids find their origin in the mucous membrane and are not encapsuled or rendered distinct in any way. The size of both the adenoids and the tonsils varies with age. In the first few years of life rapid hypertrophy occurs. These structures usually reach their maximum bulk at about the age of six, by which time the child is usually facing repeated infections in his environment. At puberty involution begins, and by the age of twenty little trace of the adenoids normally remains.

The diagnosis of adenoids is usually made by posterior rhinoscopy. The appearance in the mirror is that of vertical ridges which fill up a large part of the space of the nasopharynx and may completely obscure any view of the choanae. The enlargement may be due to infection, or the hypertrophy may be due to chronic nasal congestion, to lack of aeration and to inefficient nasal breathing. Dietetic error and faulty metabolism have also been blamed for the enlargement of adenoids.

Infection of adenoids in babies may be of very serious significance, for in consequence of the obstruction to the nasal airway feeding may be so interfered with that the life of the child is endangered.

Babies appear to be particularly prone to infection, and in a number of cases there is more than the normal amount of adenoid tissue present at birth. The excess of this tissue becomes a ready soil for the multiplication of organisms. Familial infection plays a greater part in these cases than is generally realized. It can be understood how a person with an acute coryza can infect a child, and it is important that anyone suffering in such a way should never approach a young baby.

A degree of infection, unnoticed by an adult, can be a virulent infection when encountered by a child. It is not unusual for puzzled parents to seek the advice of the specialist on account of persistently recurring nasal infection in their child. To cure this so-called tendency, operations may be performed upon the child, which, more properly, might be carried out upon the parents. Even dental caries is believed, in certain instances, to be able to infect a child's nasopharynx. If a baby is in contact with anyone – relation or nurse – who suffers from chronic rhinitis or chronic sinusitis, the child runs a constant risk of infection.

Acute infection of adenoids may occur without obvious involvement of the tonsillar region, and the infection is usually a sequel to nasal inflammation. It is diagnosed by posterior rhinoscopy. The adenoids will be seen to be acutely inflamed, and here and there small yellow spots of pus exude from the spaces in the adenoids, in similar manner to the points of exudation seen in follicular tonsilitis. Inflammation, however, is more often subacute or chronic.

Symptoms may be considered under the following headings: those arising from (*a*) local effects, (*b*) effects on the ears, (*c*) effects on the sinuses, (*d*) more remote effects.

(*a*) **Local effects**

These are primarily those of nasal obstruction. They are the result of a mass placed in this particular anatomical position. If the mass is sufficiently large it will obstruct the nasopharynx, but in many instances the determining factor of the obstruction is inflammatory enlargement consequent upon infection. Mouth-breathing is the result, and there is snoring at night. The nares become narrowed, the palate becomes high and is arched, being known as the 'Gothic' palate, and there is an undershot jaw with ever-open mouth. The mental faculties are dulled, the expression is stupid, and the so-called 'adenoid facies' is produced.

(*b*) **Effects on the ears**

The mass of adenoids may, by its bulk, obstruct the Eustachian tube and thereby give rise to deafness. On the other hand, deafness, which is a very common accompaniment of adenoids, may be due not so much to the adenoids themselves as to the chronic infection which accompanies them. This sets up in the Eustachian tube a chronic inflammation without bacterial invasion, which is responsible for the obstruction and leads to middle ear deafness. The effects of this Eustachian inflammation may be serious. Failure to arrest it may result in permanent damage; in many of these patients the drum is scarred, collapsed and adherent. Today there are many adults suffering from deafness which might have been avoided by adenoidectomy in childhood.

An acute infection of the nasopharynx in such cases will readily set up an otitis media; and in children the width of the Eustachian tube, its shortness and horizontal direction, are all conducive to the entry of infected material into the middle ear. These effects happily tend to disappear with the removal of the adenoids. In the majority of cases of sinusitis the removal of the adenoids results in a proper aeration of the nasopharynx and this is one of the most important factors in producing a healthy sinus system. The result almost invariably is a complete disappearance of the symptoms. Similarly, with the Eustachian catarrh; in the majority of cases the deafness presents before the removal of the adenoids disappears spontaneously or with simple treatment.

(*c*) Effects on the sinuses

These are important in that the inflammation in the adenoids travels via the nasal mucosa into the neighbouring sinuses, so that in the majority of cases a sinusitis of more or less severity accompanies the adenoids. The effect of this sinusitis is that the child presents a typical nasal discharge from the anterior nares. This is not due to actual obstruction of the nasopharynx by the adenoid mass, as is commonly supposed, since inspection of the nasopharynx, by means of posterior rhinoscopy, will reveal an adequate airway beside the mass of adenoids. The cause of the anterior nasal discharge is that the sinusitis results in a chronic inflammatory condition of the nasal mucosa in the posterior part of the nose. It is this inflammatory condition which causes the blockage of the nose and forces the secretion to find another pathway. Owing to the inflammatory condition which is present, sinus secretions are more copious than normal, so that there is a free flow of mucus and mucopus from all the air cells surrounding the nose. This appears anteriorly as nasal discharge.

(*d*) Remote effects

These are also described. Difficulty in swallowing may lead to poor appetite and stunted growth. Frequent attacks of nasopharyngitis predispose to chronic lower respiratory infections, and may aggravate asthma and bronchitis in a child who is prone to such illness.

Diagnosis of adenoids

It does not always follow that a child who is a mouth-breather is suffering from adenoids, and it is a common mistake to assume that adenoids are present in all cases where the mouth is kept open or where there is evidence of obstruction.

Enlarged adenoids in adults is a rare condition. Adenoids, therefore, must be a positive diagnosis, which is made by posterior rhinoscopy, as previously described (p. 16). X-rays of the nasopharynx are helpful in cases of difficulty. If a nervous child is brought with tonsils which obviously require to be removed, the diagnosis of adenoids should be left until the operation for removal of the tonsils, when, under the anaesthetic, careful examination can be made.

Treatment. Adenoids may be treated by either conservative or operative methods. The former may be of help in mild cases and consists of correction of any dietetic error, adequate exercise in the fresh air, and most important instruction in correct methods of breathing and nose blowing. Adequate nasal aeration is essential for restoration of nasopharyngeal health. Exacerbation of symptoms may call for the temporary use of nasal decongestants and antibiotics, but if recourse has to be made frequently to such a treatment or if ear symptoms develop it is almost certain that surgical treatment is required. This consists of the operation of adenoidectomy.

REMOVAL OF ADENOIDS

Adenoidectomy by itself is indicated if the patient suffers from symptoms due only to adenoids. In children admitted for tonsillectomy, however, it is always good practice to deal with the adenoids at the same time. In this case it is best to do the adenoidectomy as the first stage of the combined operation. When the nasopharynx has been cleared, a gauze pack is inserted and the surgeon proceeds to the tonsillectomy. The nasopharyngeal pack is removed at the end of the tonsillectomy and almost invariably it will be found that the bleeding in the nasopharynx has ceased. If the tonsils are not being removed the pack should be inserted in the same way and the surgeon must wait at least five minutes for bleeding to cease before removing the pack.

Anaesthesia is generally by means of halothane. The mouth is opened by a gag and the tongue is depressed, showing the soft palate. The soft palate is then lifted forward with the forefinger of the left hand and the curette is slipped under the soft palate, which is protected by the left forefinger. The curette is passed up to the roof of the nasopharynx and is pressed into the adenoid mass at its highest part. The curette is drawn down the nasopharynx, with the handle vertical for a short distance, then the handle is swung forwards, sweeping the adenoid mass off the posterior pharyngeal wall. Two or three curettes are used for the operation – a large one to remove the bulk of the mass and smaller ones to clean off any tags which remain. The forefinger is useful in identifying the position of these, but should not in any circumstances be used for scraping off the adenoids.

Post-operative bleeding is a troublesome complication and is usually due to a tag of adenoids remaining. In rare instances it will be necessary to insert a post-nasal pack under general anaesthesia.

Correct diagnosis and removal of adenoids renders the child able to take full advantage of normal breathing through the nose, freedom from recurring, prolonged nasal infections, as well as relief from ear complications. As far as the latter are concerned, however, it is important to stress that although the majority of patients are cured or much improved, a number of children continue to have recurring ear troubles because of associated Eustachian tube insufficiency.

Thornwaldt's bursa

This is a pocket or fold which is produced in the nasopharynx by the adenoids. Sometimes it is full of mucus and at other times it becomes the site of suppuration. The treatment is simple and satisfactory, and consists in removal of the mass by the usual methods for removal of adenoids.

EXAMINATION OF THE OROPHARYNX

This is preceded by inspection of the mouth, teeth and gums, as well as tongue, palate and floor of mouth. The contents of the oropharynx are then inspected systematically according to the description of the anatomy given on page 97 and illustrated in Fig. 32.

As inspection proceeds downwards the epiglottis often comes into view, especially in children. The lateral wall of the pharynx on each side should be inspected, lymphoid tissue, known as the lingual tonsil, can be seen in many patients.

THE TONSILS

The tonsil is a large body of lymphoid tissue, only a part of which is visible on inspection. It consists of an upper pole, a body and a lower pole. There is frequently a constriction between the lower pole and the main body of the tonsil. The upper pole is usually 'buried' in the muscle of the soft palate. The fold of mucous membrane which conceals the upper pole of the tonsil is known as the *plica semilunaris*.

The tonsil is enclosed on its deeper aspects by a dense fibrous capsule. Outside this is a loose layer of areolar tissue separating the capsule from the pharyngo-basilar fascia covering the muscles of the tonsil bed. This loose areolar layer renders possible complete removal of the tonsil without damage to surrounding structures. The bed of the tonsil is formed by the *palato-pharyngeus* muscle, separating it in the upper part from the *superior constrictor* muscle, while the lower part of the tonsil is separated by the *stylopharyngeus* and the *styloglossus* muscle, from the same muscle.

The blood supply of the tonsil is chiefly from the tonsillar branch of the facial artery through the tonsillar and the ascending palatine artery above, and from the carotid artery through the ascending pharyngeal branch in the lower part. The dorsalis linguae artery may also send branches to the tonsil from below, and the descending palatine from the region of the soft palate.

The nerve supply is twofold. The fifth nerve supplies sensation in the upper part through the spheno-palatine ganglion, and the glosso-pharyngeal nerve supplies the lower part.

The tonsil contains what are known as *crypts*. These are prolongations of the epithelium into the body of the tonsil in the form of tortuous channels. The glands empty into the crypts, into which are extruded bacteria and waste products. There is one particularly large crypt in the upper pole of the tonsil, called the *supratonsillar fossa*. In health the tonsils should present the same colour as the remainder of the mucous membrane of the throat; they should not protrude to any extent between the pillars of the fauces.

The function of the tonsil. The exact function remains unknown, but the tonsils are part of the lymphoid system and accordingly have a role in the production of immune bodies against bacterial infection. This function probably becomes insignificant later when the tonsil normally atrophies. Moreover, as part of Waldeyer's ring of lymphoid tissue around the pharynx, they provide also a more local role as a barrier against bacterial invasion. Unfortunately, however, this local barrier often breaks down so that the tonsil becomes in itself a focus of infection.

Inspection of the tonsils. In a great many cases it is difficult to carry out an adequate inspection of the faucial tonsil owing to its recessed nature behind the anterior pillar, and to its being largely invisible to casual examination. Tonsils may be so far buried or covered by mucous membrane of the pillars as to be completely concealed, and when they are covered in this fashion they are known as 'submerged' tonsils. In order to inspect this type of tonsil properly the mucous membrane covering of the anterior pillar must be drawn back and the tonsil made to project. This is best done with a blunt hook or some instrument specially made for the purpose. The hook is made to draw the pillar forward and is then pressed gently in behind the pillar, thus tending to dislocate the tonsil forward. This will also help to express any pus or other accumulation of debris present in the crypts and will enable an opinion to be formed regarding the condition of the tonsil. In examining the lower part of the pharynx it is necessary in most cases to use a laryngeal mirror.

ACUTE TONSILLITIS

This is a generalized inflammation of the mass of the tonsil and is usually accompanied by a degree of inflammation of the fauces and pharynx. The tonsils enlarge and project, and there is an excess of secretion of the pharynx.

The causes are various. Exposure to cold or local irritants may temporarily lower the body's natural resistance and permit infection by a variety of viruses and bacteria with virulent organisms may be the determining factor in tonsillitis, while irritation by gases, etc., also leads to inflammation.

Symptoms. The first symptom may be rawness at the back of the throat. This can cause acute pain, or pain may be felt only on swallowing. There may be a sensation of constriction at the back of the throat, and the patient has a constant desire to swallow owing to the excess of secretion, and the swallowing is extremely painful. The glands below the jaw draining the tonsillar area are frequently enlarged and tender. There are chills, malaise, headache, rise of temperature and a general feeling of illness. If the attack is very acute the patient may be prostrated and have to take to bed.

Appearance of the tonsils. The tonsils are swollen and project from between the pillars of the fauces. The mucous membrane of the fauces is bright red, and there is usually a generalized inflammation of the whole of the pharyngeal wall. The uvula may be oedematous, and the soft palate may give the appearance of being thickened. As the condition progresses it passes into an acute follicular tonsillitis. The crypts become filled with debris, desquamated epithelium and pus. The pus exudes from the surface, producing the follicular appearance which is characteristic of a well-established tonsillitis. As this stage is approached swallowing becomes still more difficult. The patient may be unable to swallow saliva, this having to be expectorated owing to extreme pain on movement of the pharynx. At times these follicles will coalesce, forming a patchy membrane on the surface of the tonsil. This appearance is characteristic of a very severe infection.

Resolution takes place with the disappearance of the membrane and follicles, and the tonsil gradually reverts to its previous condition. This may be expected within one or two weeks, but in a large number of cases resolution is incomplete and signs of infection can be detected in the tonsil. So common, indeed, is this residual infection, one might almost say that in older people complete resolution rarely takes place after severe infection.

Differential diagnosis. Glandular fever often causes confusion and is to be considered in those patients in whom ulceration or glandular enlargement are marked features. Serological tests and a blood film will help towards the diagnosis. Vincent's Angina, especially in its acute form, pneumococcal pharyngitis and agranulocytic angina must be considered. Thrushes and similar infections may be encouraged by the indiscriminate use of lozenges containing antibiotics, and may produce conditions almost indistinguishable from the original infection for which the antibiotics were used. In countries where it is still encountered, diphtheria must be kept constantly in mind.

Complications. Peritonsillar abscess (p. 126) is the most common complication of acute tonsillitis. Occasionally an abscess may form within the tonsil itself and the resulting deep sloughing of tissue may give rise to dangerous haemorrhage.

Laryngeal oedema may follow the downward spread of severe infections.

Treatment of tonsillitis

General treatment is of the utmost importance. If there is rise of temperature the patient should be treated in bed. The diet given should be light but nourishing. Fluids and soft solids will be all that the patient can take, and the intake of fluid should be encouraged. Sulphonamides and antibiotics limit secondary infection and help prevent complications.

Local treatment is directed towards soothing the affected membrane. Gargles are popular, and in their effects are largely mechanical. In the acute stages gargles should never be strong and should never nip or hurt the patient in any way. It is impossible for a gargle to reach the site of infection in the crypts of the tonsils, and so anything which is sufficiently strong to hurt the throat will merely damage and devitalize the surface membrane. Gargles should be mildly antiseptic and should be given warm. Antibiotics lozenges are to be avoided, but various proprietary lozenges which have slight anaesthetic properties are helpful. Aspirin gargle also can be useful. If very severe surface inflammation is present much comfort can be obtained by the use of a simple spray of warm bicarbonate solution. Antipyretics and analgesics are given as necessary, in the more severe cases it is usual to give antibiotics especially if complications are feared. If it is deemed essential, and this applies particularly to children, that treatment should reach the back of the throat, it will have to be given in the form of a spray.

CHRONIC TONSILLITIS

Chronic tonsillitis may be caused by repeated attacks of acute tonsillitis. Acute attacks of tonsillitis may have ceased many years before the patient comes under examination and the primary acute inflammation may have been forgotten. Resolution after acute tonsillitis may be incomplete and repeated slight inflammatory reactions may produce eventually marked chronic sepsis. For these reasons patients may be surprised by the diagnosis of septic tonsils and they frequently insist that there have been no previous attacks.

The tonsils in these cases are often deceptive. They may be very small and they may be fibrosed. In many cases the patients will state that they have no tonsils at all. But experience shows, in quite a number of instances, that when the tonsils are smallest often the greatest benefit results from their removal. The fact that tonsils cannot be seen easily using the spatula is no evidence that they are healthy.

With a chronically infected tonsil flushing of the anterior pillar is often seen. In front of the anterior pillar is a band of redness which appears to be an injection of the mucous membrane. This curves upwards and disappears just above the upper pole of the tonsil where the anterior pillar merges in the soft palate. It is in the examination of tonsils such as these that experience is required to form an accurate estimate of the condition of the tonsil. The pillars must be drawn back. If necessary, the crypts of the tonsil must be compressed and gently massaged so that the contents of the crypts can be examined properly.

Treatment. The most satisfactory method of treatment of chronically infected tonsils is removal. Tonsils may be removed by the dissection method or by the guillotine method. The dissection of the tonsil under full anaesthesia is the most reliable method, and the method of choice, because in employing this operation the operator can deal with any and every type of tonsil, and by the nature of the anaesthetic is adequately prepared to meet every difficulty, anticipated or otherwise.

In dealing with children, however, there are still some surgeons who use the guillotine method of removal, and in suitable cases the guillotine operation, in the hands of an expert, will give just as good results as the dissection method of removal, but it demands proper training.

The guillotine operation requires a high degree of skill from both surgeon and anaesthetist and on no account should be attempted by anyone unfamiliar with the technique. The operation is not suitable for patients who have had repeated peritonsillitis or a quinsy. In such patients the loose layer of areolar tissue outside the capsule is probably obliterated and separation is thus difficult.

OPERATION OF TONSILLECTOMY

Preparation. Unless the patient has been free of tonsillar or other respiratory infections for two to three weeks operation should not be undertaken, otherwise complications may result from the anaesthetic, or haemorrhage may follow. When a child is seldom free from infections antibiotics should be given for two to three weeks and then operation can be carried out more safely. The presence of poliomyelitis in the locality is an absolute contraindication to tonsillectomy. Where immunization is practised, this should be given, but at least six weeks should elapse between the giving of the vaccine and the operation. Heart, lungs and urine should be examined and enquiry should be made regarding previous illnesses, and particularly any tendency to abnormal bleeding. The patient should be admitted to hospital so that preparation and post-operative treatment can be properly supervised. On the morning of operation nothing should be given except a cup of milk, tea, beef tea, or other hot drink, not less than two hours before the hour fixed for the operation.

Premedication. The object of premedication is to avoid emotional trauma and to ensure that the child should have no memory of the experience. The anaesthesia should be light and the recovery quick and complete. Phenobarbitone can be given at 60 mg per 6 kg of body weight without danger, but 50 to 150 mg is usually sufficient for young children. If preferred sodium pentobarbitone or chlorpromazine hydrochloride may be used in dosage according to body weight and atropine should always be given. In adults the problem is usually simpler as oblivion before operation is demanded by comparatively few patients. When this is desired an intravenous barbiturate such as thiopentone can be administered while the patient is in bed.

Guillotine operation

For the sake of completeness a short description of the guillotine operation is included.

This operation is a blunt dissection of the tonsil in which the guillotine is used as a snare to grasp and fix the tonsil. The anaesthesia employed is usually halothane and should be administered by an experienced anaesthetist. When the child is sufficiently relaxed the mouth is opened widely and the guillotine is inserted into the pharynx. The tongue is depressed with the finger, with a spatula or with the blade of the guillotine, so that the tonsil is clearly exposed. The guillotine is passed below the tonsil and the ring of the guillotine is made to engage the lower pole from below. The guillotine is then rotated until the ring of the guillotine is immediately below the bulk of the tonsil, and the handle in the opposite side of the mouth. The flat aspect of the blade is then in the same plane as the anterior pillar. By elevating the ring and at the same time depressing the handle of the guillotine the tonsil will be made to bulge through the anterior pillar. The thumb of the other hand is then used to press and massage the tonsil through the ring of the guillotine. As soon as the whole tonsil is felt to have been pressed through the ring of the guillotine, the blade of the guillotine is pressed home just behind the anterior pillar. The handle of the guillotine is then drawn towards the patient's chin. This exposes the soft tissues just above the upper pole of the tonsil, and the forefinger is used to break into the soft tissue just above the upper pole, and with one or more sweeps of the forefinger the tonsil is dissected out of its bed. The expert operator becomes accustomed not only to sweep his forefinger round the tonsil, but at the same time to pull the tonsil upwards across the finger, the double motion resulting in the clean peeling of the tonsil from the fossa. If desired, the adenoids are removed with the curette. The patient is turned on the face. This allows the blood to run out of the mouth, and cold sponges on the face materially aid recovery. Bleeding quickly ceases, and after inspection of the throat the patient is returned to bed.

Dissection operation

The removal of the tonsils by dissection can be carried out either with a *local* anaesthetic or with a *general* anaesthetic, and a well-trained surgeon should be able to undertake both operations with equal facility. He should be able to select the method which will best suit the patient under treatment.

In experienced hands both methods are equally effective and dissection under local anaesthesia is just as complete as dissection under general anaesthesia. The operations in principle are identical.

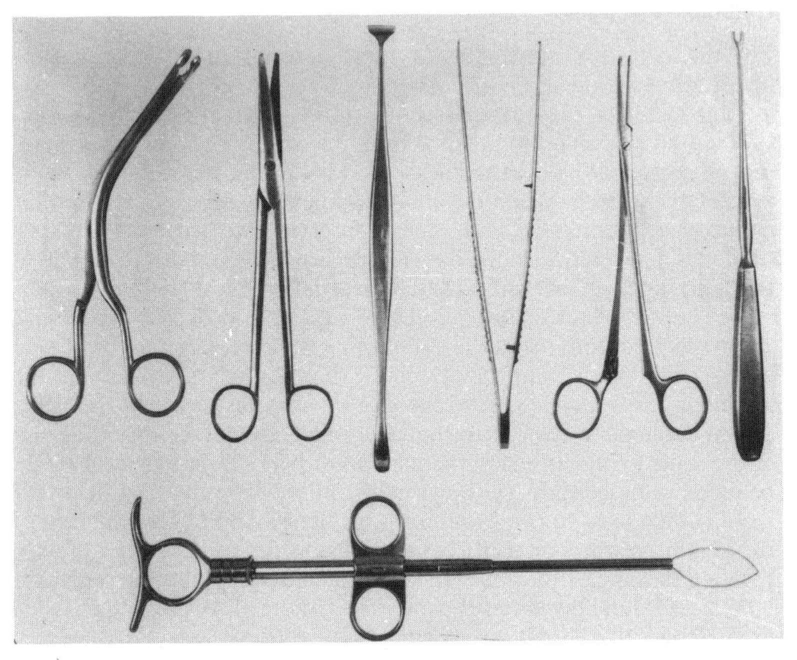

Fig. 33. Instruments for tonsillectomy. These include vulsellum forceps, straight scissors, snare; toothed forceps and artery forceps; dissector and pillar retractors.

Operation with local anaesthesia

The advantages of this method are that general anaesthesia is avoided, bleeding is minimal and the patient usually recovers more quickly. The method is not suitable for the type of patient who is intolerant of manipulations carried out within the mouth and throat. It is also better to reject those who have much peri-tonsillar fibrosis, as may occur after quinsy. In these cases complete anaesthesia may be difficult to achieve with a local anaesthetic.

After suitable medication the throat is sprayed with cocaine (2–4 ml of 10 per cent). After a short wait procaine is injected into the anterior and posterior pillars, as well as into the tissues external to each tonsillar capsule; 50 ml of 0.5 per cent procaine can be used safely. Adrenalin may be added but must not exceed the final concentration of 1 in 200,000. The tonsil is drawn medially with a pair of forceps while the injection is being made behind the tonsil. The patient should be sitting upright in a chair, and after a ten-minute interval the operation is carried out with the patient in this position. The surgeon is seated immediately in front or on the left side of the patient: good illumination of the operation field is of paramount importance.

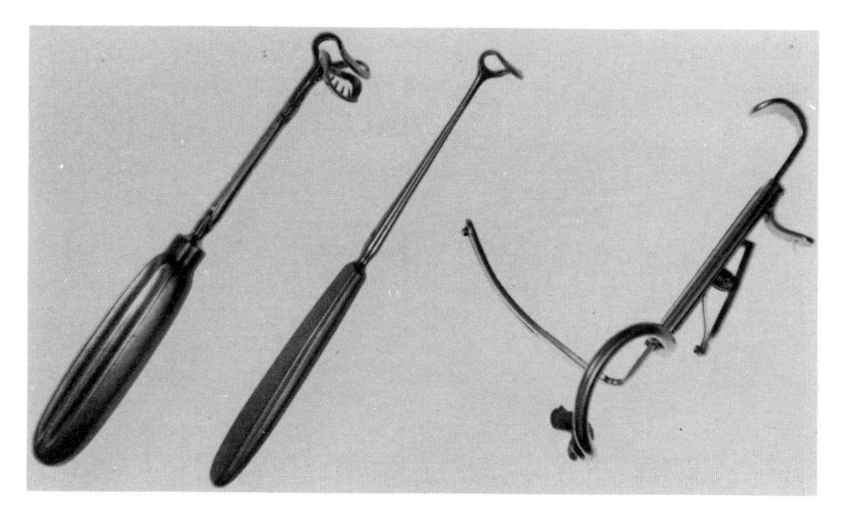

Fig. 34. Adenoid curettes and Boyle-Davis mouth gag for dissection of tonsils.

Tonsillectomy with general anaesthesia

The selection of anaesthetic may be left to the choice of an experienced anaesthetist, but it should be given by intratracheal insufflation as this permits a pack to be inserted in the lower part of the pharynx to prevent blood entering the trachea. Intubation is usually carried out through the nose by means of a soft plastic tube.

No preliminary preparation of the throat is required, although some surgeons inject the fauces to diminish the amount of bleeding. Usually the patient is placed with a sandbag behind the shoulders and with the head extended. The surgeon seats himself at the end of the table and a gag is inserted. It should provide control of the tongue and it should be as suitable for the endentulous as for the patient with teeth (Fig. 34). When the gag is inserted the tonsil is grasped by a vulsellum or other instrument and drawn towards the operator so as to put the pillars on the stretch. This enables the preliminary incision to be made around the upper pole as close to the body of the tonsil as possible (Fig. 35). The preservation of the mucous membrane of the pillars is an important factor in the appearance and the function of the pharynx after operation. The tonsil is then stripped from its bed by a combination of sharp and blunt dissection (Fig. 36). The vessels are caught with clamp forceps as they are exposed or divided, and the dissection is carried down to and, if necessary, below the lower pole of the tonsil (Fig. 37). If desired a snare can be used to finish off the lowest part of this operation, but the snare should not be used to take the place of dissection (Fig. 38).

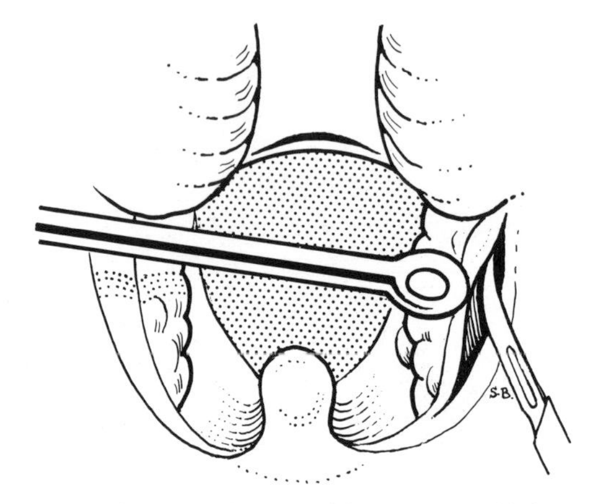

Fig. 35. Shows incision of anterior pillar. Tonsil is drawn out with forceps putting pillar on the stretch to define the attachment to tonsil.

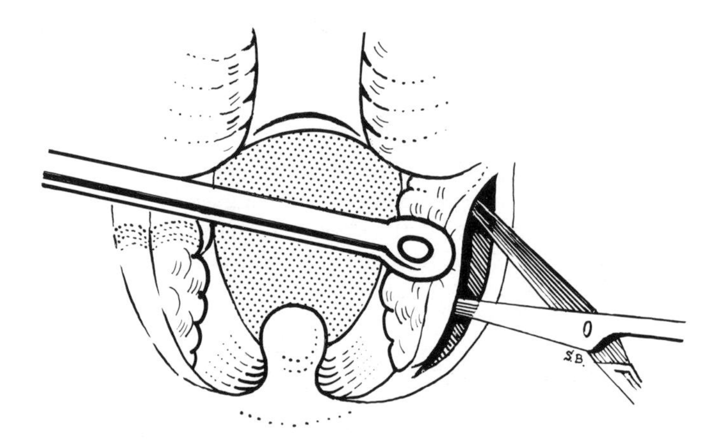

Fig. 36. Blunt dissection of tonsil by scissors inserted through incision in anterior pillar. Dissection is done by forceps, dissector or scissors.

It is essential to define the capsule of the tonsil as the identification of the capsule greatly simplifies the operation. The haemorrhage can be controlled by haemostats or suction, or the fossa may be packed with dry gauze as the dissection proceeds. When the tonsil has been finally removed the bleeding points are caught with forceps and tied off with with silk or catgut or, if desired, can be under-run with catgut and tied off. Various haemostatics are used to control oozing, but the surest method of preventing haemorrhage is the proper ligation of the bleeding points. As an alternative to ligatures the surgeon can employ electro-coagulation. Special insulated forceps are necessary, and the method obviously cannot be used if explosive anaesthetic agents are

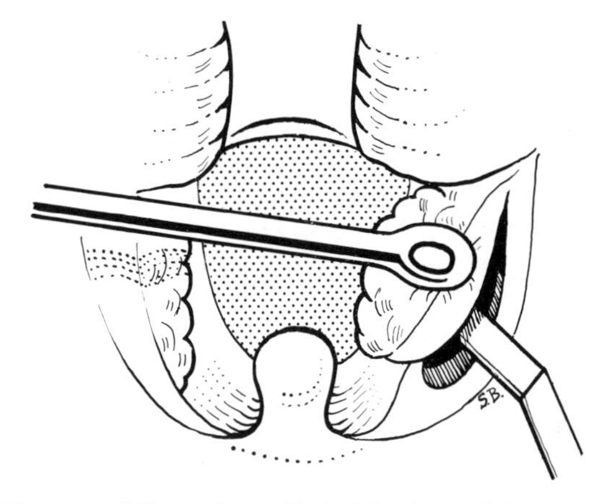

Fig. 37. Shows tonsil dissected out of its bed, leaving pedicle below lower pole.

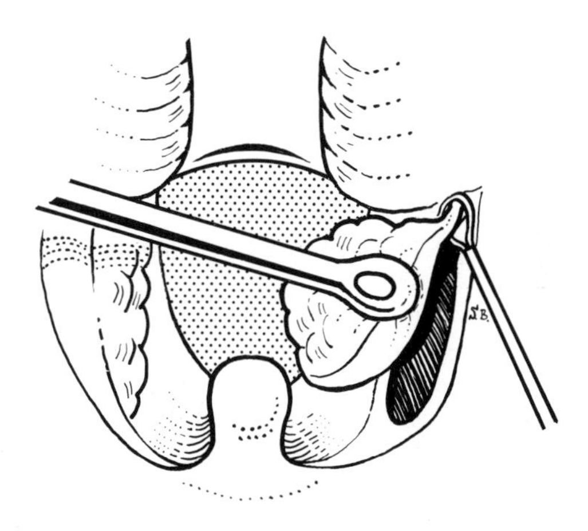

Fig. 38. Snare placed round the pedicle.

being given. Control of bleeding by this method is usually more complete and more rapid. If properly used the method does not increase the risk of haemorrhage or excessive sloughing, and seems to give the patient less post-operative pain.

After-treatment. For the first few hours after operation the patient should be given nothing by the mouth, but after four or five hours, when the risk of reactionary haemorrhage has passed, the patient should be encouraged to use the throat. This prevents stiffness of the pharyngeal muscles and prevents the patient starving himself of fluid by refusing to swallow. The more the patient swallows the easier it becomes and the more rapid is the progress. A sedative is usually required on the night of the operation. Drugs such as codeine and aspirin are frequently of greater value than morphia and other similar hypnotics. However, if pain is excessive, pethidine can be given. The morning after operation a normal diet should be started. With encouragement even children can usually manage this and quickly realize that the painful stage is soon passed. Aspirin in warm water swallowed a few minutes before each meal is of great benefit. Frequent, simple gargles are freshening and soothing. The use of chewing gum or boiled sweets to suck also helps by cleansing the throat and keeping musculature working. On the day after operation the patient should be able to get out of bed. Children can usually go home the following day if they are eating satisfactorily, adults may need to stay in hospital one or two days longer depending upon home conditions On the day after operation a laxative should be given if required.

Relief of pain. Various sprays and powders have been recommended for the relief of pain. Soluble aspirin is one of the best remedies. It can be used as a gargle or blown into the throat from a powder blower. A combination of aspirin and codein e.g. Mist A.P.C. administered shortly before meals will ease the feeding problem. In children it may be necessary to use a spray with a weak solution of peroxide of hydrogen. Syringing with warm solutions, such as sodium bicarbonate solution or 1 in 80 carbolic, is helpful.

COMPLICATIONS FOLLOWING TONSILLECTOMY

Haemorrhage

This is the most frequent and the most dangerous complication following tonsillectomy. The haemorrhage usually falls into one of two classes – *reactionary haemorrhage* and *secondary haemorrhage*. Reactionary haemorrhage occurs within two days of the operation. It is due to the effects of a local injection wearing off and the subsequent dilatation of the vessels, or to incomplete haemostasis or the slipping of ligatures. Secondary haemorrhage occurs five to ten days after operation, and is due to the separation of the slough which forms on the surface of the bed of the tonsil. In some cases the slough is deeper than in others and may include a superficial vessel. When the slough separates the vessel is opened and the haemorrhage may be brisk.

To deal with the haemorrhage in the reactionary stage is a comparatively simple matter. A sedative, in dosage proportional to the age of the patient, can be given, provided the risks (p. 115) are fully realized This allays anxiety, produces a certain degree of analgesia, and permits freer manipulation and treatment. If bleeding persists in spite of adequate treatment the possibility of an abnormality of the clotting mechanism should be considered. Should this be found, arrangements for blood transfusion must be made immediately.

To examine the throat properly, adequate illumination is essential.

Forceps for removing clot, mops, peroxide of hydrogen, the materials for ligaturing the bleeding points – all of these may be required and should be ready. If on inspection the tonsillar fossa is found full of blood clot, the clot should be completely removed. In the majority of instances this is sufficient to cause cessation of the haemorrhage. If not, mops or balls of cotton-wool moistened in peroxide of hydrogen are placed in the tonsillar fossa, and pressure is made upon the fossa for several minutes. If this does not control the haemorrhage or if a spurting vessel can be seen the blood vessel responsible must be ligated. In the case of a tolerant patient and a skilled surgeon a ligature can sometimes be put on in the patient's bed without the need for further anaesthesia.

Where the bleeding point is difficult to see, or adequate skill is not immediately available, continuous pressure should be made on the tonsil bed using a large pad of gauze held in a Luc's forceps, or the special forceps made for the purpose. This will control the situation until the surgeon is available.

When blood loss is serious the patient must be returned to the operating theatre for ligation of the bleeding point under general anaesthesia. Otherwise the problem quickly becomes more difficult with increasing blood loss, deterioration in the patient's general condition and collapse. A blood transfusion should be given at the same time. It is a grave mistake to persist with half-hearted and ineffective attempts to stop the haemorrhage until the loss of blood has placed the patient in real danger. Continued close observation is essential in these circumstances.

In *secondary haemorrhage* treatment is usually straight-forward. Removal of the clot and application of pressure with a peroxide swab generally suffice. Sedation is helpful but must be given with care. If bleeding continues an anaesthetic is given and an attempt made to ligate the vessel. The presence of infection and granulations make this difficult. Deep understitching or suturing the pillars together over a pack may be needed. An antibiotic is given to control the excessive infection which is present in these patients. This type of haemorrhage is almost entirely confined to those patients who have been unwilling to use the throat properly in eating and drinking.

Tonsillar haemorrhage must always be regarded as a serious complication, for if half-hearted and inadequate attempts are made to stop the haemorrhage the patient may lose so much blood in a short space of time as seriously to endanger life. It must also be remembered that the practice of giving an injection of morphia carries a considerable danger if the local bleeding point has not first been dealt with, as, under the influence of the hypnotic, bleeding will continue, the blood going down into the stomach. Thus, the first warning of severe haemorrhage may be the emptying of the stomach of a large quantity of altered blood, an occurrence which is usually followed by the collapse of the patient.

Sepsis

Some infection in the exposed tonsil fossa is inevitable after operation. Severe sepsis following tonsillectomy occurs most frequently in those patients who refuse to swallow. This lack of movement produces muscular stiffness, and allows the slough to spread to a depth and extent which would not occur if the proper muscular action were maintained. It is the precursor of secondary haemorrhage. In addition to the septic absorption from this surface, the lack of fluid is a serious factor particularly in children.

Antibiotics are of use. The patient must be encouraged to swallow, and if necessary the throat should be sprayed with antiseptics, such as peroxide of hydrogen; this causes movement of the muscles as well as cleansing of the throat. To accomplish this patience and ingenuity may be required. If the lack of fluid is serious, intravenous fluids may be given to correct the fluid balance.

Abscess

The glands may become enlarged, and the enlargement may precede infection and abscess formation. This is most commonly encountered in children in whom the tonsillectomy has been undertaken because of the presence of enlarged glands. It is always wiser to warn parents in such cases that the operation may be followed by an exacerbation of the gland inflammation.

Otitis media

Pain is often felt in the ears after tonsillectomy, being referred from the fossae. True otitis media occurs if infected material is forced up the Eustachian tube. This is rare.

Chest complications

Chest complications include atelectasis, broncho-pneumonia, and lung abscess. They are usually the result of aspiration of blood clot, but with modern anaesthetic techniques they are very rare.

Symptoms. There is usually pain in the chest, some cough and shortness of breath, pyrexia, and there may be some cyanosis. The patient often has an anxious expression. The physical signs include impaired chest movement, dullness on percussion and impaired air-entry. X-rays are of great assistance.

Treatment. Re-expansion and aeration are encouraged by energetic physiotherapy. Chemotherapy should be provided. If re-expansion does not occur rapidly then bronchoscopy is indicated in order to remove the obstructing clot.

Lung abscess is the most serious pulmonary complication and has been regarded as embolic in nature. Swinging temperature and an unproductive cough are common, but if rupture occurs into a bronchus much foul sputum is produced. X-rays are essential for diagnosis. Repeated bronchoscopic aspiration combined with intensive chemotherapy and physiotherapy may control early abscess formation. Repeated aspiration via the chest wall may obliterate others. Lobectomy may be needed for a chronic abscess with extensive damage in the involved segment.

RESULTS OF OPERATION

After the removal of tonsils and adenoids there should be certain well-defined results. Assuming that the operation has been satisfactorily and expertly performed, tonsillitis is an impossibility, so that where tonsillitis formed the initial reason for the operation it should cease to give trouble. Nasal discharge should also disappear almost immediately. As has been pointed out, this is due to the relief of post-nasal congestion and sinusitis. Where nasal discharge persists, following removal of adenoids, the surgeon has not completed his treatment until the sinuses have been fully investigated.

Adeno-tonsillectomy will not of itself protect against respiratory infection. On the other hand, where respiratory infection follows nasal catarrh or frequent episodes of adenoiditis, in a descending pharyngeal process, the elimination of the primary infection tends to lessen the incidence of respiratory troubles.

Otitis media

In otitis media the removal of the adenoids removes the most common cause of this disease in children, and it will help to protect the child from sepsis of the nasopharynx. In many cases this sepsis is the starting-point of otitis media. Experience shows that otitis media often fails to clear up until the adenoids have been effectively dealt with. In adults the influence of tonsillectomy is considerable in this respect. Otitis media frequently commences with an attack of tonsillitis, and removal of the tonsils will give at least a certain degree of protection.

Acute rheumatic fever

A great deal has been written regarding rheumatism and its relation to streptococcal throat infections. Tonsillectomy has probably been carried out with excessive enthusiasm in the past and much controversy remains. Tonsillectomy cannot benefit established rheumatic heart disease, but it is becoming generally accepted that the operation is advisable in children who have suffered rheumatic fever and in whom persistent streptococcal infection occurs in the tonsils. Further heart damage can be prevented by operation in these circumstances; antibiotic cover is essential.

Infective fevers—measles, scarlet fever, etc.

The incidence of diphtheria is lowered in the tonsillectomized child, and removal of tonsils and adenoids is recognized by public health authorities as the surest method of eliminating a carrier. It is agreed that tonsillectomy should not be undertaken when poliomyelitis is in the locality, as the incidence of bulbar paralysis is high when the disease follows tonsillectomy. It is wise, therefore, to ensure, as far as possible, that children submitted to tonsillectomy have been inoculated against poliomyelitis. Tonsillectomy has no proved influence on the incidence of other fevers.

Nephritis and pyelitis

These diseases appear to have small connection with the tonsils and adenoids and the benefit of adeno-tonsillectomy remains difficult to prove. The remarks made above in relation to acute rheumatic fever apply here also. Operation may be advisable in patients who are suffering repeated episodes of renal damage consequent upon attacks of streptococcal tonsillitis.

Effects of tonsils and adenoids on nutrition

Malnutrition is a frequent sequel of infected tonsils and adenoids, and the results of their removal in certain of these cases are dramatic. There is marked improvement in weight, and rapid progress is made until the normal weight of the child is reached. Removal of tonsils and adenoids, however, does not of itself increase weight.

SUMMARY OF INDICATIONS FOR TONSILLECTOMY

Recurring attacks of acute tonsillitis. This is by far the most common indication.

Prolonged glandular enlargement in the neck which does not subside with recovery of the tonsillar infection. The possibility of tuberculous adenitis must be kept in mind.

The occurrence of a quinsy (peritonsillar abscess), or of a lateral or retro-pharyngeal abscess initiated by an episode of tonsillitis.

Acute rheumatic fever. The place of tonsillectomy is disputed, but there seems good evidence that the risk of further attacks is lessened by tonsillectomy if tonsillitis has been responsible for recurrences.

Acute nephritis. The same remarks apply.

Enlargement of the tonsils is not itself an indication for tonsillectomy in a child, though it is often for this reason that children are referred to hospital. The tonsils are very variable structures in childhood and their size can alter almost from week to week. Moreover, some tonsils are submerged and appear small, whereas others are almost pedunculated and appear extremely prominent and large. Having said this it must be stated that very occasionally sheer bulk may be an indication for tonsillectomy if it is felt that obstruction is resulting.

Bronchitis and chest troubles, if initiated by a sore throat, may benefit from tonsillectomy by limiting the incidence of upper respiratory infection.

Various skin and eye diseases have been reported to be helped by removal of septic tonsils, but the exact relationship is uncertain.

Improved appetite and growth often follow tonsillectomy in children, but the operation can seldom be recommended purely on such grounds.

Tonsillectomy in singers. This is by no means contraindicated, but the patient should be warned that it may be some time before the voice will be fit for professional engagements, and that some degree of retraining may be necessary after the operation.

SUMMARY OF INDICATIONS FOR ADENOIDECTOMY ONLY

In some cases it is desirable to remove adenoids only. If the tonsils are healthy and producing no symptoms they should be left alone. Adenoidectomy only is indicated in the following situations:

Recurring ear symptoms such as earache, episodes of conductive deafness, or of acute otitis media, or repeated mucous otitis.

Recurring nasal symptoms such as 'colds', nasal obstruction, mouth-breathing, and discharge, possibly accompanied by sinusitis. In many cases these indicate episodes of adenoiditis and such attacks must not be confused with nasal allergy.

15. Acute Diseases of the Pharynx

PHARYNGITIS

Nasopharyngitis

Nasopharyngeal inflammation is, as a rule, part of an acute inflammation in the pharynx proper, or in the nasal cavity. It may be said in many cases to be the starting-point of acute rhinitis, laryngitis, tracheitis, etc. Chronic infection may also occur, and in these cases it is usually due to lymphoid hypertrophy, that is to overgrowth of the small follicles of lymphoid tissue previously referred to and their subsequent inflammation. Cigarette smoking, alcohol and exposure to irritating fumes are frequent causes of nasopharyngitis. Douches and sprays are sometimes of value in treatment, and any source of irritation should be eliminated. When it is part of another inflammatory condition, such as rhinitis, the treatment of nasopharyngitis is properly that of the primary disease.

Simple acute pharyngitis

Pharyngitis may be caused by cold, by irritation such as results from fumes, by certain fruits or severe digestive disturbance.

There is injection of the mucous membrane of the posterior pharyngeal wall and the lymphoid nodules stand out prominently, enlarged and of a darker red than the surrounding membrane.

The patient complains of irritation and rawness of the throat with possibly slight pain on swallowing. This pain is usually less when swallowing food than saliva. There is a constant desire to swallow which aggravates the symptoms.

Infective pharyngitis

This is a further stage of the last condition. It is generally streptococcal, but staphylococci and pneumococci can be responsible. Not infrequently cases are encountered of an infective pharyngitis in which one particular organism appears to be responsible for the spread of what may amount to an epidemic. This is sometimes known as 'hospital sore throat', and occurs not only in those possessing tonsils, but sometimes in those without.

Symptoms. The condition is characterized by severe dysphagia, pain and toxaemia, and the glands on each side of the neck are usually swollen and tender.

Appearance in the throat. There is acute inflammation of the posterior part of the fauces, involving the pillars of the fauces, the soft palate and the posterior pharyngeal wall. The mucous membrane is uniformly red and oedematous, but as a rule the lymphoid tissue immediately behind the posterior pillars stands out as a ridge on each side of the pharynx. If there is any enlargement of the lymphoid nodules on the posterior wall of the pharynx these will be seen as brighter patches of inflammation. This condition is seen most frequently in cases in which tonsillectomy has been carried out, but if the tonsils are present they will share in the superficial inflammation, though as a rule they do not show any actual enlargement.

Membranous pharyngitis

This is a further stage in inflammation of the pharynx, and is due to infection by virulent organisms such as streptococci or pneumococci. A thin greyish membrane is seen spreading over the fauces and the posterior wall of the pharynx and downwards towards the larynx. The membrane is patchy and does not peel off as does a diphtheritic membrane. It gives one the impression that it is a discoloration of the surface of the mucous membrane rather than a patch of exudate.

Symptoms. This form of the disease is characterized by very severe constitutional symptoms. There is obvious toxaemia and the patient is extremely ill. The condition is a serious one, and if unchecked may have very grave results. The spread in a downward direction towards the larynx is to be feared and every effort must be made to prevent this, as it may cause oedema of the larynx or septic broncho-pneumonia.

Treatment. In mild cases simple antiseptic lozenges and antipyretics often suffice. Antibiotic lozenges should be avoided. Gargles, however, have their own place in treatment, as they induce movement of the throat and secretion. If the glands are involved, immobility and local heat are soothing and help to reduce the swelling. In the more acute forms antiseptic sprays should be used in order to ensure cleansing of the pharynx. Copious irrigations of the throat give great relief. These can conveniently be given by placing a basin on a chair by the side of the bed over which the patient can hang his head. In this position the throat is douched by means of a Higginson's syringe with one to two pints of warm solution of sodium bicarbonate. Steam inhalations are comforting to the patient, particularly when the inflammation is tending to spread into the larynx. Chemotherapy or antibiotics should be given at once, even before the organisms have been identified by the usual throat swab. If pain in the pharynx prevents the proper absorption of fluids, intravenous glucose saline should be given early.

LUDWIG'S ANGINA

This condition is cellulitis and eventually abscess formation in the floor of the mouth extending downwards into the planes of the neck. A brawny swelling forms under the chin without fluctuation. There is intense pain on tongue movement, and the patient may be severely dehydrated owing to inability to take anything by mouth.

Treatment. Chemotherapy or antibiotics, in full doses, should be administered. Should incision be required it should be carried out under general anaesthesia with intubation.

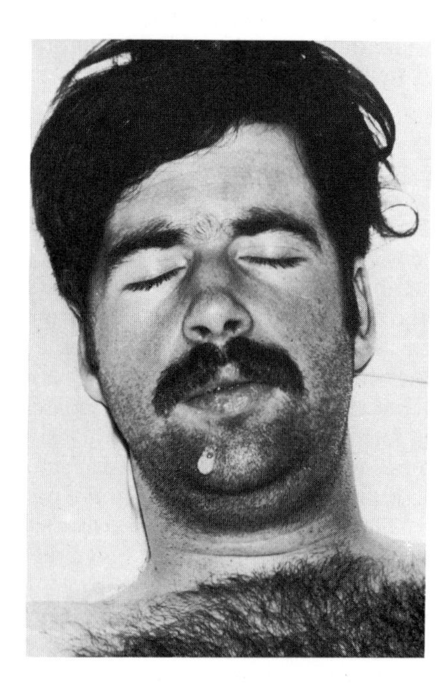

Fig. 39. Ludwig's Angina:—Note the brawny neck swelling, the ill appearance of the patient and the saliva drooling from the mouth.

DIPHTHERIA

Although this disease has virtually disappeared in many countries, it is still present where measures have not been taken for widespread protection of the population. A description must therefore be retained in this section.

Diphtheria is an infection due to a specific organism—the Klebs-Loffler bacillus. It is characterized by the formation of a membrane upon the mucous membrane of the upper air passages. In appearance the membrane is a yellowish grey, is patchy and is usually seen at the pillars of the fauces, the tonsils and the base of the uvula. It is fairly sharply defined. The membrane bleeds in characteristic fashion when it is removed from the mucous surface. There is usually a tender enlarged gland at the angle of the jaw, and there is also, as a rule, some febrile disturbance. While the patient may be extremely ill, in the majority of cases the amount of membrane formation does not impress one as being accompanied by the same degree of constitutional disturbance as would be the case were the membrane that of a streptococcal infection.

So far as the laryngologist is concerned, the chief problem lies in the differentiation of the cases – between membranous pharyngitis of the diphtheritic type and other types. It is advisable to be able to make the distinction, as the one case may be treated without special precautions, and the other must be isolated. As the disease progresses there is extension of the membrane formation which may involve the larynx, leading to serious complications such as obstruction of the airway.

Diagnosis. A knowledge of the clinical appearances described above is essential for the early diagnosis of diphtheria, as valuable time may be lost in treatment while awaiting the bacteriologist's report. The most important part of the diagnosis, however, is the bacteriologist's examination of the throat swab which should include part of the membrane, if present.

In every case, therefore, in which any suspicion exists, a swab should be taken; slight and atypical cases are sometimes seen and this renders reliance on clinical signs alone dangerous.

Treatment. Early administration of antitoxin should be the aim. The average dose for an adult varies from 8,000 units to about 100,000 units according to the severity of the attack. For nasal or laryngeal diphtheria 8,000 to 10,000 units will suffice, and all doubtful cases should receive a dose of 4,000 units pending the laboratory report upon the throat swab. In addition antibiotics should be administered.

Careful watch should be kept where involvement of the larynx is suspected, and aspiration, intubation or tracheotomy employed, if obstruction of the airway demands these measures.

VINCENT'S ANGINA

Vincent's angina is the name given to a disease characteristically causing local ulceration of the tonsils. The organisms responsible are *Vincent's spirillum* in symbiosis with a fusiform bacillus. These organisms may be isolated from a swab. The disease can take either an acute form or a chronic form, and may be localized to the tonsil or be widespread throughout the mouth and pharynx.

The acute form. The acute form is the more diffuse, and as a rule there is reddening of the mucous membrane of the gums and fauces, with the formation of small patches of greyish membrane. Though the patient may feel ill, it is rare that anything is felt other than a sore throat, together with some general disturbance.

The chronic form. The more chronic form consists of ulceration, which is found most commonly on one or other of the tonsils. The ulceration may be unilateral and is of a deep, ragged character. There is a dirty greyish membrane on the floor of the ulcer, but there is no special characteristic such as raising or rolling of the edges. It is frequently associated with a membrane on the gums and around carious teeth.

Symptoms. Occasionally the throat is painful, but the patient does not as a rule show much general disturbance.

Diagnosis. Diagnosis lies chiefly in the hands of the bacteriologist. The identification of the characteristic organisms in a direct smear is the most important point. The differential diagnosis lies between syphilis, tuberculosis and other ulcerations of non-specific character. Histological examination will show only subacute inflammatory tissue, but should be done in any case of doubt, as an early carcinoma may harbour the specific organisms.

Treatment. At the outset bacteriological sensitivity studies should be made, but penicillin administered by injection will usually eliminate the infection. Isolation and bed rest are advisable until the ulcerations are healed. Healing is also promoted by the use of peroxide gargles and by the administration of Vitamins B and C. When complete recovery has taken place the patient should be advised to have the tonsils removed, as the possibility of recurrence is considerable.

In those cases in which the infection has spread to the gums a valuable form of treatment is local application of 30 per cent chromic acid solution. The thorough treatment of this form is best undertaken by the dentist.

During treatment feeding utensils must be sterilised and afterwards infected toothbrushes must be discarded.

HERPES OF THE SOFT PALATE

This is a painful condition accompanying acute infective conditions of the nose. The patient may complain of an acutely sore throat, particularly high up around the soft palate. On examination of the fauces there is little or nothing to be seen beyond slight oedema of the uvula. Close examination will reveal the herpetic vesicles usually on one side or the other about the base of the uvula.

Treatment. The best treatment is the administration of a soothing paint such as boroglycerin, and bland gargles.

ERYSIPELAS

This disease sometimes spreads from the face to the pharynx, and when it does so it is a serious complication. The characteristic bullae are formed, and there is marked oedema and inflammation of the mucosa. The chief danger is oedema of the glottis.

AGRANULOCYTOSIS

Agranulocytosis is a condition of leukopenia in which neutrophil polymorphonuclear cells are reduced in number or disappear from the circulation. There are marked pharyngeal and buccal lesions of ulcerative and necrotic type.

Aetiology. There are indications pointing to two types of disease: (1) that in which there is no known origin, and (2) that which is due to the action of some drug. The drugs concerned are amidopyrine, the arsephenamines and some sulphonamides. Certain antibiotics may be responsible at times for this blood disorder, *e.g.* chloromycetin and aureomycin. Other drugs which must be kept in mind are thiouracil, butazolidine, and cytoxic drugs used in cancer chemotherapy. Many of the agents listed are in common use and their toxic effect on the marrow has constantly to be borne in mind.

Symptoms. Irregular pyrexia and sore throat occur. Sometimes there is recurrence of sore throat with rising temperature in a patient to whom treatment has been given for tonsillitis. Rapid progressive weakness and haemorrhage may take place. The blood picture shows diminution of polymorphonuclear cells with comparative increase of mononuclear cells. The white cell count is usually reduced.

Pharyngeal signs. In the pharynx there is a diffuse greyish membrane, sometimes with superficial ulceration. This involves the tonsil as a rule, but may extend on to the pillars and posterior wall or forward to the cheek or the alveolus. The glands beneath the jaw and in the cervical region may be enlarged and there may be glandular swellings elsewhere in the body.

Treatment. Immediate withdrawal of the drug causing the disease is essential. Occasionally this is sufficient to effect a cure, but energetic treatment may be required.

Local treatment. Applications appropriate for acute infections of the pharynx should be used. In particular, irrigations are recommended and anaesthetic lozenges if dysphagia is great. In some instances bacteriological investigation shows the presence of large numbers of Vincent's organisms and in such cases swabbing with Fowler's solution of arsenic or chromic acid solution (30 per cent) will assist recovery.

Treatment of the blood condition. Where immediate improvement does not follow withdrawal of the drug concerned the outlook is serious. A swab should be taken for bacteriological culture and sensitivity studies and large doses of penicillin combined with streptomycin given. If staphylococcus is present methycillin should be substituted for penicillin. Since Chloramphenicol and sulphonamides have been known to produce agranulocytosis they should be avoided. Pentneucliotide, liver extract and Vitamin B_{12} are sometimes recommended but are not of proven value. Fresh blood transfusion may be of help. Steroids are inadvisable.

PERITONSILLAR ABSCESS (QUINSY)

Peritonsillar abscess generally arises as a complication of acute tonsillitis. Infection passes through the tonsil capsule into the loose peritonsillar layer of areolar tissue where it produces a cellulitis and then an abscess. The organisms causing peritonsillar abscess are usually those associated with the infection of the tonsil – staphylococcus or streptococcus.

Symptoms. There is acute pain in the throat with a feeling of tension. There may be an enlarged tender gland behind the angle of the jaw. As the abscess develops the throat becomes more painful; it is reddened and there may be considerable trismus. Speech becomes difficult, and the saliva may run out of the mouth owing to the inability to swallow. General disturbance is usually severe, and the patient may suffer from lack of food. If the trismus will permit detailed inspection the soft palate on the affected side will be seen bulging downwards and forwards so that the uvula may be pressed against the opposite tonsil. The mucous membrane is red and oedematous; the tonsils may protrude from behind the pillars. On the other hand, the tonsil may appear to be even more recessed than previously.

Treatment. In the early stages hot fomentations over the painful glands, and gargles and sprays together with antibiotics are used. If energetically carried out this treatment may abort the condition; if not, the abscess will have to be opened. There are two methods of opening the abscess. In the first method the abscess is opened through the supratonsillar fossa and the tonsil is partially freed from the anterior pillar. In the second method the abscess is opened by a guarded knife or by sinus forceps being thrust into the most prominent part of the soft palate. Of these two methods, that of opening the abscess behind the anterior pillar is the better, as the abscess is opened throughout a large extent of its cavity wall. A special pair of forceps or a pair of turbinotomy punch forceps is pushed upwards and outwards in the superior tonsillar crypt, and is opened when the abscess cavity has been entered. The withdrawal of the forceps open enlarges the opening. Then the forceps are re-inserted open. The one blade is passed into the abscess cavity and the other is applied just behind the anterior pillar. When the forceps are closed a further cut is made in the abscess wall, and a large drainage opening is provided. If this method is employed, reopening is very rarely required. Where no obvious point of fluctuation can be found a vertical line is taken from the point at which the anterior pillar joins the tongue, and a horizontal line through the base of the uvula; at the intersection of these two lines will be found, approximately, the best point for opening the abscess. Tape is wound round the blade of a knife about half an inch from its point and the abscess incised.

Anaesthesia is sometimes a problem in dealing with these cases. The opening of an abscess may be an exceedingly painful procedure, and, in certain cases, to open it without an anaesthetic of some kind may do considerable harm. Spraying with cocaine solution or injecting procaine gives little real anaesthesia, but does help to a certain extent to relieve the trismus. If a general anaesthetic is used great care, effective suction, and all the facilities of a proper operating theatre are essential. Accidental rupture of the abscess and inhalation of pus can be dangerous and it is for this reason that incision is usually made with a local anaesthetic. When general anaesthesia is being used it is wise to tilt the table with the head well downwards and be ready to turn the patient onto the side at a moment's notice if necessary. An experienced anaesthetist, however, is usually able to pass a naso-tracheal tube without great difficulty. The surgeon can then gently insert a pack to protect the larynx after which the abscess is opened and pus sucked out.

In all cases the patient should be advised to have the tonsils removed because quinsy is frequently recurrent. If the quinsy is being drained under general anaesthesia there is much to be said for tonsillectomy at the same time. With full antibiotic cover this is a perfectly safe procedure for the great majority of patients and avoids the inconvenience of a second admission to hospital with consequent loss of working time.

RETROPHARYNGEAL ABSCESS

The most frequent type of abscess is due to infection of the retropharyngeal lymph nodes in the posterior wall of the pharynx anterior to the prevertebral fascia. This is the type usually found in infants, and as these nodes may be low down in the pharynx the abscess may not be obvious on superficial examination. As these nodes tend to atrophy after the age of two years the frequency of this type of abscess decreases when the child grows older. In adults the abscess as a rule is higher in the pharynx and may be above the level of the soft palate. Retropharyngeal abscess occasionally occurs in a chronic form, behind the prevertebral fascia. This type is caused by tuberculosis of the cervical spine and presents as a painless swelling in the posterior wall of the pharynx. A lateral X-ray film of the soft tissues and cervical spine is always a wise precaution.

Symptoms. The symptoms are usually pain and discomfort on swallowing. There may be nasal obstruction in the case of abscesses situated high up and occasionally, obstruction of the larynx in those situated low down. There is no trismus in this form of abscess. In an abscess occurring in the lymph nodes the organism is usually the

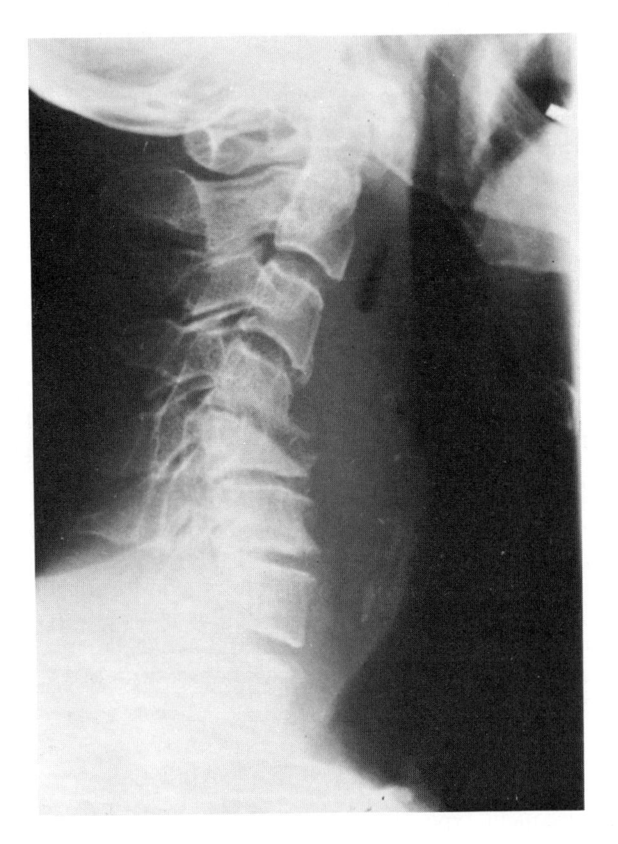

Fig. 40. Retro-pharyngeal abcess: – Without knowing the history one would probably diagnose this as tuberculous because of the destruction of the cervical spine. In fact it was an acute condition following severe tonsillitis.

streptococcus, whereas aspiration of a chronic abscess is likely to reveal Koch's bacillus.

Treatment. The abscess due to lymph node infection should be opened through the pharyngeal wall. If possible, the use of an anaesthetic is avoided, and in children the head is held dependent. The assistant should be ready to turn the patient over quickly when necessary. The best method of opening the abscess is by Hilton's method or with a guarded knife. In caries of the vertebrae the abscess should be opened by dissection behind the sternomastoid, from the outside.

Abscess due to otitic infection may be encountered in the pharynx. This is a rare complication and is due to pus from the ear or mastoid infection finding its way through the planes of the neck around the

Eustachian tube, through the jugular foramen or other route. The treatment of this form of abscess is that of the primary infection and evacuation.

LINGUAL TONSIL ABSCESS

Lingual tonsil abscess is formed by infection in the lymphoid tissue on one side or the other at the base of the tongue. This is most frequently caused by the streptococcus.

Symptoms. The symptoms are extreme dysphagia. There is difficulty in speaking; there is a tender swelling in the submaxillary region just below the angle of the jaw. When these patients are first seen, the expectation in the mind of the examiner is that a peritonsillar or retropharyngeal abscess will be discovered; but when the mouth is opened, and it is opened easily for there is little trismus, a normal pharynx is seen. Examination with a laryngeal mirror, however, will reveal a swelling on one side of the base of the tongue. Lingual tonsil abscess is frequently opened by pressure from the spatula when the examiner is endeavouring to examine the lower part of the pharynx. The opening of these abscesses is easily carried out by means of a curved probe or forceps. In cases of difficulty the best method of attack is by means of a laryngoscope and a long straight guarded knife.

Abscesses are also found in other parts of the pharynx – in the vallecula, etc. These are treated on general principles as outlined.

After-treatment. After-treatment of these abscesses consists in gargles, fomentations to the outside of the neck to reduce the glandular swelling and reopening should the cavities close before complete drainage has taken place. Where tonsils have been suspected as the entering point for infection they should be removed after the infection has subsided.

Antibiotics or sulphonamides will probably have been given as part of the after-treatment to combat toxaemia and prevent recurrence.

FUNGUS INFECTIONS

These are commonly called *thrush*, and the usual organism is *Candida albicans*. It is a disease chiefly of weakly infants and debilitated adults. Scattered patches of whitish membrane are seen in the mouth and pharynx which may resemble diphtheria, but which are as a rule lighter in colour and are not accompanied by the general symptoms associated with the more serious disease. On removal of the membrane there is a tendency to bleeding.

Treatment. The areas may be painted with an aqueous solution of gentian violet (1 per cent) and in severe infections nystatin suspension should be used at a dosage of 4 ml four times daily. Downward spread into the oesophagus can be a serious complication, but generally can be controlled by Nystatin.

16. Chronic Infections of the Pharynx

CHRONIC PHARYNGITIS

This troublesome condition may occur in a wide variety of types but is basically chronic inflammation of the mucous membrane of the pharynx with hyperplasia of its various elements including the lymph nodes. When these nodes are the most noticeable feature the disease is called granular pharyngitis or chronic hypertrophic pharyngitis.

Aetiology. The cause is frequently an extension of nasal obstruction and inflammation. The mucous membrane being continuous from the nose into the pharynx, it not infrequently happens that while infection is localized in the nasopharynx and the posterior parts of the nares, the pharynx suffers from the general inflammation. Sinus infection, possibly unsuspected, may cause irritation by the passage of infected secretions. Climatic conditions may produce the irritation, while gases, smoking, alcohol and dietetic indiscretion are other factors often encountered. The condition is probably more frequently a cause of complaint in women than in men. This trouble sometimes follows tonsillectomy, and it seems to be Nature's attempt to replace the lymphoid tissue which has been removed by operation, and in certain cases the reinfection or inflammation of these lymph nodules is as troublesome to the patient as the previous tonsillitis. The appearances may follow nasal operation, particularly those operations in which there has been rather too enthusiastic removal of tissue, and where there is left a tendency to atrophy. Patients suffering from rheumatism and gout are frequently subject to this affection.

Symptoms. The description given of the symptoms varies greatly with individuals. It may be simple sore throat, a pricking or irritation as of a foreign body, or an accumulation of mucus causing a constant necessity to swallow.

Appearances. In the simple form there is a general redness of the posterior pharyngeal wall; the mucous membrane is thickened and reddened; the fauces usually share in the congestion, and a degree of oedema of the uvula may be found. The pharyngeal mucous membrane may suggest a rubbery consistency.

In the hypertrophic types there is increase in the size of the lymphoid islands in the mucosa of the posterior pharyngeal wall and of the lateral band behind each posterior pillar. In such patients examination shows reddish elevations in the mucosa, and the lateral band may amount to a column of tissue standing out markedly behind each posterior pillar.

Treatment. The general condition of the patient is of the greatest importance. Anything which tends to prolong the inflammation must be eliminated as far as possible and this frequently involves altering a patient's habits; it may be in regard to food, tobacco, alcohol, etc., or it may be necessary to eliminate some source of sepsis. This sepsis may be found in the sinuses, teeth or tonsils. Tonsillectomy, unless carried out only after careful consideration, may aggravate the condition.

Local treatment consists in gargles and paints, of which paints are probably the most valuable, as few can gargle behind the anterior pillar.

Mandl's paint may be efficacious but should be discontinued immediately if it is found to have an irritant effect. In the hypertrophic types of the disease cautery or diathermy can be applied to the hypertrophic lymphoid tissue in the lateral pharyngeal bands and on the posterior wall.

The condition is very intractable, and treatment for the most part is unsatisfactory owing to the constant tendency to recurrence and relapse.

ATROPHIC PHARYNGITIS

This condition is most frequently an extension of an atrophic disease of the nose; occasionally it is encountered without obvious nasal change. Sometimes it follows drastic nasal operations, but may be part of a general atrophic process which can be traced from the nose to the larynx or even trachea.

Symptoms. The most usual symptom is irritation of the pharynx, with a burning sensation or dryness. There may be a constant desire to hawk, owing to the stickiness of the secretion or crusting on the posterior wall of the throat.

Appearances. The posterior pharyngeal wall appears glazed, and it may be reddened in small patches where lymphoid follicles have become irritated. The outstanding characteristic, however, is the absence of moisture.

Treatment. Treatment is palliative only. If possible the primary condition should be treated, while locally the greatest benefit will be obtained from the use of oily sprays.

KERATOSIS PHARYNGIS

This condition consists of the presence of yellowish-white excrescences on the mucous membrane. These are small conical masses of keratinized epithelium, which are most commonly found at the mouths of crypts or near follicles of lymphoid tissue. The usual sites are the tonsils and the lingual tonsils, but they may be seen also in the nasopharynx, on the posterior pharyngeal wall and over the dorsum and base of the tongue.

Symptoms. For the most part symptoms are absent, and the condition is usually diagnosed in the course of a routine examination. Occasionally symptoms of irritation and tickling cause advice to be sought. It is characteristic of these masses that they are difficult to remove by swabbing.

The aetiology is doubtful, but is ascribed by some to the presence of *leptothrix* in the pharynx.

Treatment in the absence of symptoms is not demanded and the condition may undergo spontaneous cure in the course of a year or two. If irritation is being caused, the masses responsible may be removed with forceps and the part painted with iodine, salicylic acid or silver nitrate 10 per cent. Where the tonsils are chiefly affected they may be removed.

TUBERCULOSIS OF THE PHARYNX

This is encountered as an *ulceration*, *tumour formation (tuberculoma)* or as a *fibrotic condition (Lupus)*. The ulceration is rarely primary and most frequently accompanies or follows tuberculosis elsewhere. The ulcer may involve the tonsil and the fauces, may erode the soft palate and cause considerable destruction of tissue. The ulcer usually commences as a nodule, which breaks down and causes involvement of the deeper structures. Tuberculosis is sometimes found in the tonsils. In children, if the glands of the neck are enlarged, the tonsils when removed should be submitted for histological examination. In a percentage of cases these tonsils will be found to contain tuberculous foci.

Tuberculoma

This form may be found in the vallecula, on the anterior surface of the epiglottis or on the pharyngeal wall. It may closely simulate cancer by forming a large fungating mass and by producing early localized enlargements of the glands of the neck. The mass is apt to break down and may cause much destruction of the epiglottis and surrounding parts. In such cases there is sometimes no laryngeal lesion; the cords are normal, but the lung shows a fibrotic condition of slow progress, which may pass unnoticed even after careful investigation. (See Tuberculosis of the Larynx.)

Diagnosis. Diagnosis is made by discovering the lesion in the lung, and by taking a portion of tissue from the fungating mass and submitting it for histological examination, when tuberculous nodules will be found.

Treatment. This should be carried out in a sanatorium. It consists of the usual tuberculosis regime. Diathermy is of value, and also the cautery, in limiting the local lesion.

Dysphagia may be serious and require careful management. (See Tuberculosis of the Larynx.)

SYPHILIS

Primary form

Chancre of the tonsils is occasionally met with, but is very rare. It appears as a superficial ulcer on an enlarged tonsil. The tonsil is seen to be slightly inflamed, and there is a certain amount of induration around the ulcer. The glands behind and below the angle of the jaw are enlarged.

Secondary form

This is more frequently seen, the complaint usually being that of sore throat. Mucous patches are found and superficial ulceration, which may take a form resembling snail tracks.

Tertiary form

This is a gummatous ulceration caused by the breaking down of the gumma. It is a punched-out ulcer with a wash-leather base and induration of the edge. There may be perforation of the soft palate or of the hard palate and considerable destruction of surrounding structures. Although there is usually some discomfort, it is surprising how little general trouble results even from an extensive lesion in the fauces.

Diagnosis. Diagnosis in the primary form as to be distinguished from simple ulceration, from Vincent's Angina, from tuberculosis and from diphtheria.

Serological tests are essential at any stage and should always be done for ulcerative conditions around the mouth and pharynx. A biopsy should be made to exclude any coexistent disease.

Treatment is that of the systemic infection combined with local hygiene.

PEMPHIGUS

This is characterized by a bullous eruption on the soft palate and fauces. The bullae are greyish white in colour, and patches of erosion show where they have broken down. The local symptoms are those of burning sensations and general discomfort in the throat. As a rule, lesions can be found elsewhere, as in the eyes or in the gastro-intestinal tract.

Prognosis. The condition is fatal for there is no known specific. The disease is slowly progressive and it may be eighteen months or two years before the patient dies.

GLANDULAR FEVER

Also known as infectious mononucleosis, this virus infection occurs in three forms: anginous, glandular and hepatic. They often overlap. The patient has pyrexia and malaise, associated with a throat infection and glandular enlargement which may resemble tonsillitis or pharyngitis with adenitis, but which fails to resolve on treatment. Splenic enlargement may provide the clue to diagnosis. This is made by examination of the blood picture and enables the differentiation from leukaemia to be made. Serological tests, such as the Paul-Bunnell test and the tests used in syphilis, are often positive.

Treatment is non-specific and it may be several weeks before the patient regains normal health.

17. Chronic Diseases of the Pharynx

THE NASOPHARYNX

FIBROMA

Apart from fibromata benign tumours are very rare in the nasopharynx. Fibromata usually take their origin in the periosteum of the roof of the nasopharynx, but they may also be found taking their origin from the choanal borders. They consist of fibrous tissue covered with epithelium. Many are highly vascular and are really fibroangiomata. The tumour may be sessile or pedunculated.

Symptoms. The chief symptoms are those of slowly increasing obstruction of the nose. When obstruction becomes more marked, should sinus infection take place, discharge and headache are prominent. Epistaxis occurs and can be dangerous. As the tumour grows, pressure symptoms and signs may become extreme, for though histologically benign the tumour is clinically malignant on account of its persistent growth.

Treatment. The aim of treatment should be complete removal. It has been maintained that these tumours undergo spontaneous recession after the age of twenty, but recent investigations seem to throw doubt upon this belief, and it is not recommended that treatment should be delayed in expectation of this taking place. Hormone treatment may aid regression, but treatment is usually a combination of electro-coagulation, external irradiation and surgery. The introduction of cryosurgery has made the management of these tumours much less dangerous. Preliminary radiotherapy does much to reduce the degree of vascularity and also usually results in some diminution in the size of the tumour. Although the response may be slow, occasionally remarkable reduction in bulk is obtained. The surgical approach to the residual tumour is obtained by the transpalatal route, supplemented by a lateral rhinotomy if necessary. Induced hypotension has substantially simplified the difficulties and dangers of surgery which in the past has usually consisted of piecemeal electro-coagulation of the lesion. Cryosurgical destruction, however, is preferable and almost bloodless. It is important that in removal all fragments of tumour should be examined histologically. The histological appearance often varies greatly from one part of the lesion to another and sarcomatous change is sometimes present.

When the growth can be removed completely the outlook is good.

In a disease that formerly was always dangerous this improvement is due to modern methods of treatment.

MALIGNANT TUMOURS

The histological classification of tumours of this region still requires some clarification. One of the most logical systems is that of Eggston and Wolff and the following descriptions are based upon their work. Tumours can be referred to their tissues of origin.

1. Those which come from the outer or inner embryonic layer.
   e.g. Benign papillomata, mixed salivary tumours.
   Malignant epidermoid epitheliomata or glandular adenocarcinomata.
2. Those tumours which come from the middle or mesodermal layer.
   e.g. Benign osteomata, fibromata, chondromata, myomata.
   Malignant fibrosarcomata, lymphosarcomata, etc.
3. Embryologically undifferentiated tumours such as lympho-epitheliomata, transitional cell tumours and melanomata.
4. Teratomata including dermoid cysts.

The majority of tumours encountered in the nasopharynx are of epithelial origin and are anaplastic in character. Lympho-epitheliomata are also not uncommon, and it is in the differential diagnosis of these difficult types of tumour, particularly in their confusion with lymphosarcomata, that most of the variations in classification have arisen. Cancer of the nasopharynx is extremely common in the countries of south-east Asia. If seen in the early stages these tumours may appear as spreading sessile ulcers in the neighbourhood of the Eustachian tube. They have been seen in the choanal border and at times they may be more vegetative or fungating in character. Unfortunately attention is not attracted till overt signs elsewhere indicate that the tumour has spread within the cavity of the skull or to other structures outside the nasopharynx.

Symptoms. Almost a third of these patients show enlargement of the cervical nodes, usually bilateral and high up. A similar number have a nasal voice and epistaxis, possibly also with nasal obstruction. About 20 per cent first complain of deafness due to Eustachian tube involvement. The remainder notice fifth or sixth nerve symptoms or proptosis as the first indication of the disease. It should be noted that even in cases showing these advanced signs slight thickening or swelling of the mucous membrane may be the only local sign. Immobility or distortion of the soft palate may be caused by direct infiltration or by involvement of the muscles controlling its movement.

Treatment. Recurrence of disease is still common whatever treatment is used. External irradiation from a linear accelerator or cobalt source offers the best chance of relief. The field must include glandular areas in both sides of the neck. Infusion of cytotoxic drugs into both external carotid arteries can produce dramatic and prolonged remission. Its use in combination with radiotherapy is still being assessed.

THE OROPHARYNX

BENIGN TUMOURS

Angiomata and myomata are described, but the only benign tumours seen with any frequency are papillomata. Two or three such warty and often pedunculated growths may be seen on the soft palate or anterior pillars. They are usually small and discovered accidentally. They generally produce no symptoms until the patient happens to notice their presence. They show no tendency towards malignant degeneration and are readily snipped off with scissors. Myomata can be dissected out.

Pleomorphic salivary adenomas ('Mixed Salivary Tumours') are best regarded as lesions of borderline malignancy and accordingly are considered in the next section.

MALIGNANT TUMOURS

The classification already detailed (p. 136) applies here also. Carcinomata are the most frequent type and they are more differentiated than in the nasopharynx, being usually squamous epitheliomata. The tumour not infrequently arises from the pillars of the fauces. Commencing at the junction of the anterior pillar and the tongue it may spread up the pillar, back on to the tonsil, or into the substance of the tongue. It may also spread forwards along the alveolus. The tumour sometimes takes origin on the edge of the tongue, far back, and spreads on to the lateral wall. The lower part of the pharynx and the base of the tongue are also occasionally the site of the primary growth, and masses there may involve the valleculae and the epiglottis, and spread to various parts of the larynx.

Symptoms. The symptoms occasioned by these growths are often slight until the growth has made considerable progress. Then slight difficulty in swallowing, or some swelling, or excess of secretion and irritation in the tongue, sends the patient to the doctor or specialist for advice. In the lower part of the pharynx difficulty in swallowing, or a change in the voice, is often the first sign of disease. There may be pain, and it is frequently referred to the ear; and glandular enlargement is a sign which is of serious significance from the point of view of prognosis. Frequently the patient first seeks advice because of a swelling in the side of the neck, which on examination is found to be a hard, possibly fixed, gland a little below the angle of the jaw. When this gland is found in an elderly man, unilateral, and without apparent cause for origin, the most careful search must be made of the pharynx and laryngo-pharynx by palpation as well as by inspection for the possibility of primary focus. The significance of the glands is that the disease has almost certainly extended beyond the limits of the pharyngeal wall, and the results obtained from treatment in these cases with glandular involvement are less successful than in cases in which the growth is purely local.

Local appearances. These vary with the site and type of the lesion. There is usually ulceration and destruction of tissue, and at the same time there is formation of a reddish granular fungating tissue which may form a mass, or, on the other hand, may creep over the surface of the membrane in a thin sheet. On touching the tissue it bleeds readily, and is frequently exceedingly tender to touch. In advanced cases there may be destruction of all the landmarks of the part affected. The tonsil may be lost in the fungating mass of new growth. The soft palate and uvula may be destroyed and the tongue so firmly fixed by infiltrating growth that adequate examination is rendered difficult.

Histological examination is an essential step in diagnosis, the Wassermann reaction and a chest X-ray must also be done routinely.

Squamous-cell carcinomata occur in various grades of differentiation and are the most frequent tumour of the oropharynx; lympho-epithelioma is not uncommon.

Sarcomata are of various types and occur especially in the tonsil. Unilateral enlargement of a tonsil in a patient, irrespective of age, should always arouse suspicion. Lympho-sarcoma is the commonest, but reticulo- and embryonic sarcomata are seen occasionally in this region.

Mixed salivary tumours occur in the palate and around the tonsil. In the latter situation the swelling is sometimes mistaken for a quinsy, but there is no trismus and no evidence of acute inflammation. Although sometimes classed as benign these tumours differ only in their degree of malignancy. Some may appear histologically benign but they have a great tendency to recur and cause difficult problems in management. (See also p. 183).

Treatment of malignant tumours of the pharynx

These may be treated by surgery, by surgery plus radiation or by radiation alone. Results from surgery alone are, however, extremely disappointing, especially in advanced cases. Surgery followed or preceded by radiation has given fair results in the hands of some operators. The most promising form of treatment for small isolated growths is external irradiation. For larger lesions many surgeons prefer to radiate first and then operate. Others excise first and irradiate any possible extension afterwards. Of these two methods the former is probably the more popular. The type of radiation treatment will depend upon the equipment available, but cobalt or super-voltage irradiation is preferred.

Recent developments in chemotherapy may assist in treatment of these forms of tumour, but more experience is needed in their use.

Interstitial irradiation is useful for small recurrences. Patients with large fungating tumours or recurrences can be greatly helped by cryosurgery.

LEUKOPLAKIA

This is a chronic thickening of the epithelium which appears as whitish patches on any part of the mucous membrane of mouth or tongue. Its aetiology is obscure, but sometimes it is considered to be due to irritation, by smoking, excessive drinking, syphilis or dental sepsis. It may be a pre-cancerous condition and therefore must be kept under regular supervision.

LEUKAEMIA

Leukaemia and other diseases of the reticulo-endothelial system occasionally present as a pharyngeal disorder. In ulcerative or hypertrophic conditions of the pharynx therefore it is often wise to examine the blood film and white cell count.

CYSTS

Thyroid remnants and thyro-glossal cysts occasionally occur in the pharynx. Mucous retention cysts are not unusual, especially in the vallecula. Retention cysts in the tonsil are common and sometimes cause unnecessary alarm to a patient who happens to notice one.

FOREIGN BODIES IN THE PHARYNX

These are most commonly fish bones, but a large number of articles, including artificial dentures, may lodge in the pharynx.

Fish bones lodge in the tonsil, the lingual tonsil or the tongue. In locating a foreign body, the patient's sensations are sometimes a valuable guide. If the patient points to the side of the throat to localize the discomfort, then the foreign body is, or has been, in the pharynx. If, on the other hand, the patient points to the mid-line, then the foreign body is probably below the level of the pharynx and is beyond the reach of spatula and forceps.

One of the most common sites of lodgment being in the base of the tongue, the use of a spatula may help to conceal a bone from the observer. In these circumstances it may be more easily identified with the mirror. To aid the removal of foreign bodies the use of a cocaine spray (10 per cent) is frequently of assistance.

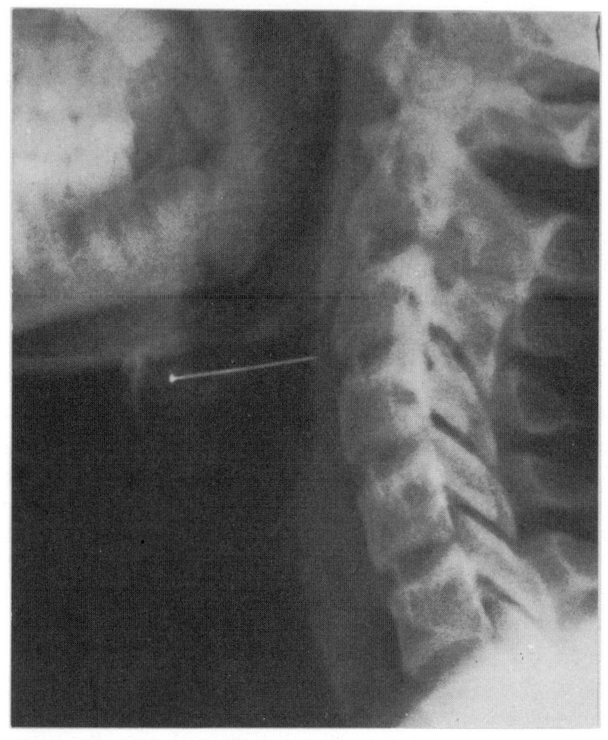

Fig. 41. Foreign body in lower part of the pharynx. A great variety occurs. All foreign bodies in the pharynx and oesophagus are potentially dangerous, especially bones.

NEUROLOGICAL DISORDERS – SENSORY

Anaesthesia

This is most frequently seen as a symptom of bulbar paralysis, or thrombosis of vessels in the posterior fossa, or diphtheria. It may be due also to hysteria. It is unilateral or bilateral, and may be accompanied by laryngeal paralysis.

Diagnosis is made by touching the parts with a probe, when the usual reflex will be found to be absent.

Hyperaesthesia

This is comparatively common, and it is difficult to say when it becomes abnormal. It may be due to pharyngeal irritation by alcohol, etc.

Paraesthesia

The sensation as of a small foreign body in the pharynx is common amongst females, and frequently there will be found some point of irritation such as an inflamed lymphoid nodule. Treatment of this, combined with a tranquillizer and reassurance, often produces relief.

Glossopharyngeal neuralgia

This is a rare condition similar to that in the trigeminal nerve in which the trigger point is usually around the anterior pillar of the tonsil. It is treated by section of the glossopharyngeal nerve external to the tonsil.

MOTOR

Paralysis

Paralysis of the soft palate, especially in young patients, should give rise to suspicion of poliomyelitis. It may also be a sequel to diphtheria. Various syndromes arise from paralysis of the lower four cranial nerves, from lesions in the brain stem, posterior fossa, jugular foramen and upper part of the neck. Bulbar palsy, vascular lesions such as posterior inferior cerebellar artery thrombosis, multiple sclerosis and tumours are possible causes.

Examination in bilateral paralysis of the palate shows it to be immobile in speech and not to retract on touching with a probe. In unilateral palsy the palate rises up to the healthy side (curtain movement). Associated paralysis of the tongue, pharynx and larynx must always be looked for.

Treatment depends on the cause. Except in certain cases due to neuritis the outlook is not good and severe difficulties in feeding may occur if food tends to enter the airway. Tube feeding may be necessary to maintain nutrition, protection being provided for the respiratory tree by means of a tracheostomy and use of a cuffed tube.

Very occasionally when a slowly progressive neurological disorder is going to lead to the patient's premature death from starvation and repeated aspiration pneumonia, division of the crico-pharyngeal sphincter or laryngectomy may provide great relief from the patient's difficulties.

Spasm

Tonic spasm is most frequently functional but is encountered in tetanus and rabies.

Clonic spasm, sometimes called *pharyngeal nystagmus*, consists of rhythmical movement of the soft palate and pharyngeal wall. It indicates a central nervous lesion.

THE HYPOPHARYNX (LARYNGOPHARYNX)

Disorders of this region generally require endoscopic means for diagnosis and therefore are discussed in Chapter 26.

SECTION IV THE LARYNX

18. Anatomy

The larynx consists of a cartilaginous framework which is bound together by ligaments and covered with muscle and mucous membrane. The cartilages of the larynx are usually spoken of as 'paired' and 'unpaired' cartilages.

The unpaired cartilages. The *epiglottis* is a leaf-shaped piece of cartilage which is attached both to the base of the tongue and to the upper part of the thyroid cartilage. The *thyroid cartilage* (the largest cartilage of the larynx) is that which makes the prominence upon the front of the neck known as 'Adam's apple'. It consists of two wings or alae which are joined together in the mid-line anteriorly and extend backwards. In the front, at the junction of the alae, is a notch which is called the 'thyroid notch'. On the posterior edge of the alae, above and below, there are two processes – superior and inferior. Below the thyroid cartilage, and articulating with it posteriorly, is the *cricoid cartilage*. In front it is joined to the thyroid cartilage by the crico-thyroid membrane. The cricoid cartilage is a closed ring of cartilage in the form of a signet ring, of which the signet or large portion of the cartilage is the posterior part.

The paired cartilages. First and most important are the *arytenoid cartilages.* These are pyramidal-shaped bodies which are placed upon and articulate with the posterior part of the cricoid cartilage, and which play an important part in the movement of the vocal cords. They consist of solid pieces of cartilage in the shape of a three-sided pyramid. At the base are two processes, the one anterior and the other lateral.

The anterior process is spoken of as the *vocal process*; the lateral process as the *muscular process.* To the vocal process, in front, are attached the vocal cords, while the muscular processes form the main attachment for those muscles activating the vocal cords in phonation and respiration.

On the top of the arytenoids are found two small cartilages called the cartilages of *Santorini*; while two other small cartilages – the cartilages of *Wrisberg* – are found in the fold of membrane, the ary-epiglottic fold, which connects the arytenoid with the base of the epiglottis and forms the upper edge of the laryngeal space (Fig. 42).

THE LARYNX FROM ABOVE

Looking down upon the larynx, the epiglottis is seen first of all. In front of the epiglottis and attached to the base of the tongue, a ridge of

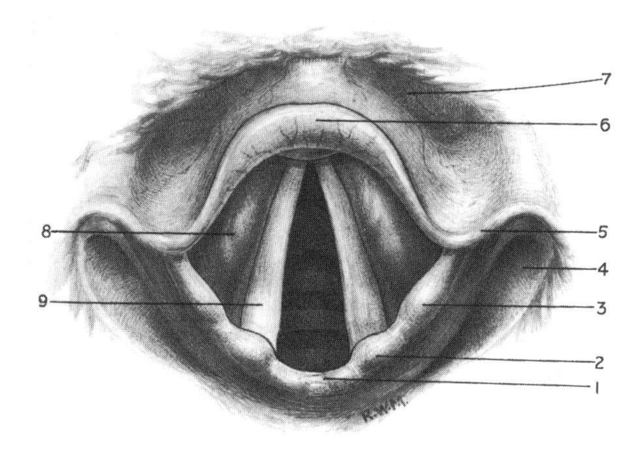

Fig. 42. View of larynx from above, showing: (1) interarytenoid region; (2) arytenoid cartilage; (3) ary-epiglottic fold; (4) pyriform sinus;(5) pharyngo-epiglottic fold; (6) epiglottis; (7) rallecula; (8) false cords; (9) true cords.

mucous membrane can be seen stretching to the anterior wall. This is known as the *glosso-epiglottic* ligament, and on each side of it is a hollow which is called the *vallecula*. The posterior border of this hollow is another fold called the *pharyngo-epiglottic* ligament. This separates the vallecula from the pyriform sinus. The pyriform sinus is the lowest part of the laryngo-pharynx, and is formed by the division of that part of the laryngo-pharynx into two by the body of the larynx. From the base of the epiglottis two folds curve posteriorly. The *ary-epiglottic* folds curve round until the arytenoid cartilages are reached, and behind the arytenoid cartilages the posterior walls dips to the inter-arytenoid space.

INTERIOR OF THE LARYNX

In the interior of the larynx two folds of mucous membrane are stretched from front to back. They are rounded and pink in colour, and are called the false cords or *ventricular* folds. Inferior to them is an opening into the space known as the Sinus of Morgagni or *laryngeal ventricle*. This space runs upwards and outwards behind the ala of the thyroid and ends in a small saccule or appendix. The lower lip of the ventricle is formed by a muscular bundle which is the true vocal cord. Seen from above, the cord looks narrow and white. It looks like a band of white fibrous tissue stretching from front to back, but in reality all that is seen is the upper edge of a triangular bundle of muscular tissue, of which the outer edge is a thin condensation of fibrous tissue.

The *true cords* are attached anteriorly in the mid-line to the posterior surface of the thyroid cartilage. Posteriorly they are attached to the body of the arytenoid cartilages and to the vocal process. Between the vocal cords and the inter-arytenoid space there is frequently thickening of the mucous membrane. Below the vocal cord is the *subglottic space*, which is the narrowest part of the larynx. The subglottic region lies behind the cricothyroid membrane, so that a tracheotomy tube introduced by the stab method of laryngotomy will lie in the subglottic space. The fact that this part of the larynx is narrow must be kept in mind, and the tube should be removed at the earliest opportunity, or transferred to some other more suitable part of the trachea.

MUSCLES OF THE LARYNX

There are two chief muscle groups of the larynx – the adductor and the abductor.

The crico-thyroid muscle. This is the chief tensor of the cords. This muscle is attached to the lower edge of the thyroid cartilage and to the upper part of the cricoid cartilage. Its function is to increase the tension of the cords by rocking the cricoid cartilage backwards, or, alternatively, pulling down the thyroid cartilage. This increases the length of the vocal cords, and in so doing increases their tension.

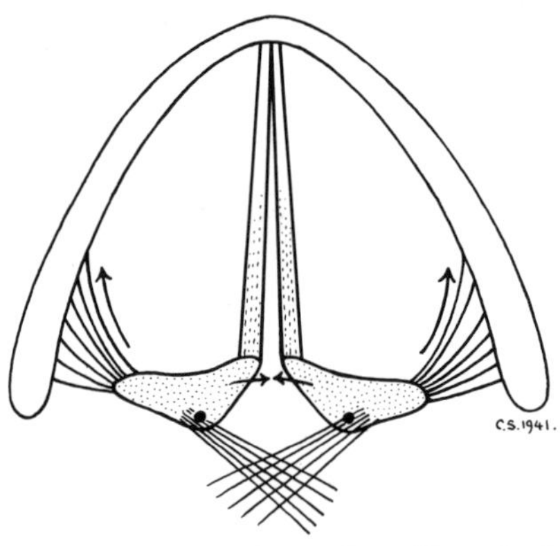

Fig. 43. Adduction of vocal cords, showing action of lateral crico-arytenoid and the transverse arytenoid muscles.

The thyro-arytenoid muscle. This muscle is attached anteriorly in the mid-line to the thyroid cartilage. It runs backwards as a muscular bundle to be attached into the vocal process and the body of the arytenoid cartilage. Its medial edge is sometimes separated into another muscle – the *musculus vocalis*. The chief function of this muscle is preservation of uniform tension of the vocal cord.

The lateral crico-arytenoid. This muscle is attached to the lateral side of the body of the cricoid cartilage and to the arytenoid cartilage, and by pulling on the muscular process it rotates the vocal process inwards, bringing the cords into apposition in the part anterior to the vocal process.

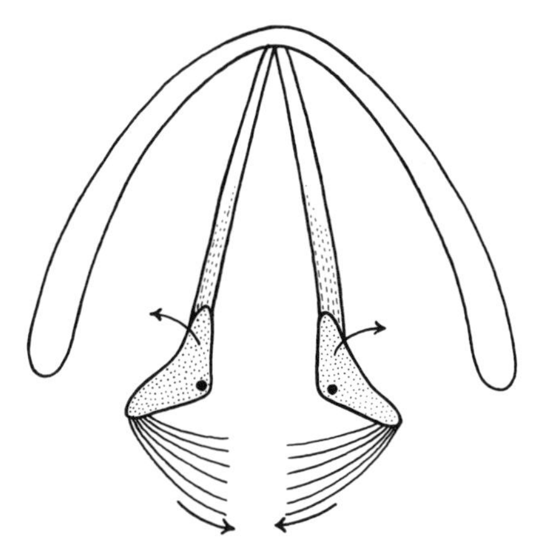

Fig. 44. Abduction of vocal cords, showing action of the posterior cricoarytenoid muscle.

The transverse arytenoid muscle. The posterior chink between the vocal cords is eliminated by the action of the *transversus muscle*, which is attached to the bodies of both arytenoids and draws the arytenoid cartilages together (Fig. 43).

The posterior crico-arytenoid. *The Abductor Group* contains one muscle – the *posterior crico-arytenoid* – which is attached to the mid-line of the posterior part of the body of the cricoid cartilage. It runs outwards and upwards to be inserted into the posterior part of the muscular process of the arytenoid. By pulling on this process it rotates the vocal process outwards, thus separating the vocal cords.

NERVE SUPPLY OF THE LARYNX

The nerve supply is from two nerves only, the recurrent laryngeal nerve and the superior laryngeal nerve.

The motor supply. The motor nerve supply with the exception of the nerve supply to the crico-thyroid muscle is from the *recurrent laryngeal* nerve.

The *left recurrent* laryngeal nerve leaves the vagus nerve at the level of the aortic arch and after working round the arch passes through the mediastinum, between the trachea and the oesophagus, to reach the neck.

Here it travels beneath the common carotid artery, the inferior thyroid artery and the thyroid gland successively, and then it enters the larynx beneath the lower edge of the inferior constrictor muscle.

On the *right* side the course differs in the lower part, the origin of the nerve being at the level of the sub-clavian artery below which it passes to enter the neck.

As the nerves enter the larynx they are called the *inferior laryngeal nerves*.

The crico-thyroid muscle takes its motor supply from the external branch of the superior laryngeal nerve.

Sensory supply. The sensory supply is chiefly by the *superior laryngeal* nerve. The superior laryngeal nerve takes origin from the ganglion nodosum of the vagus nerve. From this it runs down behind the great vessels of the neck until it reaches the superior border of the inferior constrictor muscle where it divides into *internal* and *external* branches.

The *external branch* is the nerve already referred to which supplies the crico-thyroid muscle. The *internal branch* supplies sensation to the larynx, to the level of the vocal cords. Below that level sensation is supplied by the inferior laryngeal nerve.

Blood supply. The laryngeal branches of the superior and inferior laryngeal arteries supply the larynx from above and below. The crico-

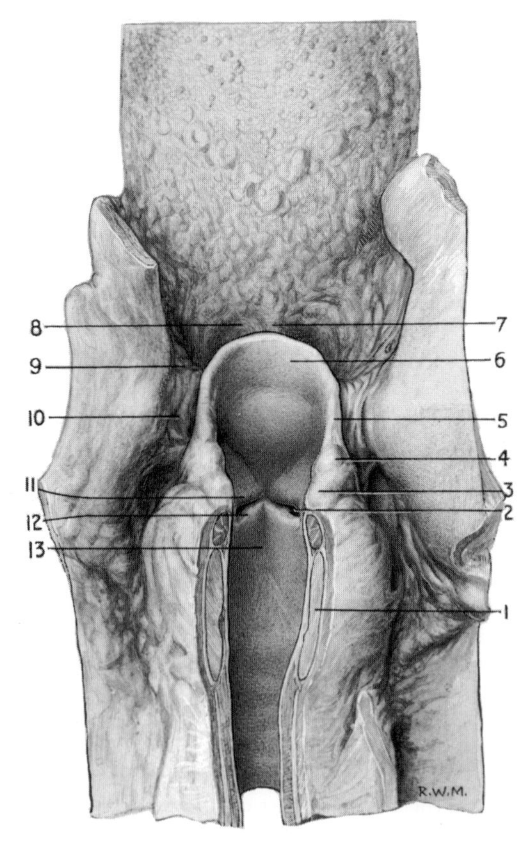

Fig. 45. Larynx viewed from behind, showing: (1) cricoid cartilage; (2) laryngeal ventricle; (3) arytenoid; (4) and (5) accessory cartilages in ary-epiglottic fold; (6) epiglottis; (7) glosso-epiglottic fold; (8) vallecula; (9) pharyngo-epiglottic fold; (10) pyriform sinus; (11) false cord; (12) true cord; (13) subglottic space.

thyroid artery sends a branch across the mid-line to anastomose with that of the opposite side.

Lymphatic system. The portion of the larynx above the vocal cords drains to the upper deep cervical nodes, and that below the cords through the crico-thyroid membrane to the pretracheal nodes and thence to the deep cervical chain. The vocal cords themselves are virtually without lymphatics.

Functions of the larynx. The functions of the larynx are respiration, phonation and fixation of the chest in severe muscular effort.

Development of the larynx. In the child the larynx is found to differ considerably from that of the adult. The epiglottis in the child is long and is frequently folded on itself to appear almost tubular. The upper orifice of the larynx appears to be elongated and the aryteno-epiglottic folds are relatively shortened. This form of larynx is encountered occasionally in adults, and renders adequate examination of the larynx extremely difficult.

19. Examination of the Larynx

Indirect laryngoscopy

Indirect laryngoscopy is a simple procedure within the capabilities of any well-trained practitioner prepared to give some time to its practice. Gentleness on the part of the examiner and confidence and relaxation on the part of the patient are essentials for success.

Good illumination is absolutely necessary, and for this a head lamp or head mirror may be used. Also there should be at hand, laryngeal mirrors, a spirit lamp and squares of cloth or gauze with which to control the tongue. The position of the patient and the examiner is important. The patient should sit upright with the head bent slightly forward, and the examiner sits in front of the patient or on the patient's left side, assuming the examiner to be right-handed.

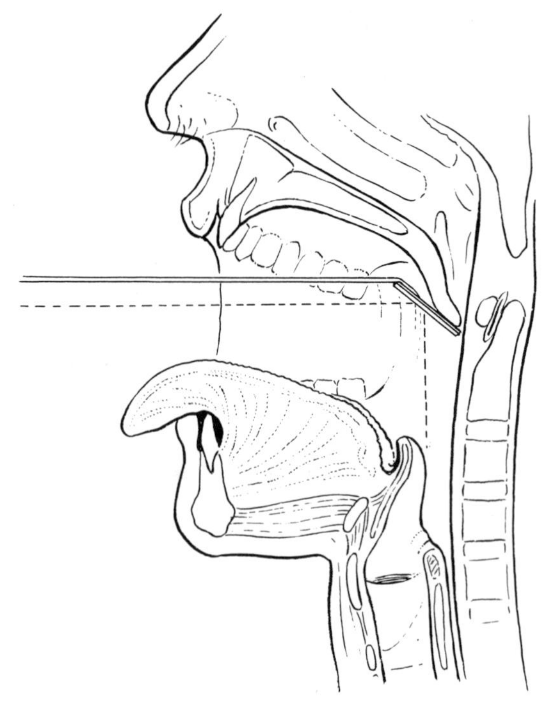

Fig. 46. Indirect laryngoscopy. Showing projection of light beam upon the larynx.

The patient is asked to put out the tongue, any dentures having been removed, and it is grasped with the tongue cloth or gauze as far back as is conveniently possible. The thumb may be above or below the tongue according to the preference of the examiner, but one finger should be able to raise the upper lip during the examination if necessary. The grip should be firm but gentle and the tongue should on no account be pinched but rather rolled over the finger below it as the superior surface is longer than the inferior. Care must be taken to protect the frenum from damage by the lower teeth (Fig. 47).

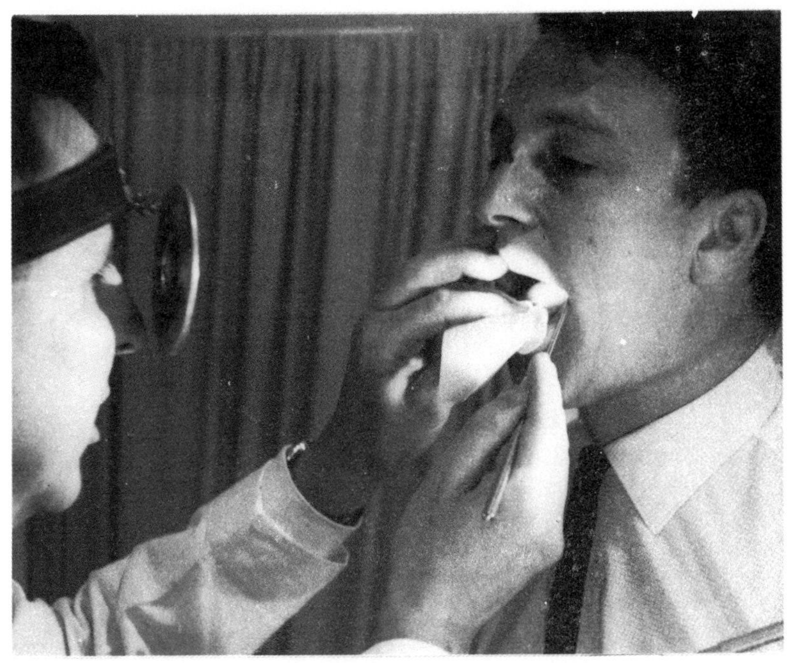

Fig. 47. Indirect laryngoscopy. Note that the image in the mirror is a reversed one.

A large size of laryngeal mirror is warmed, and after testing to ensure that it is not too hot, it is placed firmly but gently on the soft palate just above the base of the uvula. The light is then directed to the various parts of the laryngo-pharynx by tilting the mirror, but the mirror should not be moved from its place on the soft palate or the patient will probably 'gag' and close the throat. The patient, the while, is told to breathe easily and steadily, and it is better to make several short examinations than try to see everything during one attempt.

The same routine should be followed each time, as in all clinical examinations, since only in this way will the chance of missing important changes be minimized.

The first structure to come into view is the epiglottis, which usually overhangs the interior of the larynx. Then the valleculae are seen, the ary-epiglottic folds, and part of the pyriform sinuses. Each structure is examined in turn and note is made of any redness of the mucous membrane, swelling or oedema, any excess of secretions, ulceration or other abnormality.

The interior of the larynx is examined next. This may be impossible owing to the overhang of the epiglottis, but if the patient is asked to say 'ee' or 'eh' the epiglottis will rise and the anterior of the larynx will come into view.

The interior of the larynx

Having exposed the larynx it is possible to examine the structures within it.

The *ary-epiglottic folds* are first examined, and then the arytenoids themselves. They should be smooth and symmetrical, and of a healthy pink colour.

The *false cords* are next examined. They should appear equal, and should not overhang or conceal the true cords below. If they do they are abnormal, probably owing to disease. Their surface should be smooth, without ulceration or nodule formation. This observation is important, as some diseases may be discovered first in this region.

The *true cords* themselves may now be seen; they should be white in appearance. They should be smooth, glistening, with a slight degree of moisture, but there should be no appearance of secretion lying on the cords. Any irregularity of the edges, nodule formation, or anything suggesting ulceration is noted. In some cases glistening irregularities are seen and these are probably lumps of mucus. The patient gets rid of these by coughing, and then the examination is repeated. It may be difficult to see the anterior part of the larynx clearly, but if the patient is asked to say 'ee' this part is usually exposed adequately. The inter-arytenoid region is the last to be inspected. A certain amount of thickening may be regarded as normal, but any marked heaping or vegetation is of pathological significance.

In many instances the upper part of the trachea can be seen below the larynx, and the presence of blood on the posterior wall may be important where there is haemoptysis of uncertain origin.

The movement of the vocal cords

The final part of indirect laryngoscopy is the inspection of the movement of the larynx and the vocal cords. It is important to ascertain if the vocal cords are moving normally or if there is any fixation or paralysis, for interference with function may be the first sign of malignant disease in the area.

A knowledge of the normal movement of the vocal cords is essential before a reliable diagnosis can be made, and also of errors which can be caused by incorrect technique. It must be remembered that the image, being a 'mirror image', is reversed.

The first abnormality which may appear to the inexperienced examiner may be an inequality in the excursion of the cords, which, however, is more apparent than real. This is due to the tilting of the mirror, which gives a distorted view of the cords. The mirror, therefore, must be held so that the image is centralized and vertical as far as possible.

The first position examined is that of quiet respiration. In this the cords should lie moderately separated, and equidistant from the mid-line. On inspiration they move outwards a small distance, and on expiration they move in again, but do not reach the mid-line. On forced inspiration the outward excursion is much greater, the cords moving out till they are close to the sides of the larynx, a position which is seen in cases suffering from extreme lack of oxygen. Phonation brings the cords together, though a slight chink can still be seen, and the cords vibrate rapidly or more slowly according to the note produced.

In the act of coughing the cords come closely into apposition before the air is expelled.

(For abnormalities of movement see Paralysis of Larynx, p. 175.)

Difficulties in examination

Nervousness or irritability of the pharynx may prevent even the most skilled examiner making a proper inspection, and in such cases a local anaesthetic, used as a spray or a lozenge, may help. Where symptoms render an exact diagnosis essential the surgeon should examine the larynx by the direct method. There are, however, disadvantages in this, for where laryngeal movement is involved the laryngoscope may cause abnormalities by its introduction. Also if a general anaesthetic is being used the patient cannot co-operate in phonation or coughing.

Children are more likely to tax the patience and ability of the examiner than adults and more frequently require a general anaesthetic.

Quality of the voice

'Mirror examination' of the larynx is often difficult even to the experienced laryngologist. Much can be deduced from listening to the voice and it may be possible to differentiate paralysis of the vocal cord from a lesion of the cord itself by the difference in quality of the voice. Both types of change cause what is often described by the patient as 'hoarseness'.

In some patients the voice is of poor volume, breathy, but not rough. Owing to excessive air-wastage much energy goes into the production of comparatively little sound. Such patients may be found to have a paralysis.

In other patients the voice is truly rough in quality and its roughness often corresponds to the degree of irregularity of the vocal cord on which the lesion is situated. It is in these instances that the voice may properly be described as hoarse.

20. Acute Diseases of the Larynx

ACUTE LARYNGITIS

Aetiology. Acute laryngitis may occur as an isolated disease or it may form part of a general reaction in the upper air passages.

In the former case sudden exposure, excess of tobacco or alcohol, or even over-use of the voice may be the cause. When due to infection in the air passages elsewhere, it forms part of a general inflammation, but in itself is very easily precipitated by straining the voice in presence of a mild catarrh. This form is comparatively common amongst actors, singers and others who use their voices in a professional capacity.

Symptoms. Laryngitis may cause symptoms varying from very slight hoarseness to complete loss of voice, with pain and general disturbance. The ordinary acute attack is usually accompanied by pain in the throat. The patient frequently complains of a feeling of constriction around the region of the thyroid cartilage, and this is sometimes described as a string tied round the throat. There is pain on swallowing and on speaking. The voice may be completely lost, but normally a husky tone can be obtained. Cough from the irritative condition is frequently present and may be very painful. There is a febrile reaction owing to the general infection, and the patient may be confined to bed feeling extremely ill. The temperature as a rule is not high, but there may be some rise of temperature from the coryza which is responsible for the laryngitis.

Appearances. On examination of the larynx the epiglottis will be seen to be acutely inflamed. There is reddening of the tip of the epiglottis and there may be some slight oedema. The arytenoids are reddened and also show some swelling. Oedema and flushing of the false cords may be one of the most marked features of the infection. The false cords may be so swollen that they conceal the true cords beneath. The true cords will appear watery. They are thickened and rounded; their colour may vary from a slight pink to a bright red, the reddening being most marked at first at the part of the cord farthest from the free edge. Movement of the cord may be restricted owing to the swelling of the surrounding parts, but the movement is equal and there is no paralysis. The whole larynx shows the presence of hypersecretion, and the vocal cords may be covered with mucus.

Treatment. During the acute stage the most important principles of treatment are rest of the voice and an even atmospheric temperature of about 65 to 70° F (20° C). This is most easily achieved by putting the patient to bed. It must be noted that a warm atmosphere does not imply lack of ventilation. This is important as it is necessary to ensure a fairly moist atmosphere. In circumstances in which central heating or electric fires are used, one steaming kettle is sufficient to humidify a small room.

Applications to the larynx must be soothing in character. Steam inhalations containing Friar's Balsam are helpful. Hot gargles are useful to treat the accompanying pharyngitis as they assist the flow of mucus which lubricates the larynx and pharynx.

Direct application to the larynx by sprays are sometimes suggested, but considerable skill is required, and the effects while comforting are transitory.

Where pain is severe hot fomentations to the throat, or applications of heat in other forms, give great relief. A sedative can be given for the painful irritating cough.

ACUTE EPIGLOTTITIS

This disease of infancy is frequently described as part of acute laryngo-tracheo bronchitis, but there are so many important differences that it is advisable to look upon them as separate diseases. Epiglottitis is less common than laryngo-tracheo bronchitis but is more fulminating and dangerous.

Symptoms. There may be little warning of the onset: a slight sore throat or upper respiratory infection is common but there is little to indicate the commencement of a dangerous disease. Difficulty in swallowing, one of the main symptoms, occurs early. A change in the cry or voice is characteristic and resembles that caused by a foreign body in the throat. Inspiratory stridor develops rapidly and may terminate in sudden fatal obstruction. It must be emphasized that the duration of symptoms may be only a few hours, so that speed in diagnosis and treatment is essential.

Clinical signs. Apart from a slight pharyngeal inflammation the chief change is the swelling of the epiglottis. This is caused by oedema of the loose tissues on the upper surface, which may later spread to involve the supra-glottic region more widely.

Diagnosis. Other causes of stridor and difficulty in swallowing such as foreign body, diphtheria and congenital malformation must be excluded. Retro-pharyngeal abscess can cause dysphagia and respiratory obstruction, but a lateral X-ray of the neck will eliminate this as a cause. Direct examination of the larynx is essential for diagnosis, but as it may precipitate complete obstruction it should be carried out only when facilities for immediate tracheostomy or intubation are at hand.

Treatment. Whenever possible the patient should be treated in hospital. Tracheostomy or intubation is very often necessary and the choice of these depends upon the particular surgical and nursing skills available. Unless an experienced nursing team is in charge tracheostomy is probably preferable, but both should be regarded as elective procedures rather than measures taken in an emergency. Throughout the illness the child should be nursed in a tent with a high level of humidity. Ampicillin is the antibiotic of choice because of the frequency of *haemophilus influenzae*. The place of oxygen and of steroids in treatment is still undecided, but there is agreement that anoxia is an indication for tracheostomy or intubation and not merely for the administration of oxygen. If dysphagia and pyrexia have caused dehydration intravenous fluids may be needed, and this route can then be used for chemotherapy.

ACUTE LARYNGO-TRACHEO BRONCHITIS

This acute and serious disease is encountered in young children, rarely in adults. The organism most commonly isolated is *haemophilus influenzae*, Type b, but as it is difficult to identify the incidence is uncertain. The disease is diffuse in nature and the course may be rapid, although it is less fulminating than epiglottitis. As deaths are not infrequent it must be regarded very seriously.

Symptoms. There is frequently a preceding nasal or pharyngeal infection, but the onset of the illness coincides with a sharp rise of temperature and pulse rate and a rapidly increasing toxaemia. There is marked inspiratory stridor which soon becomes severe.

Clinical signs. The chief cause of stridor and obstruction in this disease is subglottic oedema of the mucous membrane. The inflammation frequently spreads throughout the bronchial system. This is the main difference between this infection and epiglottitis, in which the oedema is supra-glottic. Sticky secretions form crusts which may be a serious case of obstruction and which are difficult to remove.

Treatment. In less severe infections relief of symptoms may be obtained by the use of chemotherapy and by nursing the child in a tent with a high degree of humidity, but if improvement does not occur quickly and if signs of increasing anoxia or respiratory obstruction develop, then early tracheostomy or intubation is essential. These measures are not to be regarded as emergency procedures. Tracheostomy is usually preferable to intubation because it not only avoids trauma to the inflamed subglottic area, but it allows adequate tracheo-bronchial toilet. Indeed, the repeated removal of the tracheo-bronchial crusts by means of a fine suction catheter inserted through the tracheostomy and employing a sterile technique, is an essential part of treatment of the disease.

To keep the secretions loose and prevent the formation of crusts humidification is vital.

As with epiglottitis, ampicillin is the antibiotic of choice, but chloromycetin can be used as an alternative, depending on the bacteriological reports. The value of oxygen and steroids remains unproven. If dehydration occurs, intravenous fluids should be given and this will provide a vehicle for the antibiotics without disturbance to the child.

ACUTE MEMBRANOUS LARYNGITIS

This disorder occurs in both children and adults and can be differentiated bacteriologically from diphtheria. It may commence in the larynx or spread from a pharyngeal infection. The onset may be insidious but leads to increasing oedema of the larynx with obstructed breathing and severe constitutional symptoms.

Diagnosis. Pharyngeal infection may be manifest. In the larynx a thin greyish yellow membrane spreads over the arytenoids and interior of the larynx. Oedema can develop rapidly. Dysphagia is often present and leads to dehydration.

Treatment is on the same lines as in laryngo-tracheo bronchitis.

LARYNGEAL DIPHTHERIA

This disease is encountered most frequently in children. It is not easy to diagnose, and in every case of croup it must be suspected as a possible cause.

Symptoms. The early symptoms are hoarseness and cough, then stridor with spasm, which finally leads to complete obstruction of the larynx. An important point in the symptoms is the progressive character of the stridor.

As it rarely occurs primarily in the larynx the problem of diagnosis is that of the pharyngeal condition (p. 122).

Treatment. This consists in the adoption of general measures for diphtheria, including the administration of anti-toxins. Removal of the membrane is advised if possible. One of the most useful methods of doing this is by means of suction. Intubation can be considered if the necessary instruments are available. If these means of treatment are not available, tracheostomy will have to be carried out.

ACUTE OEDEMA OF THE LARYNX

This may be the result of trauma, especially in children; it may result from the inhalation of irritants or drinking hot fluids. It may be infective in origin or it may be due to some form of sensitivity, and a degree of oedema accompanies most acute infections of the larynx and acute disease in surrounding structures.

Treatment. In the early stages of oedema steam inhalations are useful and fomentations to the neck are comforting in cases of inflammatory disease. Where angioneurotic oedema or some form of sensitivity is the cause, antihistamines or adrenalin should be tried. To gain time it will be found of use at times to spray the larynx with cocaine solution, 5 per cent, containing adrenalin. This relieves the spasm which may be present and gives the patient comfort.

PERICHONDRITIS

In the majority of cases this disorder is the result of diseases such as syphilis, tuberculosis or malignancy within the larynx. It is also seen as a complication of radiotherapy.

The condition manifests itself by pain, swelling and tenderness over the affected cartilage; swallowing and talking may also be painful. Laryngeal oedema sometimes causes danger of obstruction.

Treatment consists of intensive chemotherapy, and aspiration of any abscesses. If the airway is in danger, tracheostomy is necessary. If necrosis of the larynx is extensive, laryngectomy may afford the best chance of survival.

INJURIES OF THE LARYNX

Open injuries result from cut-throat wounds and also from glass cuts in traffic accidents. Occasionally the larynx or nearby trachea may be almost transected, but such injuries are generally rapidly fatal from aspiration of blood before aid can be given. In lesser injuries the great danger is again aspiration and the nature of the injury is usually obvious. A cuffed endotracheal tube must be passed urgently, and in a wound of any size this can be done through the wound itself into the opened airway. Bleeding is controlled, and when the patient is sufficiently resuscitated a tracheostomy is established, and injury repaired according to individual circumstances.

Closed injuries result from a kick or blow, and again may result from traffic accidents. Fracture of the cartilages and tearing of the mucosa with haematoma formation and swelling occur.

The symptoms are pain on speaking, haemoptysis and stridor if much swelling is present. Laryngoscopy will reveal ballooning of the mucosa and there may be extravasated blood.

Tracheostomy is indicated if stridor is present. In case of severe injury with fracture and dislocation of cartilage, or mucosal damage with bleeding, repair through laryngo-fissure is urgent. A stent mould should be retained for several weeks to prevent stenosis. In lesser injuries observation is necessary, but no active interference should be contemplated unless symptoms demand it.

TRACHEOSTOMY

Once looked upon as an emergency measure, this operation has now acquired such a wide range of therapeutic application that it must be considered from several aspects.

Indications. The *relief of upper respiratory* obstruction remains an important reason for tracheostomy. Any condition or disease, oedema or obstruction by disease such as carcinoma, may demand tracheostomy.

Drainage of the lung. This is an important part of treatment where secretions are retained in the trachea and bronchi, particularly when the effort of clearing the secretions is exhausting the patient. Suction through a tracheostomy opening can be life saving.

Protection of the lung. In cases of neurological disorder safety of the lung can be assured when cough reflexes are inhibited, either from muscular paralysis or absence of sensation. A cuffed tracheostomy tube is the patient's best protection under these circumstances.

Comatose states, as from head injury or poisoning, will frequently benefit from tracheostomy which can ensure lung drainage and adequate ventilation.

Wounds and accidents involving the mouth or pharynx.

Assisted respiration can be carried out most conveniently through a cuffed tracheostomy tube connected to a mechanical respirator.

The lung can be safeguarded from inhalation of blood and secretion by tracheostomy with a cuffed tube.

Signs of obstruction. The most valuable of all signs, in all probability, is the reaction of the circulation to the added work thrown upon it by the oxygen deficiency. As long as the pulse remains steady and fairly low, there is little danger of immediate trouble. If a point should be selected which is necessarily arbitrary, it may be said that when, in the absence of other disease, the pulse rate in the average adult rises above 100 per minute, the patient is entering the danger zone. Up to that point the patient's colour is of comparatively little importance, for if the pulse remains steady the patient's heart is coping adequately with the obstruction. When the pulse rate rises the lack of oxygen is becoming acute and the circulation is beginning to fail.

Emergency measures. Although tracheostomy should be performed with adequate preparation and with sufficient time to do a satisfactory operation, more urgent measures may be necessary.

Intubation. This gives immediate relief and permits the surgeon to proceed to tracheostomy without haste. The instruments required are a laryngoscope and an anaesthetic tube preferably of small size. To save the patient unnecessary discomfort the patient's throat should be sprayed with 5 per cent cocaine solution containing adrenalin if time permits. If the necessary instruments are not available laryngotomy may be required.

Laryngotomy. In this procedure the larynx is opened through the crico-thyroid membrane. This may be done with a simple stab with a knife or a vertical incision is made over the membrane and, with the left forefinger marking the lower edge of the thyroid cartilage, the knife is passed horizontally immediately below the finger tip into the larynx.

The knife is twisted to obtain an airway and any convenient instrument or tube is used to keep the opening patent. At the earliest opportunity the tube should be moved to the standard tracheostomy position.

Operation of tracheostomy

The operation of tracheostomy is one which should, as far as possible, be performed with adequate preparation and sufficient time in hand to make a satisfactory operation. Two incisions are currently used for this operation: the transverse and the vertical. The first is more popular as an elective procedure, while the latter is more frequently used in an emergency when time is short.

After the skin has been incised and reflected, the steps of the operation are the same whichever approach is used. Whenever there is serious obstruction in the larynx the anaesthesia of choice is local anaesthesia, but as the majority of these operations are now interval procedures general anaesthesia is more usual, with an endo-tracheal tube in place. In extreme emergencies there may be no time for an anaesthetic of any kind. The local anaesthetic is injected in a rhomboidal form, commencing at the lower edge of the thyroid cartilage and infiltrating both sides of the neck simultaneously to a point about 2 inches on each side of the trachea. The lines of injection are made to meet again at the suprasternal notch. This form of injection leaves the structures through which the operation is to be performed in a normal condition, and does not produce the oedema which injection into the tissues immediately over the trachea will cause. The operation is thereby simplified. Deep injections are made on each side of the trachea towards the anterior border of the sternomastoid. After waiting for two or three minutes for the local infiltration to take effect the incision is made. If the midline vertical incision is chosen it should commence just above the level of the cricoid cartilage and extend downwards to the suprasternal notch. In the case of a transverse incision it should be at about the level of the second tracheal ring. It is a mistake to attempt a tracheostomy through an inadequate incision. The incision is quickly deepened through the subcutaneous tissues, and the pretracheal muscles are separated in the mid-line. As the muscles are retracted a soft red structure is brought into view overlying the trachea. This is the isthmus of the thyroid gland. To obtain free access it is wisest to divide the isthmus, as its division simplifies after-treatment. In order to free the isthmus, a small horizontal incision is made over the lower border of the cricoid cartilage. This will incise the pretracheal fascia, within the layers of which the thyroid gland is enclosed. An elevator can then be slipped down between the thyroid isthmus and the trachea, and the thyroid isthmus is divided between forceps. This leaves the trachea completely bare. The stumps of the isthmus are then ligatured with strong catgut. All forceps are removed and complete haemostasis

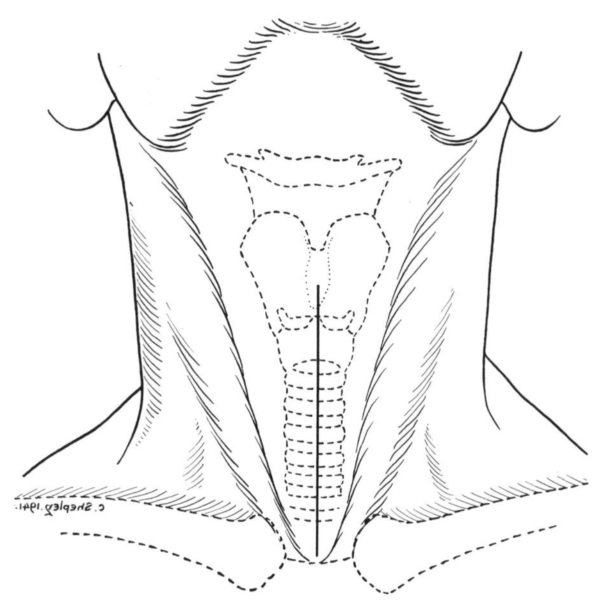

Fig. 48. Incision for emergency tracheostomy.

ensured. Five drops of 5 per cent cocaine solution are injected into the trachea, between two of the rings to minimize coughing. A strong-bladed knife is inserted under the third tracheal ring, the blade directed upwards, and a cut is made through the third and second rings of the trachea. The sharp hiss of the breath intake will then be heard and the trachea is opened. It may be accompanied by a spasm of coughing, but this quickly settles down. An oval hole is then made in the tracheal rings by cutting the edges of the incision. The object of this enlargement is chiefly to render reinsertion of the tracheal tube, if it becomes displaced, a matter of greater simplicity, also it prevents pressure damage

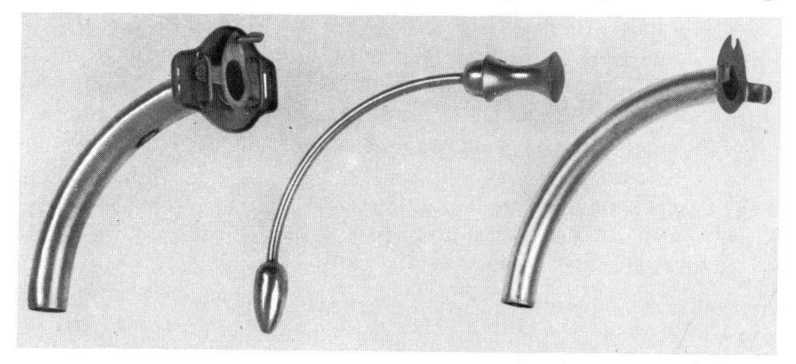

Fig. 49. Tracheostomy tube (Jackson's pattern). The outer tube, the introducer and the inner tube are shown.

to the cut tracheal rings. The tube is then inserted and the skin incision lightly sutured. Close stitching is to be avoided because it makes tube-changing difficult. A gauze square is used as a dressing between the skin and the flange of the tube, the tube is then fixed by tying its tapes behind the patient's neck. For safety and comfort it is important that the tapes should not be too loose.

After-treatment is important. These patients should be 'barrier nursed' in a warm, well-ventilated room. In certain climates arrangements may be necessary to secure adequate humidification. An oxygen tent may be required if cardio-respiratory disease is present. On returning to bed the patient should be well propped up and encouraged to move about freely in order to prevent stagnation of secretions and stasis at the base of the lung. In an afebrile case the patient should be got out of bed the day after operation; but where tracheostomy has been done to relieve the necessity of an acute inflammatory condition the movement of the patient will naturally be judged by the general condition.

The cleansing of the tracheostomy tube is of importance. The moist swab round the tube should be changed as soon as it becomes soiled. If there is excess of secretion, suction with a flexible catheter passed through the tracheal tube will give the patient great relief by removing the excess secretion, and it will save the effort of coughing. The inner tube should be removed for cleaning every four hours, and the whole tracheal tube should be removed from the neck every day and boiled.

The advantage of an adequate tracheostomy opening, properly made, will be appreciated, as, under such conditions, the whole management can be left in the hands of a competent nurse. A tray containing the following articles should always be kept beside the patient's bed:

(*a*) Efficient suction apparatus.
(*b*) A spare tracheostomy tube complete with inner tube, introducer and tapes.
(*c*) A tracheal dilator.
(*d*) A bundle of sterile pipe cleaners for cleaning the inner tube.
(*e*) A bowl containing a small quantity of bicarbonate of soda solution with which to wash the tube.
(*f*) A bowl containing sterile suction catheters (each to be used once only before re-sterilizing).
(*g*) A pack of disposable, sterile plastic gloves. These should be used for every treatment to the tracheostomy and are discarded after being used once only.

Detubation of the patient. After the tube has been worn for a considerable period it becomes a matter of great difficulty to teach the patient to do without it. For this a small cork should be cut and a progressive area of the tube should be filled in each day until finally the patient finds that he is able to breathe normally through the mouth. The tube can then be removed and the wound allowed to close. In cases in which the wound has been present for a long period considerable difficulty may be encountered in getting the hole to close again owing to the epithelization of the edges and the thin atrophic condition of the tissues surrounding the opening. This condition will necessitate some form of plastic operation.

21. Chronic Diseases of the Larynx

CHRONIC LARYNGITIS

This affection includes several clinical entities in which the mucosa undergoes change. It must be diagnosed only when malignancy, tuberculosis and syphilis have been specifically excluded.

Pathology. Repeated attacks of acute inflammation inadequately treated, and as a result incompletely resolved, are the most common cause and produce well-defined changes in the laryngeal mucous membrane. The early oedema and lymphatic infiltration if prolonged are followed by fibrosis and hyperplasia of the elements of the mucous membrane which result in permanent thickening which can vary in its distribution in different types of the disease.

Appearances. In the early stages the vocal cords are pink and have a slightly beefy appearance. Strings of sticky secretion may be seen stretching between the cords. Movement is usually normal but may be hampered later by localized accumulations of tissue. The false cords share these appearances and may be enlarged sufficiently to hide the true cords.

Symptoms. Hoarseness and at times loss of voice are the main features. The voice may be forced by conscious effort to be clear for a short time, but it quickly loses power. Irritation may produce cough and a raw sensation in the throat.

Treatment. Any predisposing cause must be sought and, if possible, removed. Careful and complete investigation of the nose, sinuses and chest should be undertaken and infection in these areas eliminated. Enquiry should be made into the working environment for sources of irritation such as dust, chemical fumes or even noise which demands continued strain of the voice. Complete cessation of the use of alcohol and tobacco must be insisted upon, as these may be irritating factors. Rest of the voice is one of the most important items in treatment, and in those who use the voice in a professional capacity it is essential. As in acute inflammation, this rest may have to include bodily rest as the vocal cords are constantly exercised in some forms of manual labour. Steam inhalations are of value, particularly in dry conditions where humidity is low, because they give comfort by encouraging secretions.

Spraying the larynx gives symptomatic relief, and alkaline solutions are helpful or aqueous solutions of ichthyol. Direct applications of colloidal silver and astringents have been advocated. Though their mode of action is not clear, practical experience has confirmed their value. A holiday in a warm climate can at times be extremely effective, and this mode of treatment is now within the reach of a very large section of the community. Speech therapy is an important part of treatment.

PACHYDERMIA

This term is usually applied to generalized thickening of the mucous membrane which has reached the stage of extensive fibrosis. Vocal cords, false cords and arytenoids share equally in the change which gives the surface a grey appearance which seems rough and dry, but which, on occasion, may show excess of moisture. Hoarseness is the outstanding symptom and treatment is as outlined above, but is often unsatisfactory.

LOCALIZED HYPERPLASIA

Thickening and heaping up of the mucous membrane may be found in areas subjected to trauma or movement. This may on occasion be sufficient to interfere with movement. Towards the posterior end of the vocal cords the thickening may cause what is known as a 'contact ulcer', where the thickened area on one cord impinges on that on the other, giving the appearance of an ulcer. In general local surgical removal is the best treatment, but a cautery point is useful at times.

VOCAL NODULES

These are a localized hypertrophy of the fibrous elements of the edge of the vocal cords. This is liable to occur at the point of most frequent impact of the vocal cords, namely at the junction of the anterior and middle thirds.

When seen the nodules are usually bilateral, one on each cord, and they are frequently caused by misuse of the voice or by bad voice production, especially in the presence of inflammation. The condition may be seen in singers and actors who attempt by extra effort to cover the deficiencies of a colleague.

Small white points can be seen to develop on the edges of the vocal cords. With rest of the voice these will respond satisfactorily and disappear completely, but when they persist in spite of voice rest, surgical removal is indicated. This is best achieved by using suspension laryngoscopy and micro-surgical techniques. Histological confirmation of the diagnosis is important. Speech therapy is advisable.

LEUCOPLAKIA

Treatment is rather unsatisfactory and biopsy can be misleading. Regular observation is nevertheless essential. Irritants such as smoking and spirits must be avoided; syphilis should be excluded. Sometimes stripping of the cord endoscopically is satisfactory; laryngo-fissure and removal of the cord have been advocated for those which infiltrate more deeply. The role of irradiation is controversial. It is capable of producing great improvement in the appearance of the larynx and quality of the voice, and may be the best treatment to provide in those patients found to have epithelial atypia on biopsy. These are the cases in which malignancy may develop. Some argue strongly against the use of irradiation on the grounds that such treatment should only be used in malignant conditions, and in any case is a treatment which should be kept in reserve for those patients who later are found to have developed early malignant change.

LARYNGITIS SICCA

In this condition there is drying of the laryngeal secretions with the formation of crusts within the larynx. It is doubtful if this should be included under the heading of chronic laryngitis, but owing to the irritation produced there is usually some low-grade inflammation.

It is invariably secondary to atrophic conditions in the nose or pharynx. The disease is sometimes found amongst cooks and laundry-maids, and there appears to be an occupational relationship. It sometimes complicates influenza.

POLYPUS OF THE LARYNX

As there appears in some cases to be an element of inflammation in the origin of laryngeal polypus, it is included under the heading of chronic laryngitis.

Polypi can occur in several different areas in the larynx but are most frequently seen attached to the vocal cords. A polypus appears as a smooth glistening body attached to one cord. It may have a pedicle or it may be sessile, and the size of a polypus can vary within wide limits. Occasionally on laryngoscopy nothing abnormal can be seen, but on telling the patient to cough the polypus is blown through the cords, and can be seen to be attached to the underside of the vocal cords. Sometimes a large polypoid mass is seen on the upper surface of one or both vocal cords, even, at times, obscuring them. This is tissue from the mouth of the laryngeal ventricle, which may constitute prolapse of the ventricle.

Diagnosis. In all such conditions the diagnosis from malignant disease must be made by histological examination.

Treatment. The polyp is removed by suspension-laryngoscopy using the operating microscope and very fine instruments. Damage to the vocal cords and other structures is avoided in this way. In the case of polypoid tissue coming from the ventricle complete removal by punch forceps may be difficult and a cautery point drawn along the edge of the ventricle may cause fibrosis and retraction of the tissue. Speech therapy is helpful.

TUBERCULOSIS OF THE LARYNX

Tuberculosis of the larynx is invariably secondary to tuberculosis of the lung. It remains a most serious complication of pulmonary tuberculosis, though now it is not necessarily fatal. The tendency is towards healing as the chest condition is controlled. The disease is still a problem in many under-privileged populations. As in the nose, tuberculosis lesions of varying activity are encountered. The disease may be rapid in its development and spread, and show the pathological characters of acute or subacute tuberculosis, or it may resemble the slower lupoid type.

The acute forms usually occur within the cavity of the larynx itself. They are associated with cavitation of the lung and other demonstrable signs of tuberculosis, while those forms occurring in the epiglottis and surrounding parts are more frequently associated with the lupoid or fibrotic type of disease.

Direct implantation is the most usual method of infection. This occurs either by infection from secretions lying in the larynx, or by implantation of bacilli in small abrasions of the mucous membrane. Infection may take place by lymphatic spread and by the blood stream.

Clinical appearances. *Early stage*. The usual sites of the disease are the posterior part of the larynx, the cords and the false cords. In the earliest stages the mucous membrane may be pale in colour but is more frequently injected owing to a degree of inflammation. This may be due to coughing and the passage of sputum. The inter-arytenoid region may be swollen and red, and this change may involve the inner side of one arytenoid and extend up the vocal cord.

Ulcerative stage. Fissuring in the inter-arytenoid region, with swelling and ulceration, gives the appearance of vegetations. Nodules or granulations may appear in the inner angle of the arytenoid and the base of the vocal cords, and may spread up the whole length of one or both cords. When nodules form they break down and form shallow ulcers, giving a whitish irregular edge to the cord which is called 'mouse nibbled'. The false cords become swollen and may conceal the true cords.

The arytenoids become enlarged and pale and may be ulcerated. The epiglottis shows thickening and reddening which may become so massive (the so-called 'turban shape') that the interior of the larynx is concealed. This swelling may cause some embarrassment to breathing, but it is rarely sufficiently severe to give rise to anxiety. Tracheostomy is unsatisfactory in tuberculosis of the larynx.

Other areas. Supraglottic disease is less common. It may consist of small nodules on the epiglottis, on the pharyngo-epiglottic fold or in the vallecula. They may be discrete, or may form masses of vegetations or even large fungating tumours. Ulceration may occur with marked tissue destruction and a slowly progressive lesion may suddenly show rapid and even fatal spread. In the earlier stages the vocal cords and the interior of the larynx are normal and laryngeal movement is unimpaired. In some cases cervical glandular enlargement may be present, possibly as one large, hard fixed gland.

In nearly all cases tuberculous lesions can be detected in the lung. With this type of tuberculosis these are sometimes of the fibrotic type without cavitation, and in the earlier stages may well be overlooked even after careful search.

Spontaneous cure may occur in some instances, but treatment should never be neglected in expectation of this. (See also Tuberculosis of the Pharynx.)

Laryngeal movement. The effects on movement are variable, but from the onset there is usually impairment of the affected cord, which progresses to fixation as the arytenoids become deeply involved.

Symptoms. The symptoms of pulmonary tuberculosis are in many cases well marked before such patients appear for examination, but in a number of instances the diagnosis of pulmonary tuberculosis is made when hoarseness is being investigated as the patient's only complaint.

In the great majority of cases the first symptom is loss of voice, but in those showing early affection of the epiglottis, pain on swallowing may be the first complaint. The loss of voice may be transient in the beginning but is most marked after prolonged use.

As ulceration is established and nerve endings are exposed, pain on swallowing becomes severe and may be a serious obstacle to nutrition. In the later stages all voice is lost.

Stridor may develop owing to fixation of the vocal cords or to the disorganization of the larynx. Obstruction to the airway may cause urgent symptoms. Enlargement of glands may be noted, and in the extrinsic form, one or two large glands are sometimes found which are fixed and hard.

Diagnosis. Owing to the unusually sensitive pharynx common in these patients, examination is not easily tolerated and it may be necessary to spray the throat with cocaine solution before the larynx can be inspected. The examination of the larynx is followed by X-ray and clinical examination of the lungs, and examination of the sputum. It is also essential that a portion of tissue is removed for histological examination.

It is important to differentiate the condition from syphilis and neoplasm, and these diseases must be kept constantly in mind. Syphilis presents a more indurated appearance with deeper ulceration. Neoplasm may be confused with the stage of granulation formation, but has origin as a rule farther forward and is more discrete, redder and more fleshy looking. Histological examination and the blood Wassermann reaction are needed because tuberculosis, cancer and syphilis not only may cause confusion but may co-exist.

Treatment. It is essential that treatment of the pulmonary tuberculosis should be instituted under sanatorium conditions with the aid of streptomycin, P.A.S. or other appropriate drugs. Constant watch must be maintained for possible effects of the treatment upon the labyrinth as total deafness has resulted from idiosyncrasy or ill-judged treatment. Vestibular symptoms of imbalance appear first and deafness follows. Immediate withdrawal of streptomycin is indicated. Under hospital conditions collapse therapy or surgical treatment should be available and applied when necessary.

Local treatment consists primarily of putting the affected parts at rest and therefore absolute silence must be enforced; this restriction applies to physical movement also, and complete rest in bed is essential. Granulations on the cords can be reduced when necessary by the use of diathermy or cautery, and fibrosis is encouraged in this way.

Pain on swallowing may be a serious obstacle to progress and can be helped if necessary by spraying the larynx with various drugs, such as menthol, chloretone, cocaine 2 per cent or by using orthoform powder in a Leduc's inhaler. In severe cases coagulation of an exposed ulcer with the diathermy button may succeed in giving great relief.

Tracheostomy is rarely advisable, but contractions or stenosis following treatment are the chief indications.

SYPHILIS

In secondary syphilis serpiginous ulcers may frequently be seen upon the epiglottis and the arytenoids. The larynx is inflamed; there is excess of secretion and some oedema.

Symptoms. The symptoms are hoarseness and some difficulty in swallowing, but this is not severe, and is described as a 'raw' sensation.

The tertiary stage is usually seen after the breakdown of a gumma. There is often considerable ulceration of the laryngeal tissues. There may be a thickening and granular appearance of the anterior part of the larynx, with some ulceration of the edge of the cord. The chief symptom is hoarseness. The diagnosis is confirmed by means of the blood Wassermann reaction, and by the exclusion of other diseases.

22. Tumours of the Larynx

INNOCENT TUMOURS

Innocent tumours are rare in the larynx. They are most frequently *papillomata* or *fibromata*. Chondromata also occur.

PAPILLOMATA

Papillomata are most frequently seen in children and cause hoarseness. They are nearly always multiple and a virus is probably the cause. Spontaneous regression and disappearance of the lesions sometimes occur at puberty.

Treatment. The papillomata must be removed as often as necessary. This can be carried out with small cupped forceps, alternatively diathermy with a fine specially insulated sucker can be used. Suspension laryngoscopy and the aid of the operating microscope are recommended with both methods. With care the lesions can be removed repeatedly without damage to the vocal cords, although in the case of multiple and rapid recurrences some scarring is probably inevitable. Cryosurgical destruction, by means of a special endolaryngeal probe, is under trial and good results have been reported. The value of ultrasound, and the application of oestrogens remains in doubt. Irradiation has no place in the treatment of papillomata.

Tracheostomy. This may be required in children and should be carried out whenever there is any indication of obstruction. The tube should be positioned in the standard way, and as it may have to be worn for a considerable period till all indications of papillomata have disappeared, decannulation sometimes presents a problem.

Recurrence. This is one of the outstanding characteristics of papillomata in children, and it may take place in any part of the larynx and even in the trachea, or the tracheostomy opening, where this is present. In children there is very little tendency to malignant degeneration, but in spite of this, all tissue removed should be submitted to histological examination.

Adults. Papillomata are rare tumours in the adult, and have to be distinguished from leucoplakia and other epithelial overgrowths. Histological examination must be carried out in all cases. Adult papillomata are often premalignant.

FIBROMATA

This is a rare form of tumour but is sometimes found with vascular characteristics, giving the appearances of fibroangioma. These growths appear as small reddish masses on the vocal cord. Differentiation has to be made from cancer of the cord, which these growths sometimes resemble. The fibro-angioma, however, will be seen to have a perfectly smooth glistening surface, differing from the rougher, granulating type of surface presented by the malignant growth. It is inadvisable, however, to rely on appearances for differential diagnosis, and in all cases the growth should be removed and submitted to histological examination.

CYSTS

Retention cysts containing the products of seromucinous glands are the most frequent. They appear as soft fluctuating swellings, yellowish in colour around the epiglottis and ventricular folds. They are usually asymptomatic and are often found during routine examination. Small cysts may be left alone.

MALIGNANT TUMOURS OF THE LARYNX

Squamous epitheliomata form the bulk of the tumours commonly found in the larynx, though sarcomata are encountered on rare occasions. The *classification* of tumours has changed frequently, and the old classification of intrinsic and extrinsic cancer, though convenient, leaves too many difficulties of definition. The usually accepted classification at present is as follows:

	Regions	*Site*
Larynx	Supraglottic	Posterior surface of epiglottis
		Ventricular bands
		Arytenoids
		Ventricles
	Glottic	Vocal cords
		Anterior and posterior commissures
	Subglottic	Walls of subglottis
	Marginal zone	Tip of epiglottis (suprahyoid)
		Aryepiglottic folds
	Laryngopharynx (hypopharynx)	Pyriform fossa
		Post-cricoid area
		Posterior pharyngeal wall

The stage of the disease is described according to the extent of the tumour, involvement of nodes, and the presence of distant metastases.

This is known as the T.N.M. classification and based on this the disease can be grouped into stages I to IV.

The *glottic tumour* most commonly takes its origin from the vocal cord. The usual site for commencement is the junction of the anterior and middle thirds of the cord. From this point it spreads in both directions until it involves the anterior commissure and the vocal process. If unchecked it will spread round the anterior commissure to the opposite cord. It spreads backwards to the arytenoid region and then tends to become supraglottic by extending upwards from the glottic edge. As well as these directions of spread, it must be remembered that a cancer of the vocal cord is probably spreading downwards,

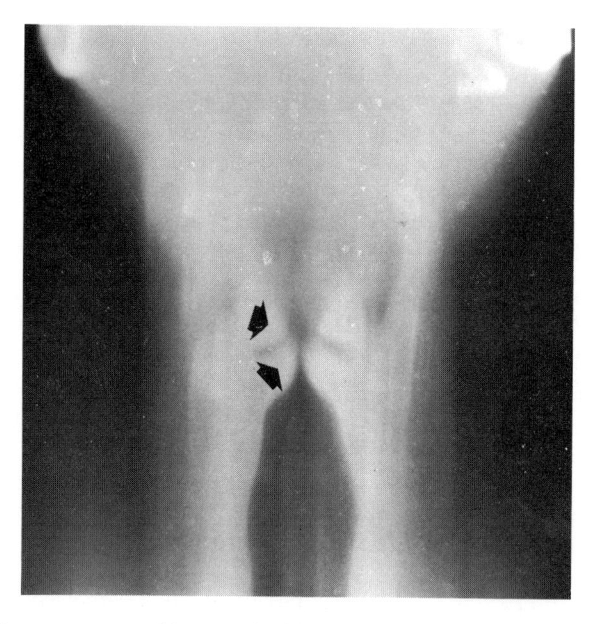

Fig. 50. Tomogram, normal larynx. The false cord superiorly, and the true inferiorly, are arrowed. The ventricle is clearly defined between them on both sides. The subglottic space is cone-shaped and symmetrical.

below the cord, and allowance in estimation of the size of growth must always be made for the probable downward extension towards the subglottic space. The movement of an affected vocal cord is one of the most important indications of the extent of the growth. Limitation of movement or immobility of the cord indicates deep infiltration and renders the prognosis less favourable. A characteristic of cordal cancer is the late occurrence of metastases. The lymphatics of the cord being few and sparse, the glands are involved late and usually are not discovered until the cancer has spread deeply.

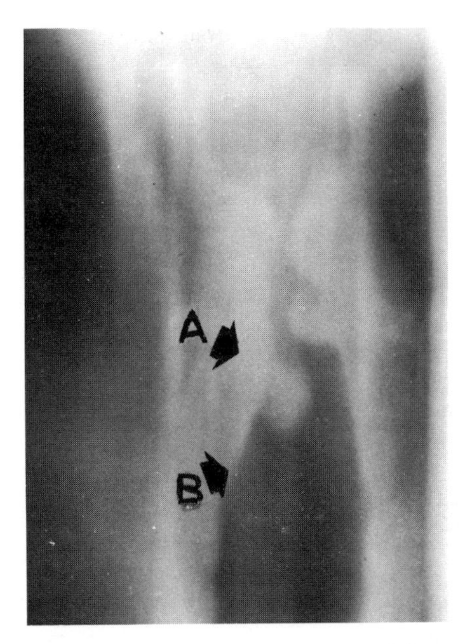

Fig. 51. Tomogram, subglottic cancer. Tomograms are especially useful for determining the extent of spread inferiorly. Note the change in contour between A and B when compared with the normal side and with the tomogram of the normal side. (fig. 50).

Symptoms of glottic cancer

The earliest symptom is hoarseness, and it should be a rule that every patient who has suffered from hoarseness for a period of three weeks without improvement should have the larynx examined by a competent laryngologist. The difficulty constantly encountered in treatment of these patients is that treatment has been delayed, and the growth has spread too far before the advice of a specialist is sought. This is especially unfortunate, as in the early stages the prognosis is excellent if treatment is properly carried out; whereas in the later stages it is frequently hopeless.

Symptoms from other sites. These are often indefinite. Local discomfort, a frequent desire to clear the throat, irritating cough, or a feeling of a lump on swallowing, may be the only complaint. Sometimes discomfort may be referred to the ear. A swelling in the neck may be the first complaint, especially with a supraglottic growth. Only later when the growth approaches the cords is the voice affected. Difficulty in swallowing or breathing results only from a very extensive growth.

Treatment of glottic cancer

The most favourable type of growth for treatment is that which is confined to one cord, does not encroach upon either anterior or posterior commissure, and in which mobility of the cord is normal. The five-year cure rate is about 95 per cent after surgery or after irradiation in expert hands with modern methods.

Irradiation leaves a normal voice and generally therefore will be the treatment of choice. It is best provided in the form of external irradiation from a linear accelerator or a cobalt source. Implantation of radium alongside the vocal cord is less satisfactory.

If an expert radiotherapist is not available then surgical treatment is indicated. This consists of splitting the larynx in the mid-line (laryngofissure) and excising the diseased cord. The resulting voice is generally better than might be expected because, with healing, a fibrous band often develops to replace the excised cord.

When the tumour has extended beyond the limits described, *i.e.* when it encroaches upon either commissure, if it involves most of the length of the cord, if there is subglottic extension, or if the cord is fixed (which means that growth has involved the underlying muscle) then laryngectomy is often advisable. Borderline cases sometimes are treated by irradiation and watched carefully for any suspicion of recurrence. This policy enables certain patients to retain the larynx, but others lose their lives.

After total laryngectomy the patient has inevitably a permanent tracheostomy and has to learn oesophageal speech. The degree of success varies, but with speech therapy most patients acquire a useful voice, and sometimes a patient develops an excellent one.

Various forms of partial laryngectomy are sometimes done to avoid the disadvantages of total removal, but these matters are beyond the scope of a book of this type. The same remark applies to those techniques which incorporate the construction of a skin-lined tube to enable speech to be produced in a more normal way.

Treatment of supraglottic and subglottic cancer

Growths outside the region of the vocal cords are silent till relatively late. Only the earliest can be treated by radiotherapy alone with reasonable hope of success. The majority of these patients accordingly have to be treated by operation, combined with preliminary irradiation.

By the time supraglottic and subglottic cancers are diagnosed there is often clinical involvement of the regional lymph nodes so that block dissection of the neck in continuity with the laryngectomy is mandatory. Difficulty arises in the management of those patients in whom the regional nodes are not clinically enlarged. It is known from pathological studies that these nodes nevertheless may contain small metastatic deposits. The tendency in the past, therefore, has usually been to carry out a block dissection as an elective procedure in such patients at the same time as the laryngectomy. Increasingly, however, in most major clinics the tendency is now towards a wait and watch policy, depending upon radio-therapy and the body's own defences to deal with such microscopic or sub-clinical metastases. When this policy is followed it is essential that the patient is seen every month and that block dissection is carried out at the first sign of any glandular involvement.

The operation on the larynx usually consists of a total laryngectomy, but to avoid the need of a permanent tracheostomy and the difficulties of learning oesophageal speech, there is a movement in certain countries towards various forms of transverse partial laryngectomies for some carefully selected supraglottic growths. These operations have not yet met with general acceptance.

23. Neurological Disorders of the Larynx

SENSORY AFFECTIONS

Hyperaesthesia, paraesthesia and anaesthesia of the larynx are encountered.

Hyperaesthesia is a common accompaniment of disease and may be found in most inflammatory conditions of the larynx.

As an example of this, one may cite the extreme irritability frequently seen in early cases of tuberculosis of the larynx.

Paraesthesia is more frequently encountered in neurotic persons, who complain of the sensation of a foreign body in the larynx, or some other symptom of irritation. In a great many of these cases a phobia of cancer will be found to be the underlying cause.

Anaesthesia may be due either to paralysis of the nerve or nerves of sensation, or it may be due to hysteria or emotional disorder. (See also Sensory Paralysis, p. 180).

SPASMODIC AFFECTIONS

Congenital laryngeal stridor

This form of stridor begins at birth or very soon afterwards and tends to disappear spontaneously at about two years of age. It has been ascribed to deformity of the epiglottis, or generalized flabbiness of the laryngeal inlet. There is now strong evidence that it is caused by incoordination of the respiratory and laryngeal musculature arising from delayed neurological development. The high-pitched inspiratory stridor is worst during crying or exertion and is minimal during sleep.

As a rule diagnosis can be made from the history, but endoscopic examination is essential to exclude certain congenital lesions such as webs and cysts.

Treatment is not usually required as the condition disappears spontaneously at the age of two and a half years, but tracheostomy may be needed in very severe cases.

Laryngismus stridulus

As a rule this, if seen in slightly older children, is a manifestation of tetany from subclinical rickets. Sudden severe attacks of inspiratory stridor occur and the terrified child has to fight for breath. Attacks typically wake the child from sleep and may end in unconsciousness. Twitching spasms sometimes occur and suggest the diagnosis.

Treatment basically is that of the causative vitamin and dietary deficiency. An actual attack can often be terminated by cold sponging or a hot bath. During the attack the tongue should be held out. Oxygen or tracheostomy may be necessary.

Acute spasm

This results from various brain-stem diseases, from tetanus, tabes and rabies, and from irritation by foreign bodies, gases or fumes. Occasionally it arises in absence of disease as such, generally in females who drink, smoke and talk too much against a 'cocktail party' background. Inspiratory stridor produces air hunger and even unconsciousness. Relief can usually be obtained by spraying the larynx with cocaine and attending to any underlying cause. If there is any possibility of a foreign body, direct laryngoscopy or tracheostomy should be done immediately.

Cough syncope

Sometimes called laryngeal vertigo, this is an unusual disorder in which an increasingly severe bout of coughing ends in unconsciousness. It occurs mainly in plethoric, elderly men. It is the result of cerebral anoxia caused by lowered cardiac output. This is secondary to diminished venous return and vagal inhibition in the presence of the high intra-thoracic pressure produced by coughing.

Treatment is on general medical lines, including control of the cough.

Functional spasm

Such spasms may be associated with overstraining of the voice or nervousness, and can result in complete loss of voice at a critical time. Pain may occur from the severity of the spasm. *Singer's spasm* and *clergyman's throat* are two forms of this disorder.

MOTOR PARALYSIS

1. Abductor paralysis.
2. Adductor paralysis.

In distinguishing between these types of motor paralysis, Semon's law gives guidance, postulating that in paralysis of organic origin, the abductor muscles of the larynx are affected before the adductor. It states also that paralysis of purely adductor type is of functional origin. This law, in common with most laws, has exceptions, but in clinical practice it is a useful guide.

With the exception of the crico-thyroid muscle the recurrent nerve constitutes the motor supply and therefore any interference with the function of this nerve will affect the laryngeal movement.

Paralysis may be unilateral or it may be bilateral; it may be partial or complete, and in certain cases it may be transient (Fig. 52).

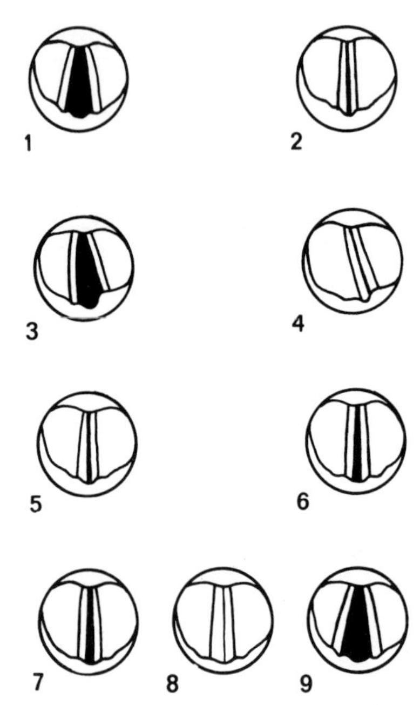

Fig. 52. Larynx on mirror examination. (1) Normal cords; inspiration, (2) phonation. (3) Paralysed left cord; inspiration (4) phonation. (5) Bilateral abductor paralysis; phonation (6) inspiration. (7) Functional aphonia; phonation, (8) coughing, (9) inspiration.

UNILATERAL ABDUCTOR PARALYSIS OF THE LARYNX

Unilateral paralysis produces few symptoms. If the cord lies near the mid-line the voice remains near normal and the condition may be unsuspected. But the farther away the cord lies and the poorer the compensation from the intact side, the more easily the voice tires or weakens as the day goes on. About a quarter of cases are idiopathic; of the remainder many are caused by serious conditions. As these include any lesion affecting the path of the recurrent laryngeal nerve, they are best considered on this basis.

Aetiology. 1. *Bulbar lesions.* Vascular lesions, locomotor ataxia, disseminated sclerosis, tumours.

2. *In the course of the nerve.* Growths or abscesses of the neck involving the vagus nerve, goitre and operations for its removal, pericarditis and aneurysm of the aorta on the left side and aneurysm of the sub-clavian on the right side, apical pleurisy affecting right or left side and cancer of the oesophagus or of the left bronchus (see Fig. 53). mediastinal tumours and glandular enlargement.

3. *Toxic causes.* A neuritis may be set up by toxins in the course of

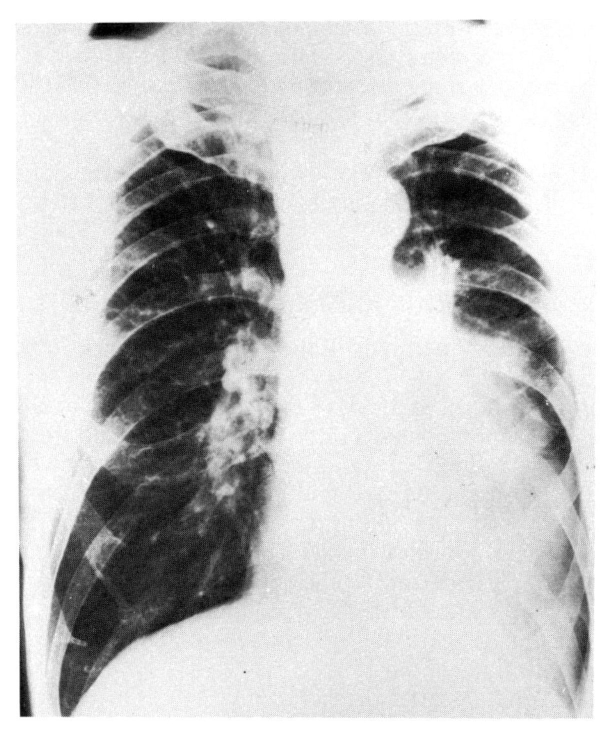

Fig. 53. Carcinoma of left lung which caused paralysis of the left vocal cord through involvement of the left recurrent laryngeal nerve.

diseases such as diphtheria, influenza, measles. Certain metals, *e.g.* lead, have been blamed.

Appearances in cases of abductor paralysis. Two stages in paralysis of the recurrent nerve are generally described, the incomplete stage, and the complete stage.

In the *incomplete stage* the paralysed cord is seen to lie in the mid-line, and there is no outward movement on respiration. Phonation causes the other cord to approach the affected cord so that there is complete apposition, and the paralysed arytenoid may be pushed aside by the active vocal process. In this stage, therefore, although there may be some weakness, the voice is not lost. The adductor muscles are still functioning.

In the *complete stage* the paralysis affects the adductor muscles, with the result that the cord moves outward and is fixed midway between phonation and quiet respiration. This is the *paramedian position*, the arytenoid tends to fall inwards, and the cord is at a lower level.

It is to be noted that every case of paralysis does not pass through these stages in regular sequence. In many cases the paralysis does not reach the complete stage, even after many months.

In examination of a case of complete paralysis, the opposite cord during phonation can be seen to swing across the mid-line, so that the voice is good, and in some cases the patient is unaware that there is any abnormality. This means that full compensation has taken place.

Treatment is that of the cause. If the voice tires easily, speech therapy is useful. If the voice is very poor owing to the cord lying far from the mid-line, injection of teflon paste can produce a better edge for phonation.

BILATERAL ABDUCTOR PARALYSIS

This is a condition of paralysis of the abductor muscles on both sides at the same time.

Aetiology. This form of paralysis may be toxic in origin, but is more often seen after operations upon the thyroid, in which case it may be due to oedema, rather than to any injury to the nerve at operation, especially if the onset is delayed for a period of hours or days after the operation. It also occurs during the course of bulbar paralysis. In a number of patients no cause is found.

Symptoms. These depend on the rapidity of onset. If onset has been very gradual, a remarkable degree of adaptation can occur and symptoms may only arise years later under stress of unaccustomed effort or respiratory infection.

If onset is rapid, as after thyroidectomy, severe inspiratory stridor develops and suffocation can occur. Quality of voice remains good but the patient talks in short staccato sentences.

Appearances. Examination will show the cords to be closely approximated in the mid-line; there is a small space between the cords which provides sufficient airway for the patient, provided no exertion is undertaken. On the smallest call for added respiratory exchange due to exertion, the cords tend to pass into spasm. They are then fixed in the mid-line. Respiration takes place only with great effort on the part of the patient.

Treatment. This condition may endanger life and urgent treatment may be necessary to provide an airway. When stridor is severe tracheostomy or intubation must be done without delay.

Intubation is useful as a temporary measure, but recovery of sufficient cordal abduction is slow after nerve injury and can seldom be expected within a matter of a few days.

It is generally advisable to perform a tracheostomy early in cases of sudden onset, where stridor is severe, especially if it occurs immediately after a thyroidectomy. When the neck has healed a valved tracheostomy tube is provided so that the patient can speak.

In less urgent cases, especially those of slow onset in older patients, a spray of 10 per cent cocaine helps relieve symptoms, especially if combined with sedation. Rest is required to diminish the oxygen needs. By these means a patient may be tided over a period of temporary difficulty.

In patients dependent on a tracheostomy, decision is taken after about a year as to whether the tracheostomy is permanent or the airway is to be improved by surgical measures. After this period of time recovery of vocal cord function is unlikely.

This decision will be decided by the habits, age and occupation of the patient. Where voice is a prime consideration it should be remembered that no operative treatment will result in as good a voice as can be maintained by a permanent tracheostomy tube and the use of a tracheostomy tube with a speaking valve. On the other hand, patients who refuse a permanent tracheostomy can now be offered a good voice with an adequate airway by the operation of arytenoidectomy. This is carried out endoscopically using suspension laryngoscopy and special micro-surgical techniques and instruments. Alternatively, the surgeon may select some form of the classical King operation, in which the vocal cord is abducted by outward fixation of the arytenoid using a neck approach. Others rely on various methods of excision of one vocal cord.

ADDUCTOR PARALYSIS

Primary adductor paralysis according to Semon's law is of functional origin. It is most frequently encountered in hysterical females, but may be induced in either sex as the result of acute shock or chronic emotional stress. Attacks often begin fairly suddenly and may be initiated by a slight throat infection. There is much air-wastage, and the voice is weak or the patient uses a whisper. The duration varies, occasionally an attack lasts many weeks. There is a great tendency to recurrence. It is customary to regard the disability as purely functional and to treat it as such, but in many cases careful investigation will reveal some slight underlying pathological condition, or some cause of irritation which will have to be treated if permanent cure is expected. As an instance of this may be mentioned interarytenoid hypertrophy which produces rapid fatigue of the voice.

Appearances. On inspection, the vocal cords will be seen lying equidistant from the mid-line, in a position corresponding to quiet respiration. They move outwards normally on deep inspiration, but on phonation they move towards the mid-line, but do not come together. When the patient is told to cough there is good approximation, and the patient is able to cough normally.

Treatment of functional paralysis. The treatment of functional paralysis requires great experience and not a little ingenuity. It is essential to make certain that the case is one of functional paralysis. This diagnosis must never be entertained while the slightest doubt remains.

The whole circumstances leading up to the onset must be reviewed. The family surroundings should form the subject of inquiry, as the circumstances leading up to the paralysis may be found within the family circle. One of the simplest methods of persuading a patient to phonate is to make him cough, and to teach him to transform the cough gradually into vocal sounds. In this condition there is a marked tendency to relapse. Hypnosis has been used with some success and is worth considering in difficult cases. Psychiatric advice seldom achieves anything useful and merely adds to the patient's anxieties, common-sense counselling is preferable.

SENSORY PARALYSIS

As the sensation of the larynx above cord level is entirely by the superior laryngeal nerve, true sensory paralysis of the larynx must be due to interference with this nerve tract, either in its peripheral or its central course.

Pressure or trauma to the nerve in its course in the neck may be due to tumour or the results of operation. Disease such as peripheral neuritis, due to diphtheria or other toxic process, may affect the nerve.

Although anaesthesia of the larynx may be found as an isolated occurrence, it is most frequently seen as an accompaniment of other diseases of a neurological character. Attention has already been drawn (p. 141) to neurological syndromes arising from lesions in the region of the jugular foramen, posterior fossa or brain stem, and these have been discussed in the section dealing with sensory paralysis of the pharynx. The aetiology, symptomatology and management of sensory paralysis of the larynx have much in common with related disorders in the pharynx.

Symptoms. Symptoms of this condition may be absent, in the unilateral case, and it may be identified only when special investigation is made. On the other hand, there may be a history of difficulty in swallowing, which the patient interprets as slight choking fits, due to food entering the larynx.

The anaesthesia is identified by careful examination of the larynx with a curved probe. Normally the larynx will not tolerate probing and insensitivity indicates anaesthesia.

As a rule the anaesthesia is unilateral, but it may be bilateral. This constitutes a serious situation, as, on swallowing, aspiration of food or fluid into the lung is liable to occur, setting up pneumonia or even causing death from obstruction. In such a case the safest line of treatment is to insert a cuffed tracheostomy tube to protect the lung. Where necessary a nasal tube is passed into the stomach for feeding purposes. In progressive brain-stem disease the prognosis is bad, but cases due to neural damage may recover after some months.

PARALYSIS OF INDIVIDUAL LARYNGEAL MUSCLES

Some authorities have stated that paralysis of individual muscles in the larynx can occur. Specific appearances are described for some of them, such as paralysis of the thyro-arytenoid or inter-arytenoid muscles, but it is seldom that they can be recognized clinically. Furthermore, it is not easy to understand how just a few fibres of the recurrent laryngeal nerve can be affected. Crico-thyroid paralysis may occur, however, as a definite entity if the superior laryngeal nerve or its external division is damaged in any way, as may occur during an operation on the neck. The voice lacks timbre and the cord is described as having a wavy outline.

FIXATION DUE TO LOCAL CAUSES

Disease in and around the larynx may interfere with the normal laryngeal movement. Apart from inflammatory conditions which have already been considered, fixation may be due to conditions affecting the joints between the arytenoid and cricoid cartilages, such as arthritis. Occasionally malignant disease will manifest itself first by hoarseness, which is caused by a limitation of movement of the vocal cords through interference with the movement of the arytenoids. Sometimes malignant disease near the cord will manifest itself by causing limitation of movement and thus a change in the quality of the voice before involvement of the vocal edge gives actual hoarseness. It is especially important that an early subglottic cancer is not missed.

Fixation and paralysis are distinguished by the fact that in paralysis the arytenoid tends to fall forwards, furthermore the active arytenoid tends to push the paralysed one sideways during phonation. If there is any doubt endoscopic examination is done. This provides a detailed view of the subglottic region and a forceps can be used to probe the arytenoid and test its movement.

24. Miscellaneous Conditions of the Neck

There are certain affections which, for reasons of anatomy and classification. do not fit conveniently into the preceding chapters. Some of the more common which lie within the province of the otolaryngologist are described in this chapter.

BRANCHIAL CYST

This is most frequently seen in young adults as a tense globular swelling postero-inferior to the angle of the jaw. This position is characteristic.

The sterno-mastoid muscle overlaps the posterior half of the swelling. The cyst is generally of slow development and arises from embryonic remnants of the second branchial cleft. The supra-tonsillar recess represents the medial end of this cleft.

The diagnosis is essentially clinical, but the condition has some resemblance to a tuberculous abscess. Aspiration of a branchial cyst produces pus-like material, but the fluid is rich in cholesterol crystals and does not contain bacilli.

Treatment consists of surgical removal, and in the absence of infection is relatively straightforward. (Fig. 41).

BRANCHIAL FISTULA

This condition is less frequently seen. It appears as a pit near the anterior border of the lower part of the sternomastoid. Owing to embryological factors the tract has a complex relationship with the great vessels of the neck and the lower cranial nerves. Its removal involves a difficult dissection between these structures.

THYROGLOSSAL CYST

Of developmental origin, these cysts occur at any position along the line of the thyroglossal tract, *i.e.* between the foramen caecum at the base of the tongue and the isthmus of the thyroid. They are always on or near the mid-line and the majority occur at about the level of the thyroid or cricoid cartilages. They move on swallowing as do thyroid swellings, but a cyst can be differentiated from a small adenoma by the fact that the cyst moves on protruding the tongue as well as on swallowing.

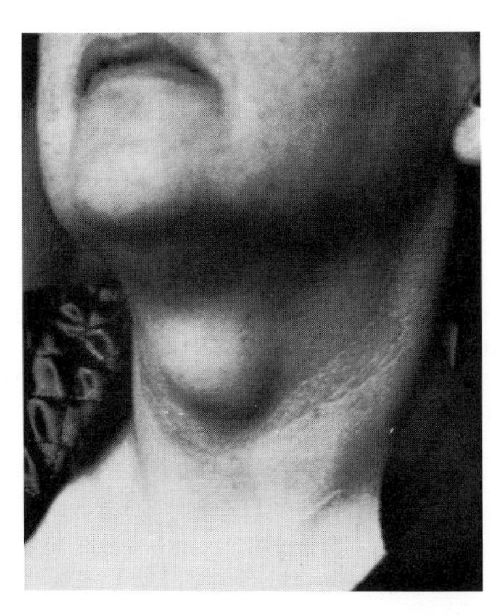

Fig. 54. Thyroglossal cyst. – This is the usual site. In addition to moving with swallowing a thyroglossal cyst also moves upwards on protruding the tongue.

When removing the cyst it is essential to remove the tract as well. This has a close relationship to the body of the hyoid, part of which must be resected as the tract is followed up the mid-line into the base of the tongue.

THYROGLOSSAL FISTULA

This is seen less often than the cyst. The patient complains of leakage of mucus from a point in the mid-line at about the level of the cricoid. The sinus and its tract are subject to recurring episodes of infection. The complete tract must be excised on the lines already described.

LESIONS OF THE SALIVARY GLANDS

The parotid gland

Tumours of the parotid are not uncommon. Most frequent is the pleomorphic salivary adenoma ("mixed salivary tumour") which should be regarded as a tumour of low-grade malignancy. Carcinomas of various types and varying malignancy are the next most numerous group and show the same clinical signs. Least common are the very benign adeno-lymphomas.

Nearly all these tumours arise in the superficial lobe of parotid near the lower pole. They present as a firm or hard swelling just antero-inferior to the lobe of the ear. As the swelling enlarges it tends to become irregular and nodular. Slowness of growth, or absence of pain and facial palsy cannot be depended upon in helping towards a diagnosis.

Biopsy is dangerous and likely to result in accidental spilling of tumour cells whatever the nature of the lesion. Aspiration or needle biopsy is sometimes employed, but again is associated with the risk of spillage, and it may provide only a small amount of unrepresentative material.

The only safe policy therefore is to carry out an excision biopsy. This takes the form of a total removal of the superficial lobe of the parotid with the contained tumour and with preservation of the facial nerve. Immediate histological examination is made and if frank malignancy is reported the surgeon will proceed to remove the deep lobe of the parotid and in appropriate cases arrange for radium implant or external irradiation.

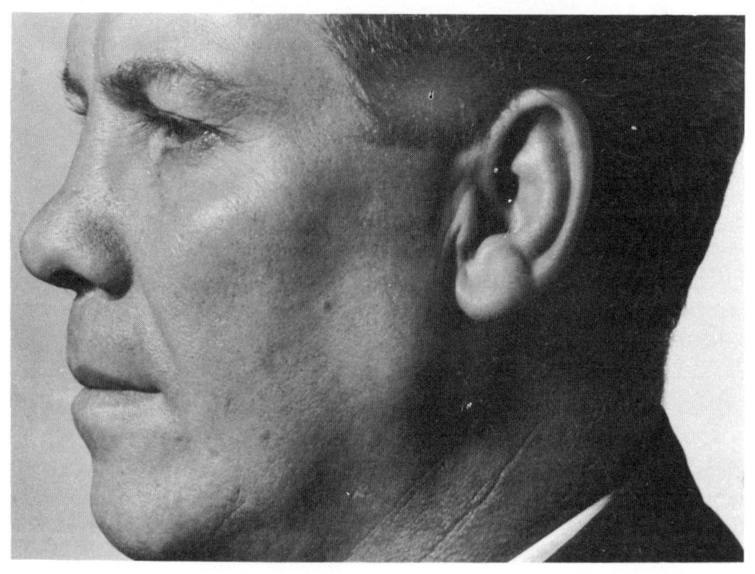

Fig. 55. Salivery tumour. This represents the typical appearance at the lower pole of the parotid gland.

The submandibular gland

Tumours in this locality are much less common, and are usually malignant, but pleomorphic adenomata do occur. They should be dealt with by complete excision of the gland.

Sialectasis is sometimes a cause of recurring or chronic enlargement of the gland, with or without calculus formation (Fig. 56).

A calculus impacted in the submandibular duct causes discomfort and swelling of the gland especially at mealtimes. Between attacks the gland resumes its normal size as its secretions escape past the calculus. This can often be palpated in the floor of the mouth.

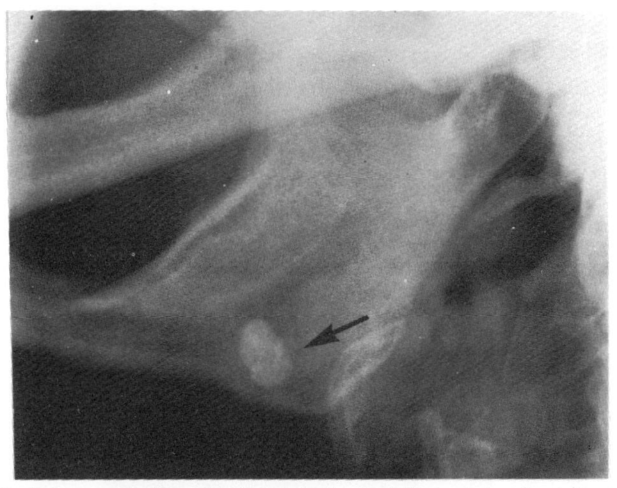

Fig. 56. Radio-opaque submandibular stone in the hilum of the gland. Patient had recurring swelling of the gland at meal times.

If there is no evidence of permanent change in the gland, the calculus can be removed through the floor of the mouth.

In patients with radiological evidence of multiple calculi in the gland itself, or of extensive chronic sialectasis, or clinical evidence suggestive of permanent damage to the gland, then the whole gland should be excised through an exterior approach.

LYMPH NODE ENLARGEMENT

Chronic swellings in the neck, of uncertain nature, may cause difficulties in diagnosis. The conditions just described, together with swellings in the thyroid gland, can usually be excluded.

Metastatic cancer

Malignant involvement of a lymph node should be suspected, especially in older patients who have a firm painless swelling in the neck. This may be the first sign of a malignant disease. It is a serious error to excise the node initially. Instead a detailed search must be made for other enlarged nodes and for a primary growth. This is usually above the clavicles and may be in the larynx, pharynx, fauces mouth, nose, nasopharynx, skin or scalp. A primary growth may be small and symptomless therefore a detailed examination under anaesthesia is usually necessary and biopsy made of any suspicious tissue. Sinuses and chest must be X-rayed and the blood picture examined. If an occult primary, especially one in the above areas, cannot be found, it is best at this stage to excise a node for histological examination by frozen section. If a reticulosis or tuberculosis is found then appropriate treatment will be initiated. The management of malignant involvement of cervical nodes is complex and beyond the scope of this book. Briefly, however, it may be said that if a frozen section shows a reticulosis or an anaplastic tumour then radiotherapy should be given, but nodes which contain a well differentiated squamous carcinoma are best dealt with by proceeding to an immediate block dissection of the neck.

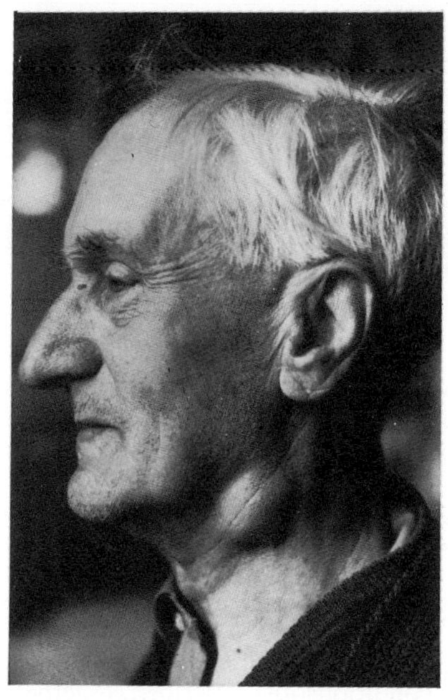

Fig. 57. Elderly patient who presented with a neck swelling. There were no other complaints. It is important that neck swellings which are thought to be malignant should not have biopsies taken from them.

In this event, one is still left with an unknown and untreated primary tumour. It is sometimes suggested that if the nasopharynx is strongly suspected then irradiation to the area should be given, but most surgeons agree that a better policy is to re-examine the patient frequently and regularly until the primary makes itself known. The primary is likely to be small when identified and amenable to appropriate surgical treatment or radio-therapy.

SECTION 5 ENDOSCOPY

25. Instruments and Examination

Endoscopy means the direct examination of those parts of the upper air and food passages which cannot be seen by means of simple methods of examination. Included under the term 'Endoscopy' is the direct examination of the larynx, trachea, bronchi, laryngo-pharynx, oesophagus and the entrance to the stomach.

Endoscopy is a highly specialized branch, and may be called a speciality within a speciality. It requires an advanced degree of technique and a lengthy training which, under most circumstances, is difficult to obtain. It should be undertaken only by those who have had the necessary training, for in unskilled hands loss of life is liable to follow accident. For these reasons only in the case of procedures which may be required in emergency, is technique described in detail. The authors will merely indicate the scope of this speciality, and under what conditions and in what circumstances a practitioner can expect help from the endoscopist.

Examination of the upper air and food passages is usually carried out by means of rigid tubes of different shapes and sizes, depending upon the part to be examined. Illumination is by artificial lighting and various systems are available. A small electric bulb mounted on a suitable carrier can be sited near the distal end of the endoscope. Alternatively the surgeon may prefer a system in which the bulb is situated in the proximal end of the endoscope. Both of these systems have their advantages and disadvantages, but they share the disadvantages of burnt-out bulbs and poor electrical contacts, also the intensity of the lighting is sometimes inadequate. One important advantage, however, is portability. The power source is obtained from low voltage batteries which are always available. Fibre-light systems are becoming increasingly popular because of the quality of illumination provided. The light can be distally or proximally situated in the endoscope, and is fed to the endoscope through a flexible tube which is plugged into the light source. Apart from the excellent quality of the illumination the fibre-light system offers freedom from breakdowns, Its only possible disadvantage is that the light source needs to be plugged in to the power supply.

The equipment required for this work is extensive. Tubes of varying calibre and length are required for the different passages; different tubes are required for the different ages to allow for the differences in lumen of the passages to be examined, and the number of forceps, suction tubes, etc., which have been devised for manipulations carried out through the tubes is legion.

Instruments for laryngoscopy

The *laryngoscope* is the shortest of the tubes. It is usually provided with a strong horizontal handle in order that the muscular tongue against which it is placed may be kept under control. The instrument is provided with a slide which enables the tube portion to be opened. If a bronchoscope is inserted through the laryngoscope the slide can be removed, thus enabling the laryngoscope to be extracted with the bronchoscope remaining in position. The laryngoscope is primarily intended for making a detailed inspection of the various parts of the hypopharynx and larynx and can also be used for taking specimens from the area for histological examination. It is used also for intubation in emergencies and as routine in intra-tracheal anaesthesia. For these purposes instruments are designed without the slide to render withdrawal of the laryngoscope simpler. Other similar instruments such as the laryngostat and the anterior commissure laryngoscope are used for examination of particular areas of the larynx and for removing histological specimens.

Suspension laryngoscopy has been reintroduced to enable the operating microscope to be used for delicate procedures on the vocal cords. It has the advantage of leaving the surgeon free to use both hands. The most recent developments in endoscopy arise from the introduction of flexible endoscopes. These are manufactured from optical fibres similar to those used in fibre lighting systems and are especially useful in oesophago-gastroscopy and in the examination of those patients in whom the insertion of a rigid tube is difficult. Flexible endoscopes carry their own fibre lighting. They give the surgeon an excellent view of the part being examined, biopsies can be made using special biopsy forceps and with the help of special grasping forceps even foreign bodies can be removed from areas which formerly might have been inaccessible except by open operation.

It might be thought that the direct view afforded by the laryngoscope would have rendered the use of the laryngoscopic mirror unnecessary, but the indirect method will always remain the chief and most important way to estimate laryngeal movement. Examination by the laryngoscope causes so much distortion of the larynx by pressure, that observations made with this instrument are unreliable.

Punch forceps have been devised for removal of tissue from the larynx. They are of various types and sizes; the best include a cage into which the specimen is caught. In using forceps without this attachment the specimen taken is frequently lost.

Instruments for bronchoscopy and oesophagoscopy

Tubes for bronchoscopy are of varying lengths and diameter; they vary from a tube of 25 cm long and 3 or 4 mm in diameter, up to the average adult size of 35 cm in length and 18 to 20 mm in diameter. Oesophagoscopy tubes are longer, and on the average are larger in diameter, 10 mm being the average adult size. The bronchoscopy tube differs from the oesophagoscopy tube in that in the lower part of the former tube holes are made in the side, so that if the bronchoscope is inserted into one lung the other lung can still breathe through the bronchoscope by means of these holes. The bronchoscope, too, is frequently provided with small tubes carried to the end of the bronchoscope for lavage of septic cavities in the lung, but these are likely to be replaced with fibre-optic systems. Telescopes are used for detailed examination.

Instruments used for the oesophagus are of great variety. Apart from the examination tube, various forceps have been introduced in order to facilitate the removal of foreign bodies from the oesophagus.

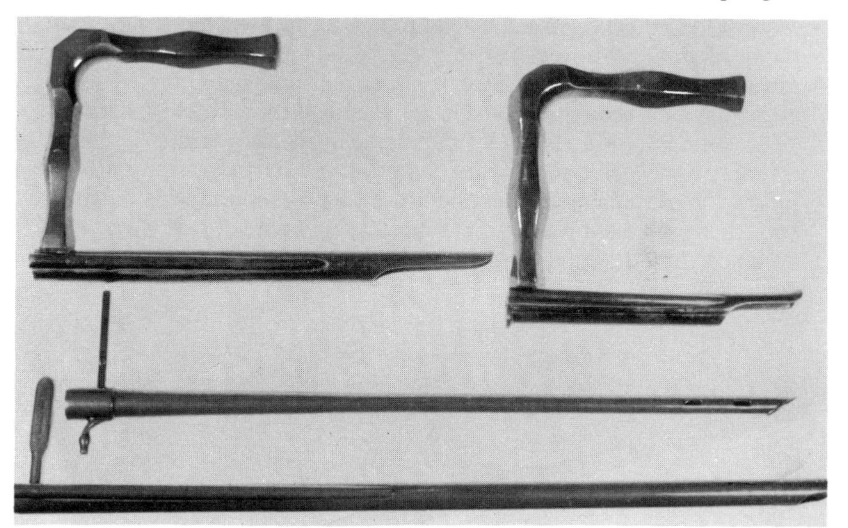

Fig. 58. Instruments for examination of the upper air and food passages. Above – Upper end oesophagoscope and laryngoscope. Below – Bronchoscope and oesophagoscope.

Forceps used with these tubes are of many different types and sizes, their use very frequently depending upon the idiosyncrasy of the surgeon. The chief essentials in forceps for this work are lightness combined with strength and a clear view. Mops on the ends of wires are used for swabbing through the tubes, and gum elastic bougies in graded sizes are provided for the dilatation of strictures.

Preparation of patient

The method of preparing the pharynx for this examination will be found in the appendix. In the first examination at least the patient should always be prepared as for a general anaesthetic. The choice of anaesthesia lies between the employment of a local or a general anaesthetic, and the method used depends partly on the skill and experience of the surgeon, partly upon the type of patient and partly on the particular necessities of the case.

The tendency is increasingly towards general anaesthesia with the use of relaxants though some surgeons still prefer local anaesthesia.

If treatment is frequently repeated certain of the preparations may to be omitted if the patient is being treated as a 'day' case.

Position of the patient

The patient is examined in the dorsal recumbent position (Fig. 59). When a general anaesthetic is used a 3-inch-thick cushion will hold the head in the preliminary position, with slight control from an assistant. For the introduction of instruments under local anaesthesia, however, more skill and experience are required from the assistant. In this case the head should project over the end of the table, with the shoulders resting on the table. The head is supported and manipulated by an assistant who sits on the right side of the patient on a level with his head. The position of the assistant is important, and he should have had some training in the technique, otherwise he will be unable to appreciate and follow the movements of the operator. Asepsis should be as complete and thorough as possible. Various types of head-rest have been designed, but the intelligent assistant is superior to any mechanical device.

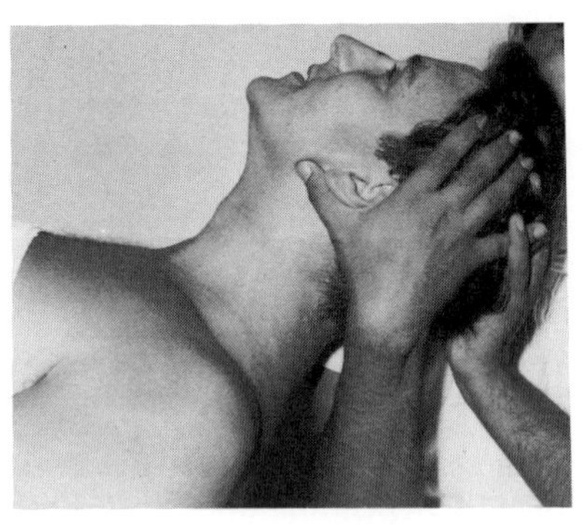

Fig. 59. Position of the patient at start of endoscopy. Note the head is extended and the neck flexed.

Introduction of endoscope

For the introduction of the endoscope the head should be flexed upon the chest. The patient is then told to elevate the chin as far as possible while keeping the head pushed forward. The assistant then, resting the left elbow on the left knee, places the palm of the hand behind the occiput, and passes the right arm under the neck, placing the right thumb under the left side of the mandible. This provides both vertical and lateral control, and brings the cervical spine into a line parallel with the pharynx. The laryngoscope is then passed into the mouth, behind the tongue. The instrument should be held in the left hand, and the right hand should be used to guard the teeth. The first two fingers of the right hand are slipped over the patient's teeth, and the thumb is placed behind the laryngoscope, so that the thumb of the right hand forms the fulcrum for any lifting movement, and the patient's teeth are guarded. If the formation of the patient's mouth permits, the instrument should be slipped into the angle of the mouth on the right side. It is not uncommon to see the inexperienced operator using the teeth as a fulcrum when levering up the point of the instrument, to the great distress of the patient. When the laryngoscope has been passed behind the tongue, it is gently pressed against the base of the tongue until the epiglottis comes into view. This is then picked up on the point of the instrument, and the base of the arytenoids will be seen. The larynx is still obscured in the anterior part of the pharynx, owing to the bulge of the base of the tongue. The laryngoscope is now pressed straight forward – that is, a lifting motion is given to the handle of the laryngoscope. This flattens out the tongue and brings the vocal cords into view. The bronchoscope or the intubation tube can then be passed into the trachea between the vocal cords, and the slide is removed to disengage the laryngoscope. The trachea can be sprayed with 5 per cent solution of cocaine if there is coughing. Secretions can be removed with the inner suction tube, and the examination commenced.

In health the mucosa should be pink and glistening and there should be no accumulation of secretions. The carina, the division between the main bronchi, like those of the lower bronchi should be thin and almost knifelike. The bronchi should move freely with respiration and it should be noted that normal movement causes widening and lengthening on inspiration and contraction and narrowing on expiration.

In the average adult the measurements from the upper teeth to the various parts of the larynx and trachea are:

From the upper teeth to the vocal cords – 11 cm.
From the vocal cords to the bifurcation of the trachea – 12 cm.

In children the measurements are relatively less. The diameter of the trachea in the adult is approximately 20 mm.

OESOPHAGOSCOPY

Within the term of oesophagoscopy is included the examination of the upper orifice of the oesophagus which lies behind the cricoid cartilage and the cardiac orifice of the stomach.

Certain anatomical facts must first of all be pointed out so that the following descriptions may be clear.

The oesophagus is a muscular tube which, unlike the trachea, is not rigid and whose lumen does not necessarily remain patent. The musculature consists of two coats – a circular coat and a longitudinal – and the tube is capable of peristaltic movement, by which food normally is passed on to the stomach. At the upper end is a muscular bundle called the crico-pharyngeus muscle, which acts as a sphincter between the pharynx and the oesophagus. At the lower end, where the oesophagus traverses the diaphragm, there is a pinching of the oesophagus, which is called the hiatus.

The nerve-supply of the oesophagus is by the vagus nerve and the sympathetic nervous system.

In the average adult the distance from the upper teeth to the opening of the oesophagus is 15 cm. The distance from the incisor teeth to the cardia is 40 cm.

Radiological examination forms an essential part of the investigation. The patient should be X-rayed in the usual positions to show the lung fields and the uppermost part of the oesophagus. A barium swallow must be carried out, and in this connection films are of less importance than the report of the radiologist regarding the oesophageal movement observed on the screen.

Preparation of the patient. The preparation is similar to that for bronchoscopy. The patient should be prepared as for a general anaesthetic, whether this is to be used or not. Also, where oesophageal obstruction is suspected, the diet should be fluid for the preceding twenty-four hours and, in cases in which X-rays show dilatation, the oesophagus should be washed out prior to the examination. This will save the examiner a great deal of time. Most examinations are carried out under general anaesthesia with a relaxant, but in some patients local anaesthesia will be advisable. Induction with thiopentone and a relaxant, followed by intubation and intratracheal anaesthesia, is usual. If the patient is intubated the operator is freed from all anxiety regarding the patient's airway, which in certain circumstances may be seriously embarrassed by pressure on the larynx by the oesophagoscope.

Technique of oesophagoscopy

It must be emphasised that oesophagoscopy should be undertaken only by those who have had proper training as it is always potentially a dangerous operation. If there is inflammation or stricture, perforation can occur even in experienced hands. Under a general anaesthetic the passage of the oesophagoscope is simpler as there are no muscular contractions to be overcome, but the use of general anaesthesia must compel the surgeon to even greater gentleness as he does not have the patient's sensations to guide him and dangerous pressure may pass unnoticed.

The position for introduction of the oesophagoscope is similar to that for laryngoscopy but the tube is passed down the right pyriform sinus.

The oesophagus is a flat tube of smooth mucous membrane which opens in front of the instrument. Movement of the lung and the aorta are clearly seen and the hiatus is marked by a stellate pinching of the mucous membrane. Just beyond the hiatus the smooth membrane changes to longitudinal folds which mark the entrance to the stomach.

Any abnormalities are noted and measured and specimens can be removed from suspicious areas.

26. Diseases of the Laryngopharynx (Hypopharynx)

The conditions included in this chapter belong more properly in the chapter on the pharynx. As the diagnosis is usually made by endoscopic methods their description has been delayed till these techniques have been described.

DIVERTICULA OF THE PHARYNX

These pouches may be lateral or central, and are due to herniation of the mucosa through weak parts of the pharyngeal musculature. This is most frequently between the oblique and the transverse fibres of the inferior constrictor muscle.

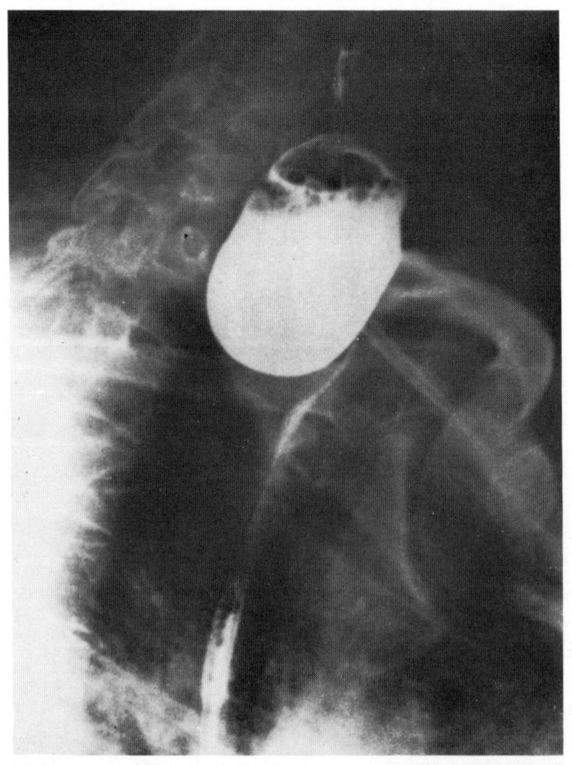

Fig. 60. Pharyngeal diverticulum. Illustrates overspill into the oesophagus.

Symptoms. Regurgitation of food, especially at night, is a common feature, and overflow of salivary secretions often produces an annoying cough. Eating and drinking are slow and noisy. The pouch increases in size, and dysphagia develops as the pouch gradually closes off the oesophagus by pressure. In the case of large pouches a swelling may occasionally be seen in the neck. (Fig. 60).

Diagnosis is made by X-rays and confirmed by oesophagoscopy.

Appearances. The oesophagoscope enters a smooth space from which no exit can be found. On withdrawing the instrument a horizontal slit or dimple can be seen on the anterior wall. This is the entrance to the oesophagus surrounded by the crico-pharyngeus muscle. Where difficulty is found in entering the oesophagus a probe can be passed first and followed as a guide by threading the oesophagoscope over the probe.

Treatment. The sac may be removed by surgical dissection in the neck, or the party wall between the oesophagus and the sac may be divided with diathermy (Dohlman's method). This is of particular value in the seriously debilitated.

GLOBUS HYSTERICUS

This occurs mainly in anxious females; the complaint is of a lump in the throat which interferes with swallowing. The condition is regarded as functional, though ciné-radiographic studies not infrequently show abnormalities in the rhythm of swallowing. Sometimes an abnormality of the cardia may produce vague 'upper-end' symptoms, frequently there is an oesophageal reflux present and it may be possible to reproduce symptoms by administering an acid barium swallow during ciné-radiographic study. Antacids are reported to be beneficial if this is the case. Globus hystericus should not be diagnosed until an organic lesion, especially a malignancy, has been excluded.

THE PATERSON-KELLY SYNDROME

Also known as the Plummer-Vinson syndrome, this is a disorder of females in which atrophic changes occur at various sites. It is probably a disease of absorption or metabolism and is nearly always associated with a microcytic hypochromic anaemia.

The major changes occur in the post-cricoid region: initially the mucosa is smooth and atrophic; later hyperkeratosis and fissuring occur, going on to fibrosis and web formation or stricture. Carcinoma occurs in certain patients. The tongue is often atrophic; frequently there are brittle nails, an angular stomatitis and achlorhydria. (Fig. 61).

The chief complaint is of dysphagia; X-ray and endoscopic examination reveal the changes in the hypopharynx.

Treatment consists of administration of iron and vitamins in high dosage. The stricture is dealt with by dilatation, after which the patient herself is taught to swallow a mercury bougie sufficiently frequently to prevent the stricture reforming. These patients should be kept under observation because malignant change can still occur even though iron and other deficiencies have been corrected.

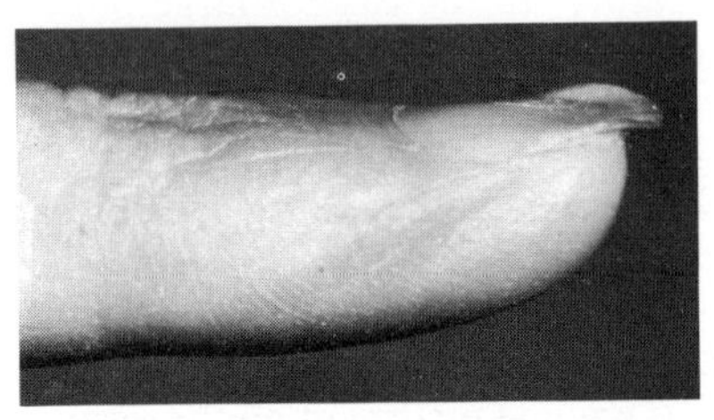

Fig. 61. Brittle spoon shaped finger nails in Patterson-Kelly (Plummer-Vinson) syndrome. (Koilonychia).

TUMOURS OF THE LARYNGOPHARYNX (HYPOPHARYNX)

Benign tumours are very rare. Squamous carcinoma is not uncommon. In females this is usually post-cricoid, in males it is commonly in the pyriform fossa. Discomfort on swallowing or a gland in the neck may be

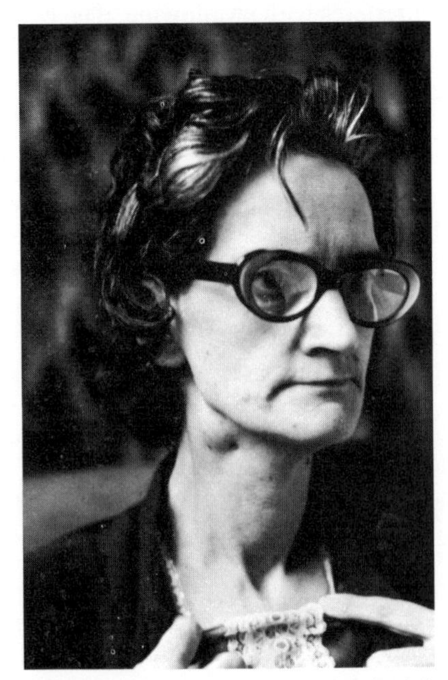

Fig. 62. Post-cricoid cancer. Patient had been aware of a glandular swelling in the neck for about six weeks but dysphagia had been present for only about three weeks. The condition was inoperable.

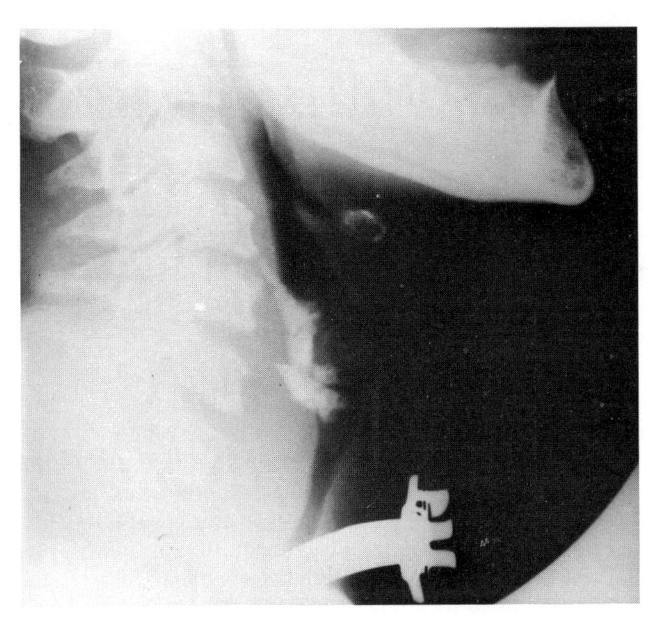

Fig. 63. Post cricoid cancer. – Note the great increase in width of the retrotracheal soft tissue. This patient had impairment of the airway as well as paralysis of both recurrent laryngeal nerves, and tracheostomy was required.

the first complaint. Pain is sometimes referred to the ear. Actual difficulty in swallowing only occurs when the growth is large. (Fig. 62).

Treatment is mainly by surgical means, though preliminary irradiation may improve the prognosis. Radiotherapy alone is extremely disappointing. Laryngectomy and partial pharyngectomy may provide adequate removal of a pyriform fossa lesion; block dissection of the neck is carried out in continuity on the homolateral side. For post-cricoid growths laryngo-pharyngectomy with reconstruction in stages by skin flaps may be adequate for some patients, but in those tumours which extend down into the cervical oesophagus complete laryngo-pharyngo-oesophagectomy is required. Repair is carried out by anastomosing the mobilised stomach to the root of the tongue. Alternatively, colon can be used. Although this is a major procedure it is done in a single stage and enables these unfortunate patients to swallow early and to return home with minimum delay.

27. Diseases of the Lung and Oesophagus

Only those conditions will be considered which fall within the province of the endoscopist.

BRONCHIECTASIS

Causes. The chief causes are unresolved pneumonia, unresolved collapse of the lung, inhalation of foreign bodies, inhalation of irritating gases, penetrating wounds and adhesions from pleural suppuration. The underlying cause of nontuberculous suppuration is interference with the normal mechanism which serves to empty the lung of accumulated secretion. Whatever be the cause – pneumonia, collapse, irritation, etc. – the essential lesion is the destruction of ciliary activity, either alone or accompanied by interference with the normal lung movement, to such an extent that cough reflex and the normal 'squeeze' of the lung are unable to expel the secretions which accumulate in the tubes. This leads to stagnation, and stagnation leads to secondary infection, so that the bronchi become cesspools of infected lung secretions. The cough consequent upon the disease leads to further weakening of the walls and dilatation of the spaces. The chronic suppuration leads again to fibrosis in the peribronchial tissue, with further fixation of the bronchi. Occasional narrowing of the bronchi may occur, so that bottle-shaped cavities are formed in which foul-smelling sputum accumulates. The ciliated epithelium in the bronchi is replaced by pavement epithelium or by granulation tissue.

Symptoms. Symptoms in the early stages are those of the primary condition. When bronchiectasis becomes established the patient usually states that a large quantity of sputum is brought up at a time. This generally occurs about two or three times a day. The patient's breath is foul, and it may be impossible for him to mix in society. The signs of chronic infection become obvious. The patient loses weight and appetite, temperature begins to swing and rigors may develop. There is blueness of the lips owing to embarrassment of circulation, and clubbing of the fingers is found in advanced cases.

Diagnosis of bronchiectasis

Physical signs depend to some extent on the primary condition. In established cases there is usually restriction of movement, diminished vocal fremitus and occasionally friction. Dullness is found on percussion, and may be patchy and not confined to definite lung segments. Breath sounds are harsh vesicular or bronchial, or fairly low pitch, and are rarely cavernous or amphoric. Vocal resonance is diminished as a rule owing to thickening of the pleura and the presence of fluid in the lung. The presence of friction indicates an active suppurative process.

The organisms found constitute a formidable list. Streptococci, haemolytic and non-haemolytic, are common. Fusiform bacilli, of Vincent's type, and spirochaetes are also met with, and saprophytes are represented chiefly by leptothrix.

Opaque media. Bronchograms are essential in assessing the extent of disease in the lung so that treatment can be planned. The opaque medium can be introduced into the lung after suitable local anaesthesia either by nasal catheter or directly through a bronchoscope. By this means cavities and dilatations can be demonstrated (Fig. 64) or the presence of a tumour indicated by the lack of penetration of the medium into the affected part of the lung.

Termination. Many of these patients die of broncho-pneumonia

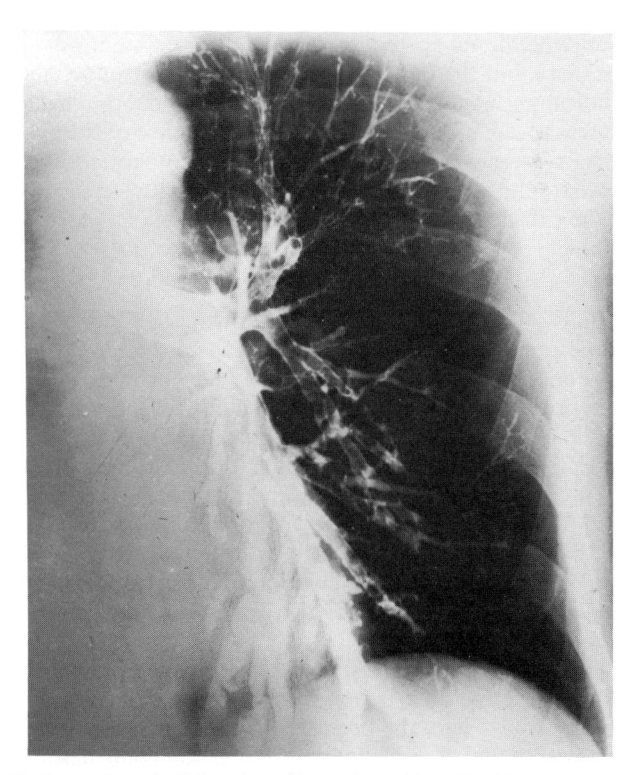

Fig. 64. Bronchiectasis. Dilatation of lower bronchi outlined by contrast medium.

during an influenza epidemic. A certain number develop brain abscesses which are frequently multiple.

Treatment. In early cases surgical excision of the affected part of the lung is the treatment of choice. In view of the close association of sinus suppuration and bronchiectasis, investigation of the sinuses should be carried out in all cases, and appropriate treatment instituted where infection is discovered. Where surgical treatment is not advisable owing to the patient's general condition, or the character of the suppuration, palliative treatment can give relief. Regular bronchoscopic aspiration can be carried out and the patient is taught the technique of postural drainage. Wide spectrum antibiotics also are of considerable value.

Bronchoscopy forms an essential part of the diagnosis as bronchiectasis may be the result of other disease such as carcinoma or of the inhalation of a foreign body.

ABSCESS OF THE LUNG

Infections such as pneumonia or virus diseases may play a part in the origin of this condition, but foreign bodies such as fragments of teeth or obstructions due to bronchogenic carcinoma may give rise to abscess. At one time operations on the upper respiratory system were blamed for the majority, but the incidence of such abscesses is now negligible.

The condition is included here because it is essential to remember the circumstances which may be masked by the presence of the abscess. In purely infective cases early bronchoscopic treatment may result in cure, but where the abscess is secondary to other disease the prognosis is that of the causal condition.

COLLAPSE OF THE LUNG

When air fails to reach a part of the lung owing to some obstruction, absorption of air beyond the obstruction causes the lung to collapse. Such obstruction may be a foreign body, a new growth, or a plug of viscid secretion which the patient, for some reason such as pain, cannot expel. In the present context acute collapse concerns us here as it is likely to follow operation or the inhalation of a foreign body. The symptoms are pain on the affected side and dyspnoea, while mechanical signs appear due to the change in the air-containing spaces of the lung. These are, flattening of the ribs on the affected side, elevation of the diaphragm on the same side and deviation of the mediastinum towards the affected side. Breath sounds are also absent over the collapsed lung (Fig. 68).

Treatment. Breathing exercises and postural coughing may be sufficient to relieve the obstruction, but in other cases early bronchoscopy is called for. Where the presence of a foreign body is suspected this should be the first step in treatment after the confirmation of the collapse by radiography.

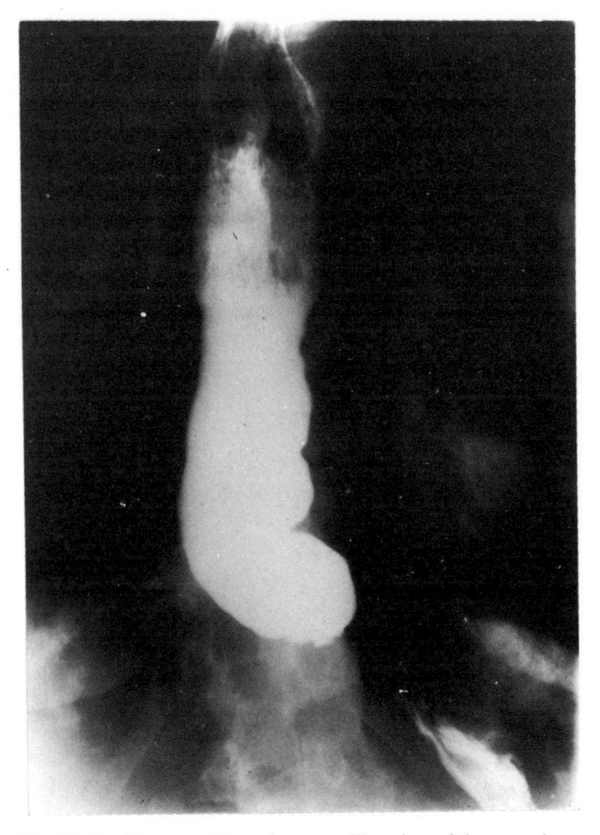

Fig. 65. Cardiospasm. Note the great dilatation of the oesophagus.

CARCINOMA OF THE LUNG

Tumours of the lung may be primary or secondary. Carcinoma anywhere in the body may produce secondary deposits in the lung.

Primary bronchogenic tumours are nearly all squamous cell carcinomata. Their degree of differentiation is variable. The frequency of this disease has increased rapidly in recent years, and it is much more prevalent in males than in females. It is also more common in smokers than in non-smokers.

Symptoms. The onset is insidious, and the earliest symptom may be cough, and where no previous lung disease has existed slight haemoptysis is of great significance. Dyspnoea may be early or late according to the degree of obstruction present, and pain may be felt if there is involvement of the pleura or the ribs. A left-sided growth may interfere early with the recurrent laryngeal nerve. The patient will have an alteration in the quality of the voice, and mirror laryngoscopy will show a paralysis of the left vocal cord.

Diagnosis. The diagnosis is made by means of radiography with lung mapping where required, and bronchoscopy. A positive diagnosis can be made by bronchoscopy in about 80 per cent of cases. Radical surgery offers the only hope of cure and that only in the earliest cases.

CONGENITAL ABNORMALITIES OF THE OESOPHAGUS

Various types of oesophageal defects are encountered. Patients with total absence of the oesophagus or those in whom both upper and lower segments end in blind pouches are very rare. Also tracheo-oesophageal fistula without atresia is a rarity. In the majority of abnormalities a tracheo-oesophageal fistula into an upper or lower stump of oesophagus is present.

This last type is the most frequent of all congenital abnormalities. It is important that all those associated with the new-born should be able to recognise this defect. It is characterised by excessive salivation, cyanosis, and the inability to swallow fluids. If an X-ray film indicates the presence of gas in the stomach whilst the passage of a catheter is prevented in the upper oesophageal segment, the diagnosis can be made with confidence. It is confirmed by introducing one to two ml. of iodised oil into the catheter and taking further X-ray photographs.

Barium must not be used in any circumstances. Once the diagnosis has been established supportive therapy, intravenous fluids and continual oesophageal suction are provided until expert help can be obtained. It should be emphasised that this is a matter of the utmost urgency.

CONGENITAL STRICTURE

Congenital strictures of the oesophagus are very rare and it is important to differentiate them from acquired strictures due to reflux oesophagitis. The diagnosis depends upon the fact that dysphagia is present at birth and that upon oesophagoscopy normal mucosa is found below the level of the stricture. These patients may be undersized and suffer from obvious malnutrition.

Treatment consists of dilatation repeated over a long period of time.

CONGENITAL WEBS

These give rise to difficulty in swallowing, possibly with slow physical development. Division of the web, preferably with diathermy, should be carried out when the diagnosis is made provided the patient is fit for operation.

CONGENITAL SHORTENING

This condition is not diagnosed as a rule until symptoms due to oesophagitis and ulceration appear. In the true short oesophagus the oesophagus terminates above the diaphragm. This can be seen in X-rays, and diagnosis can be confirmed by oesophagoscopy when the hiatus is found below the point where the oesophageal mucosa changes to the longitudinal folds of gastric mucosa. Where desired, biopsy can confirm the presence of gastric mucosa. Congenital short oesophagus is of extreme rarity. The great majority of cases diagnosed have in fact been produced after birth by gastric reflux leading to fibrosis and finally shortening of the oesophagus. Treatment is usually that appropriate to the condition of oesophagitis (p. 206).

DIVERTICULA

In the oesophagus itself diverticula are exceedingly rare and are usually due to adhesions resulting from disease outside the oesophagus. In the lowest part of the pharynx, however, they are not uncommon. Although anatomically in the pharynx, their diagnosis requires endoscopic examination, therefore the condition is included in this section (see p. 194).

NEUROMUSCULAR AFFECTIONS OF THE OESOPHAGUS

The Paterson-Kelly syndrome (Plummer-Vision).

Chapter 26 (see p. 195).

ACHALASIA OR CARDIOSPASM

Although usually known as cardio-spasm there is in fact no spasm present, but there is a failure of the cardia to open for the passage of food. The essential defect is probably in the upper segment of the oesophagus which can become enormously dilated. It seems that the failure of relaxation of the cardia is secondary to the absence of the normal neurogenic stimulus coming from this abnormal upper segment (Fig. 65).

Symptoms. Increasing difficulty in swallowing is present which may be intermittent in the early stages. Regurgitation of food occurs and there may be loss of weight and a feeling of obstruction in the oesophagus.

Diagnosis is made by X-rays, and confirmed by oesophagoscopy. Where there is considerable dilatation the oesophagus should be washed out before examination. In all cases malignant disease must be excluded.

Treatment. In early cases, dilatation by weighted mercury bougies may be very effective, as the patient can carry out the treatment himself at home. Other methods of dilatation through the oesophagoscope may be tried, and Heller's operation, in which the oesophageal coats are divided down to the mucous membrane, usually gives good results.

HIATAL HERNIA

There are two types of herniation of the stomach into the thorax.

Para-oesophageal hernia

In this there is herniation of part of the stomach and peritoneum through the hiatus of the diaphragm alongside the oesophagus. The cardia of the stomach remains in its normal position at or below the diaphragm. The general opinion is that the abnormality is congenital.

Symptoms are chiefly those of increased mass within the thorax, breathlessness, and bleeding from ulceration of the thoracic portion of the stomach, with consequent anaemia.

Diagnosis may be difficult, but X-rays will demonstrate the abnormality.

Treatment consists in surgical replacement of the viscus and repair of the diaphragmatic opening.

Sliding hernia

In this form the stomach slides upwards through the hiatus and part of it remains within the thorax with the cardia in this case within the thorax.

Symptoms are those of oesophagitis caused by reflux of gastric contents into the oesophagus (p. 206). The increased mass in the chest may lead to breathlessness if large, and increasing fibrosis may cause shortening of the oesophagus and thickening of the junction of the stomach and the oesophagus.

Treatment. This depends on the age and general condition of the patient, and while surgical treatment is the method of choice, the general condition of many of these patients precludes surgery without undue risk. In early cases and in young people conservative treatment should be fully exploited in the first place.

MALIGNANT DISEASE OF THE OESOPHAGUS

This disease is not uncommon and is one of the most disappointing forms of malignant disease to treat. The reasons for this is not only its inaccessibility, but the insidiousness of onset, which renders diagnosis difficult in the earlier and more amenable stages. It is a very rare occurrence for a surgeon to see an early cancer of the oesophagus. Consequently one cannot urge too strongly that those patients with a disability in swallowing, ought to be investigated without delay. For the most part this is a disease of advanced years, though it may be seen in fairly young people.

Symptoms. As already stated, this is an insidious affection and consists of vague discomfort, usually described as indigestion. There may be a sensation of something sticking and slight epigastric pain. Loss of weight is not an early sign, and when found, usually indicates an advanced lesion. When the disease spreads beyond the oesophagus, other symptoms may be caused such as laryngeal paralysis, from involvement of one of the laryngeal nerves. Cough may be due to pressure on trachea or bronchi, or may be caused by the overflow of secretions into the larynx. This is a late symptom.

Diagnosis. A careful history should always be obtained, and a general physical examination should be made to ascertain the presence of any complication such as glandular metastasis. The examination

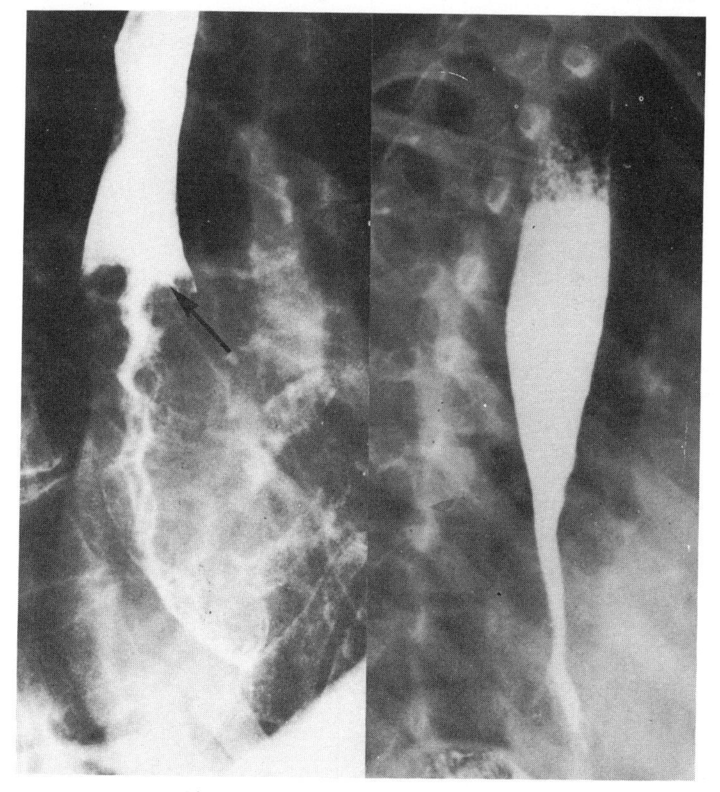

Fig. 66 Fig. 67

Fig. 66. Carcinoma of the oesophagus. Note irregularity of outline particularly the arrowed upper edge of growth.

Fig. 67. Congenital narrowing of the oesophagus. Note the smooth outline of the mucosa.

should also include the blood Wassermann reaction. Radiological investigation is essential and a barium swallow will in most cases demonstrate the lesion when present (Fig. 66). Confirmation of the diagnosis must also be obtained by oesophagoscopy, and a portion of tissue should be removed for examination by the pathologist. During the oesophagoscopy the opportunity should be taken to ascertain the exact location of the growth and its length, by actual measurement.

Treatment. Surgery offers the best chance of cure or effective palliation, especially in the lower and middle third of the oesophagus. Regrettably, however, most oesophageal cancers are inoperable, particularly those in the neck. If surgery is possible it involves removal of the oesophagus and its replacement by a suitable viscus. This usually involves bringing up either mobilised stomach or colon.

A few patients can be helped by means of radio-therapy, the source of energy being either cobalt or mega-voltage machine. Local application of radium or the interstitial use of radio-active seeds now has been abandoned.

Usually the surgeon must be satisfied with providing palliative treatment only. This may consist of insertion of a Souttar's tube through an oesophagoscope, or alternatively the larger Mousseau-Barbin tube. The latter is larger and functions better, but nearly always requires laparotomy for insertion. The tubes are not well tolerated in the cervical oesophagus, but at other sites can give useful relief of symptoms, especially when combined with radio-therapy in appropriate cases.

ACUTE OESOPHAGITIS

This can be caused by burns or direct trauma, or it may follow prolonged vomiting. It can complicate a thrush infection of the pharynx and commonly accompanies hiatal hernia.

The symptoms are those of a dull boring pain which is felt chiefly behind the sternum. The pain at times becomes acute in spasmodic fashion. There is always some degree of dysphagia.

On examination the mucosa is found to be of a darker colour than normal; it is thickened and may appear oedematous. The appearances are uniform round the circumference of the oesophagus. If the mucosa is rubbed or touched, it may be made to bleed readily and superficial ulceration may occur.

Treatment consists in dealing with the primary condition if possible, and soothing the inflamed mucous membrane. A bland fluid diet is necessary, and the administration of antacids will be of value in reducing gastric acidity. Where possible an upright posture should be maintained to prevent gastric contents flowing into the oesophagus. At night the head of the bed should be raised. Where hiatal hernia is the cause this should be treated with the appropriate surgical operation. In oesophagitis due to thrush Nystatin suspension must be given.

FOREIGN BODIES IN THE AIR AND FOOD PASSAGES

In this country foreign bodies in the air passages are rare. They occur chiefly in children, though occasionally they are encountered in adults.

In children the inhalation of a foreign body may easily escape notice, and for that reason any unexplained choking fit on the part of a child should be regarded with suspicion, particularly if any small object with which the child happened to be playing cannot be found.

Foreign bodies may be divided into two classes for the purpose of removal: those which require to be removed immediately, and those in which the surgeon can afford to study the problem and decide upon the best solution.

In the first class are those foreign bodies which are causing acute obstruction to airway. In this connection it is appropriate to remind the student that in such an emergency a tracheostomy may enable one completely unskilled in the practice of endoscopy to either grasp, or displace sufficiently, a foreign body and save a life.

Into this class fall also foreign bodies of vegetable origin as, for instance, a peanut. These produce severe bronchitis, with the disintegration of the foreign body and suppuration in the lung.

The other class includes all other foreign bodies which are not causing immediate danger to life.

Each foreign body presents a different problem which must be solved in its own appropriate fashion. There is time for proper preparation of

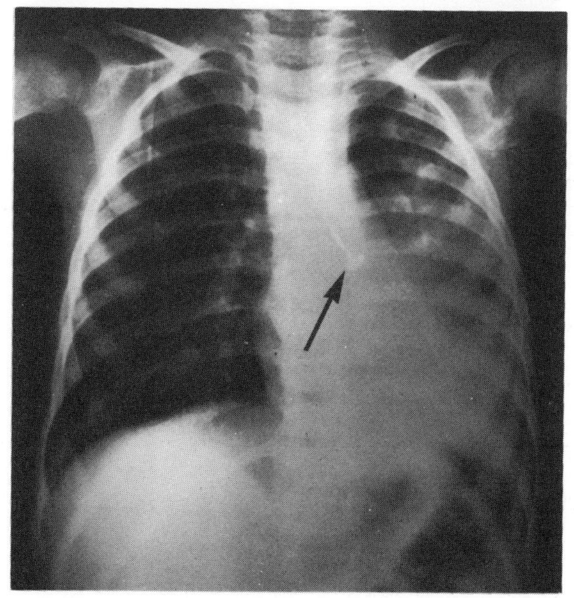

Fig. 68. Foreign body in the left bronchus; the left lung is collapsed.

the patient and careful radiographic study where the foreign body is radio-opaque. Practice of the necessary manoeuvres on a mannikin before attempting removal is advisable when difficulties are anticipated. Foreign bodies in the oesophagus may cause acute distress or obstruction, and so may demand immediate attention. Sharp bones and similar objects should be removed without undue delay. As most of these cases are now dealt with under general anaesthesia with tracheal intubation, proper preparation of the patient is essential, and the removal of a foreign body from the oesophagus is rarely sufficiently urgent a matter to justify hurried operative procedures. In dealing with radio-opaque objects X-ray studies should be made which show the foreign body in its widest diameters. The size of the foreign body is thus clearly shown.

Chevalier Jackson's dictum was that any object which can be swallowed or inhaled can be removed by bronchoscope or oesophagoscope if sufficient skill is available.

There is no limit to the types of foreign body which may be found in the oesophagus, for almost every object which can be placed in the mouth has been reported as having been removed from the oesophagus. The most common of all, perhaps, is the coin. This is encountered chiefly

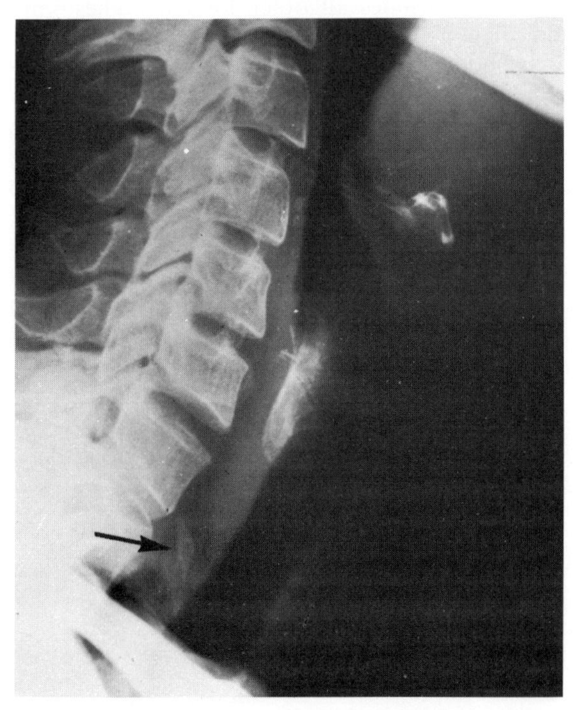

Fig. 69. Impacted meat bone at the upper end of the oesophagus.

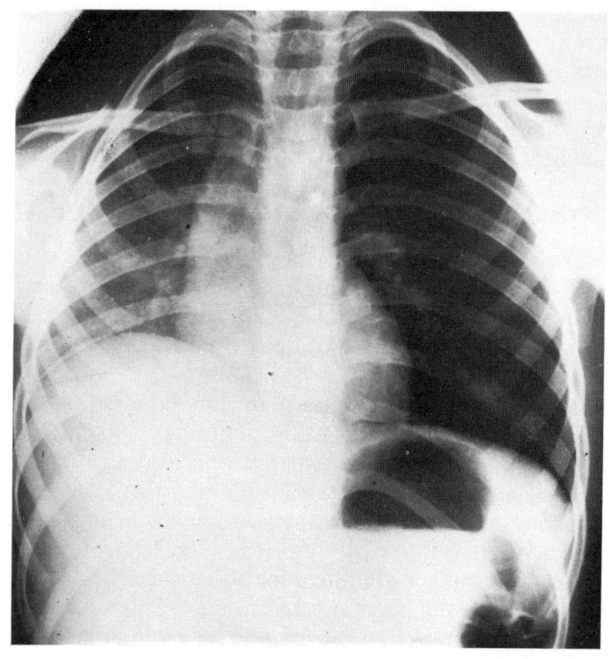

Fig. 70. Non-opaque foreign body in the left lung. Over distended left lung fails to deflate on expiration. Bronchoscopy showed a piece of apple core in the left main bronchus.

in children. This is almost always impacted at the upper end of the oesophagus, at the narrowing caused by the upper thoracic opening. Fish bones and meat bones and small dentures are the common foreign bodies encountered in adults. The removal of foreign bodies demands skill and experience on the part of the operator, and it is an operation which should never be attempted by the untrained (Figs. 68, 69, 70).

PERFORATION OF THE OESOPHAGUS

This may result from penetrating wounds of the neck, or it may come from within from a sharp foreign body which has been swallowed. Also endoscopic manipulations in the removal of foreign bodies, or in the dilatation of strictures, may cause injury. Perforation has been known to result from vomiting.

Symptoms. In the cervical part of the oesophagus rapid spread of surgical emphysema may occur, while in the lower part of the oesophagus emphysema appears more slowly but there is acute retrosternal pain. The effects of perforation are always serious and frequently fatal. There may be severe shock and early death from massive infection.

Treatment. In the cervical region immediate operation is indicated to expose the injured oesophagus and drain the fascial planes around it.

If possible the injury should be sutured and a feeding tube passed into the stomach. Heavy doses of antibiotics are given immediately. In the lower part of the oesophagus the assistance of a thoracic surgeon is required and it may be advisable to wait for a short time before advising operation. Nothing should be given by mouth; fluids are given intravenously with heavy doses of a broad-spectrum antibiotic.

CORROSIVE INJURIES OF THE OESOPHAGUS

The swallowing of strong alkalis or acids in children, or in suicide attempts in adults, is the usual cause. The immediate problem is relief of shock and pain and the administration of a suitable, weak neutralizing agent. Serious disturbance of body fluids and electrolyte control may be an early complication.

A very serious complication which appears later is that of stricture formation. It is essential to prevent this if at all possible. It can usually be achieved by gently passing an indwelling feeding tube within the first couple of days. Systemic steroids should also be started at this stage to discourage fibrosis. Oesophagoscopy can be hazardous and is of doubtful advantage.

The feeding tube must be retained for about three weeks, after which the patient can as a rule begin normal feeding. It is necessary to keep these patients under observation for several months in case stricture formation should occur at a later stage and necessitate further treatment.

SECTION 6 THE EAR

28. Anatomy

THE EXTERNAL EAR

The external ear comprises the auricle, the external cartilaginous meatus and the external bony meatus.

The auricle is composed of cartilage which is covered with perichondrium, to which the skin and superficial tissues are very closely bound down. The external cartilaginous meatus is similarly constructed, and, in addition, contains hair follicles and glands which secrete wax. The hair follicles extend only for a short distance into the ear and are not found in the deeper parts of the external meatus. Owing to the close union of cartilage and skin any inflammatory lesion, such as a boil in the cartilaginous portion of the external meatus, is an acutely painful infection.

The epithelium lining the external meatus is continued on to the surface of the drum membrane as a single layer of stratified epithelium.

The nerve supply is from the auriculo-temporal nerve. The auricular branch of the vagus supplies part of the bony meatus and is believed to include a small sensory twig from the facial nerve.

The *external meatus* varies in size and form with growth. There are also considerable variations in individuals. In the adult there is an angle in the meatus. The outer part runs upwards, forwards and inwards and the inner part runs more horizontally. This renders the use of a speculum and a certain amount of upward traction on the auricle necessary in order to expose the drum membrane. In children, on the other hand, the meatus is shorter and straighter, and the drum of a child's ear can frequently be examined quite easily without the aid of a speculum.

The tympanic membrane. The tympanic membrane consists of three layers—an outer epithelial layer, a middle layer of yellow elastic fibrous tissue and an inner layer of mucous membrane. The drum membrane is supported around its periphery by the *annulus*, which is a bone developed separately from the body of the petrous bone and forming eventually one of the component parts of the petrous bone. This ring is deficient in one small portion of the upper part of the circumference. The deficiency is known as the *Notch of Rivinus*.

The drum membrane is divided into two parts, the pars tensa and the pars flaccida. In the latter the fibrous layer is absent, hence the flaccidity.

Landmarks of the drum of the ear. The most prominent landmark is the handle of the malleus, seen as a white streak running down to the approximate centre of the drum. At its upper end is a small projection known as the short process (Fig. 80).

In the drum membrane are two folds stretching anteriorly and posteriorly from the short process. They are known as the anterior and posterior mallear folds and the part of the drum above this level is the pars flaccida.

THE MIDDLE EAR

The middle ear cleft comprises the middle ear, the Eustachian tube, the mastoid antrum and cells. The middle ear can be divided into three portions, the uppermost portion is the *attic*, the middle portion the *mesotympanum*, and the lowest portion the *hypotympanum*. The attic is that part of the middle ear above the level of the mallear folds. It is divided into a number of small pockets by the contained ossicles, their ligaments and mucosal folds. Chronic infection may localize in these spaces. (See Attic Suppuration.) It should be noted that the middle ear extends beyond the limits of the drum (Fig. 71).

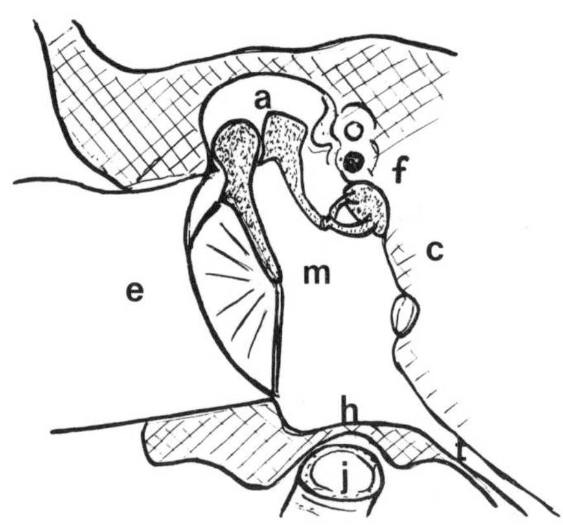

Fig. 71. Diagram showing coronal section of middle ear. (e) bony part of external auditory meatus. (m) middle ear containing the malleus, incus, and stapes; (c) position of cochlea. Note that the middle ear cleft extends a substantial distance beyond the limits of the drum. Superiorly it extends into the attic (a), above which is the middle cranial fossa. Inferiorly it extends into the hypotympanum below which are the jugular bulb (j) and the internal carotid. The position of the Eustachian tube is indicated at (t) and the facial nerve at (f).

The anterior wall of the middle ear has an opening low down in the wall. This is the opening of the *Eustachian tube*. Above it is the canal for the *tensor tympani* muscle (Fig. 72).

The posterior wall contains an opening high up which is the *aditus* leading to the mastoid antrum. Just below it is the point of attachment of the stapedius muscle – the *pyramid*.

The outer wall is formed chiefly by the tympanic membrane and the outer bony wall of the attic.

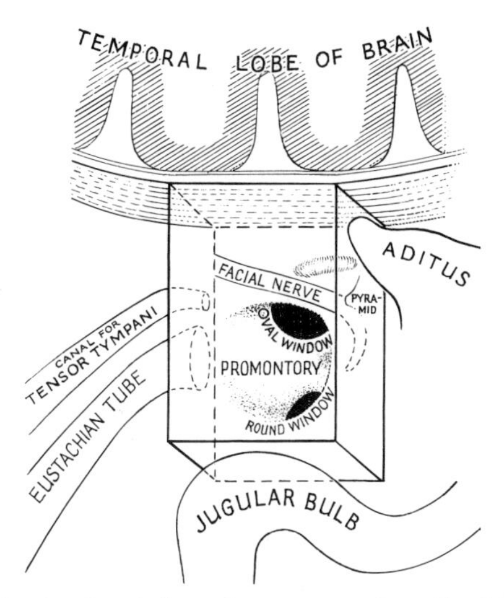

Fig. 72. Diagram showing the relations of structures to the walls of the left middle ear.

There are several important structures on the medial wall. From above downwards there is first the anterior part of the *horizontal semicircular canal*. Immediately below this, crossing the middle ear, is the canal containing the facial nerve. Below this again, posteriorly, is an opening which is known as the *oval window*, while anteriorly is seen an eminence known as the *promontory* – the lowest turn of the cochlea. Slightly posterior to the promontory is the opening of the *round window*.

Under the floor of the middle ear lies the jugular bulb, while above the middle ear is the dura mater of the middle fossa.

The middle ear contains three ossicles, the malleus, incus and stapes (Fig. 71). The handle of the malleus is firmly embedded in the middle layer of the drum and its head articulates in the attic with the body of the incus. The incus has two processes, a short process and a long. The short process is attached to the lip of the aditus, and the other, known as the long process, descends to articulate with the head of the stapes. The stapes closely resembles a stirrup and its footplate occupies the oval window, to the margin of which it is attached by the annular ligament, so forming the stapedio-vestibular joint. This joint is a simple fibrous one whereas those between the malleus, incus and stapes are synovial.

Malleus and incus move as a unit, essentially as a lever. The movement of the stapes is more complex; its footplate has a tilting movement, the axis of which alters with sound intensity under the influence of the middle ear muscles.

Muscles of the middle ear. There are two muscles in the middle ear – (1) the *tensor tympani*, inserted into the neck of the malleus and supplied by the trigeminal nerve, (2) *stapedius*, inserted into the neck of the stapes and supplied by the facial nerve. The latter comes into action in response to loud noise, the louder the noise the stronger it contracts. The effect is to restrict the vibration of the drum and ossicular chain by increasing their tension and stiffness. The sensitivity of the ear is thus reduced and the delicate structures of the cochlea are protected against damage.

Blood and nerve supply of the middle ear. The middle ear is supplied by twigs from the surrounding arteries, and the sensory nerve-supply is through the tympanic plexus and some twigs from the carotid plexus. The facial nerve has been mentioned in its course across the middle ear. The *chorda tympani* crosses the middle ear in a fold of mucous membrane between the handle of the malleus and the long process of the incus.

The mastoid antrum. This space lies just behind the middle ear. It varies considerably in size, and communicates with the middle ear by the aditus in front and with the mastoid cells behind.

This cell system may be completely absent or may extend widely throughout the mastoid bone in groups (Fig. 73).

These include:

1. *Mastoid tip cells;* these may consist of one very large cell.
2. *Perisinus cells*, overlying the lateral sinus.
3. *Petrosal angle cells*, in the angle between the dura and the lateral wall.
4. *Subdural cells*, between the roof of the mastoid antrum and the dural plate.
5. *Zygomatic cells*, extending into the zygoma.
6. *Facial cells*, running deep under the posterior meatal wall down to the facial nerve.
7. *Labyrinthine cells*, surrounding the semicircular canals.

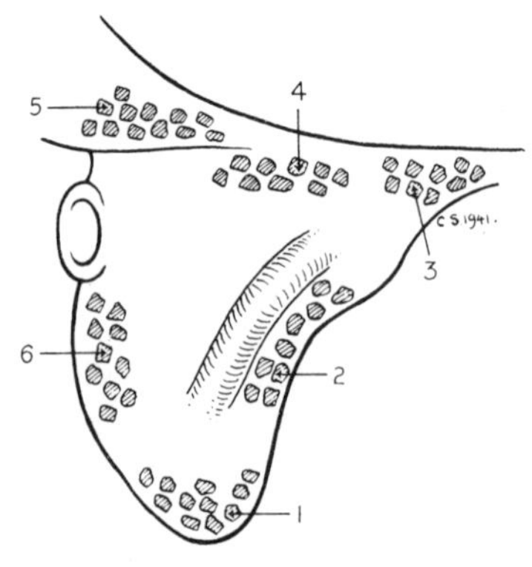

Fig. 73. Groups of mastoid cells. (1) Tip; (2) perisinus; (3) petrosal angle; (4) subdural; (5) zygomatic; (6) facial.

The Eustachian tube. The Eustachian tube communicates with the nasopharynx. It is potentially patent and may be opened by movement of the pharynx. It has a bony upper portion and membranous lower portion, and the lower end is protected by a cartilaginous structure which forms an eminence round the mouth of the tube, and is known as the Eustachian cushion. The mucous membrane of the pharynx lines the Eustachian tube and is therefore continuous with that of the middle ear.

There is a free blood-supply, and lymphoid tissue is found in the lower part.

THE INNER EAR

The inner ear or labyrinth consists of a bony capsule which is almost embedded in the petrous bone and within which is the membranous labyrinth. The bony capsule consists of three parts (*a*) posteriorly, three semicircular canals, (*b*) in the middle, the vestibule, (*c*) anteriorly, the snail-like cochlea (Fig. 74). The entire bone is hollow and contains perilymph. Suspended in the perilymph by delicate filamentous strands is the membranous labyrinth. This is a complex series of sacs and tubes containing a different fluid, the endolymph (Fig. 75).

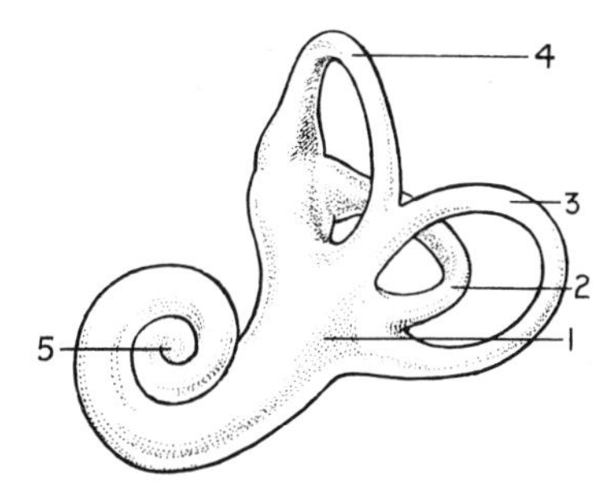

Fig. 74. The bony labyrinth on the right side, viewed from within. (1) Vestibule; (2) horizontal canal; (3) posterior vertical canal; (4) superior canal; (5) cochlea.

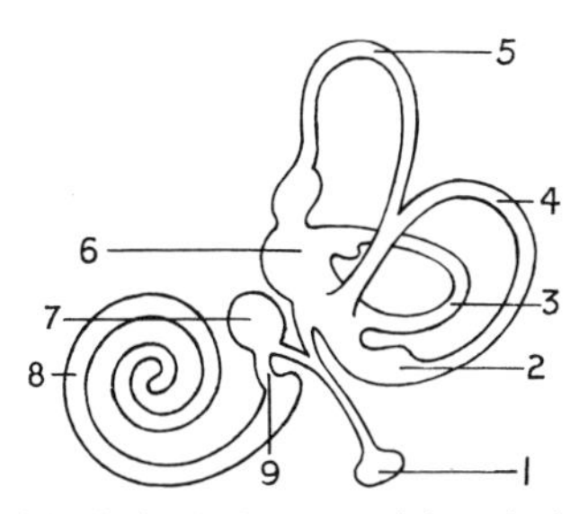

Fig. 75. The membranous labyrinth. (1) Saccus endolymphaticus; (2) ampulla of posterior vertical canal; (3) horizontal canal; (4) posterior canal; (5) superior canal; (6) utricle; (7) saccule; (8) membranous cochlea; (9) canalis reuniens.

The membranous labyrinth consists of three semicircular canals, which occupy the corresponding bony canal and are set at right angles to each other, each representing a plane in space. They are named horizontal, anterior vertical and posterior vertical (Fig. 75). The two vertical canals share a common crus. The anterior end of each canal is dilated to form its ampulla, and this region contains a patch of neuro-epithelium called the crista, the hairs of which are embedded in the overlying gelatinous cupola. This is displaced when endolymph movement occurs. The normal stimulus to excite the ampullary nerve is angular acceleration, but in clinical testing artificial currents are produced by caloric stimulation.

The five ends of the canals open into the utricle, this and the saccule both lie in the vestibule of the bony labyrinth and each possesses a patch of neuro-epithelium known as the macula. This resembles the ampullary crista except that the overlying membrane is flatter and contains particles of calcium carbonate called otoliths. The macula of the utricle is stimulated by gravitational pull and linear acceleration, the saccule probably has a similar function though experimentally it can be stimulated by sound. The utricle and saccule are joined by the Y-shaped endolymphatic duct, the stem of which extends to the saccus endolymphaticus. This lies between the two layers of dura on the posterior surface of the petrous bone, *i.e.* in the posterior cranial fossa. The saccus in man is probably concerned with absorption of endolymph.

The membranous cochlear duct is a simple tube situated in the bony cochlea and coiled for two and a half turns around its central bony modiolus. Its small connection to the saccule is called the ductus reuniens.

When seen in the bisected bony cochlea, the cochlear duct appears triangular in cross section (Figs. 76–77) in each turn. Its three sides are formed by Reissner's membrane, the stria vascularis and the basilar membrane. The cochlear duct is so situated that it is bathed by perilymph on two sides only, in the scala vestibuli on its apical aspect and in the scala tympani on its basal side. In the basal turn these two scalae end at the oval window and the round window respectively, but at the apex they are continuous with each other around the end of the cochlear duct. The scala tympani connects with the subarachnoid space, to which infection can spread from the labyrinth.

The neuro-epithelium of the cochlea is arranged as a ribbon along the entire length of the basilar membrane and is known as the organ of Corti. The particular area activated by a sound depends on the frequency, the high frequencies being represented at the basal end.

The ampullary, utricular and saccular nerves unite to form the vestibular nerve, the ganglion of which lies in the internal auditory meatus. The spiral ganglion of the cochclear nerve is situated in the modiolus. Vestibular and cochlear nerves together constitute the eighth cranial nerve.

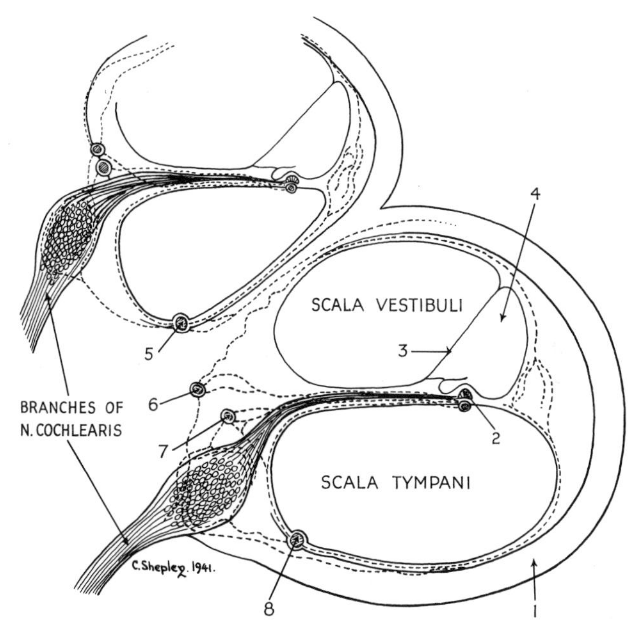

Fig. 76. Diagram of cochlea. (1) bony wall; (2) organ of Corti;(3) Reissner's membrane; (4) ductus cochlearis; (5), (6), (7), (8) auditory vessels.

The internal ear is supplied by the internal auditory branch of the basilar artery.

EXAMINATION OF THE EAR

The ear is examined by means of a projected light and a speculum, which aids in opening out the external meatus. The light may be projected upon the ear by one or more methods.

The usual method is to use the forehead mirror and an outside source of illumination, such as an examination lamp or daylight; or the light may be incorporated in the speculum as in the case of the electric auriscope. Each method has its advantages and its disadvantages. The advantages of the forehead mirror with an outside source of illumination are that there is small room for mechanical error, and it can be used with little or no preparation. Also the light can be focussed and a much more powerful illumination of the part under examination can be obtained. The disadvantage is that a considerable amount of technical skill is required to arrive at a satisfactory conclusion in the examination. The electric auriscope is simpler to use in the hands of the unskilled, as it does not require an outside source of illumination. On the other hand, it is dependent upon batteries and electric bulbs, and as these are sometimes unreliable the examiner may on occasion

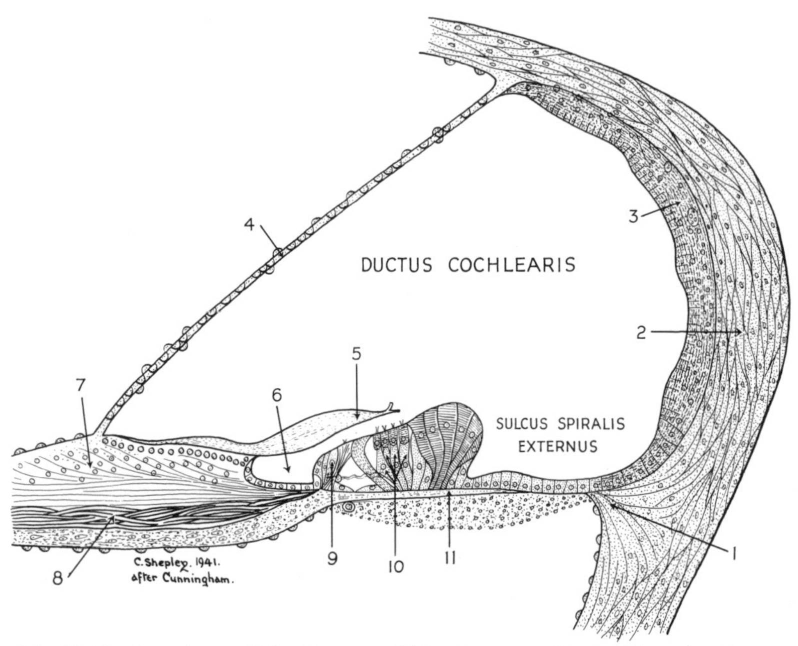

Fig. 77. Cochlear duct and Corti's organ. (1) Basilar crest; (2) spiral ligament; (3) vascular stria; Reissner's membrane; (5) tectorial membrane; (6) internal sulcus; (7) spiral lamina; (8) auditory nerve; (10) organ of Corti; (11) basilar membrane.

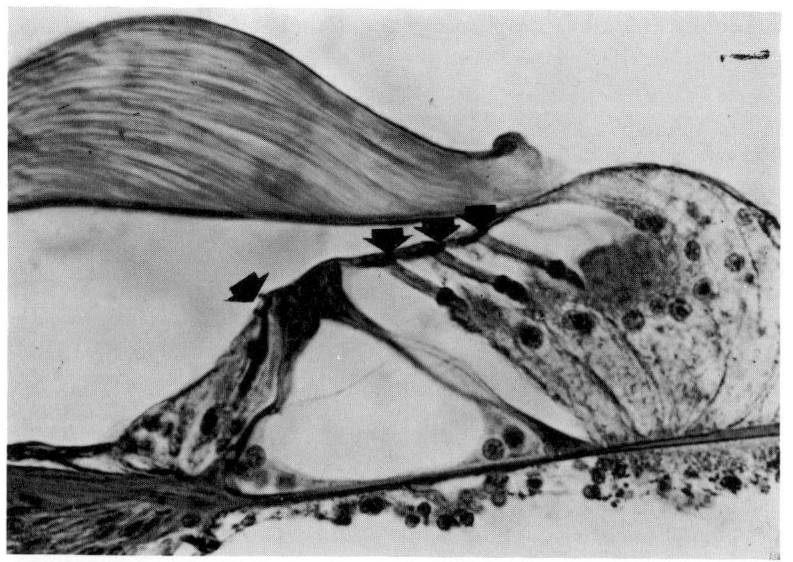

Fig. 78. Organ of Corti. The sensory hair cells are arrowed. There are three rows of outer hair cells and one row of inner hair cells along the entire length of the basilar membrane. The hair cells are responsible for the transformation of mechanical into electrical energy.

find himself without the means of examining the ear. The illumination also leaves something to be desired, and as the focus of these instruments is fixed in some instances it is found impossible to focus the tympanum properly. The usual method for examination in a consulting room is by means of head mirror and fixed illumination.

The position of the patient and the examiner is of importance. The patient faces the examiner and the light is placed a little behind the patient, on a level with the left ear. The examiner sits close alongside or in front of the patient, within easy reach for manipulation of the head. The light must be freely movable in all directions, as several different positions may be required in order to carry out the examination adequately. The light from the mirror is then focussed upon the patient's ear. The smallest and brightest spot of light should be obtained. The examiner is then ready to begin the examination.

In the examination of the left ear the patient's head is turned slightly to the right, or, if the patient is in a movable chair, the chair can be rotated a little to the right. The left hand of the examiner grasps the upper part of the pinna, the pinna being held between the second and third or the third and fourth fingers. The speculum is placed in the external meatus with the right hand, and is then taken between the thumb and first finger of the left hand so that the right hand is left free for mopping secretions, removal of wax, etc. The object of this grasp of the pinna is to enable sufficient traction to be put upon the cartilaginous meatus to draw it backwards and upwards to straighten out the angle of the meatus (Fig. 79).

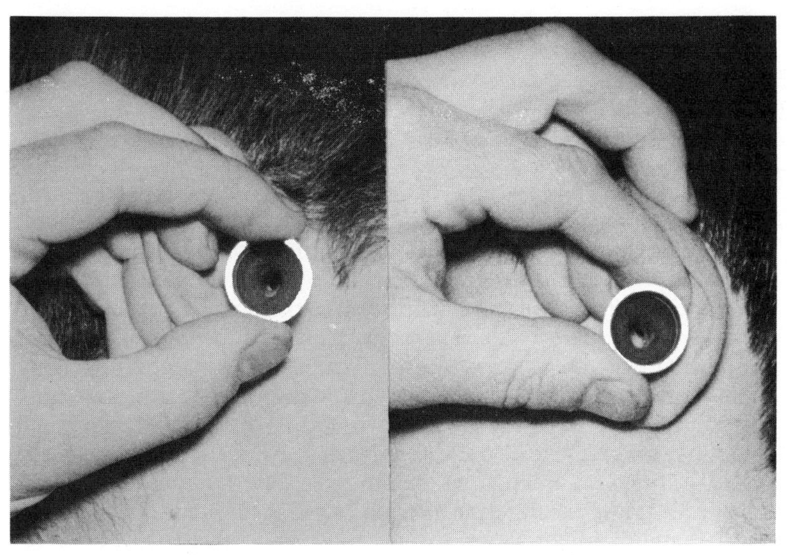

(*a*) Right ear (*b*) Left ear

Fig. 79. Method of holding speculum and retracting pinna. The right hand remains free.

With this gentle traction upwards and backwards the drum should be brought into view without trouble. One of the chief difficulties in the examination of the external meatus is the failure to ensure that the light is focussed in the proper direction. The light must be directed forwards and upwards, and in some cases the patient's head may have to be turned almost away from the examiner, whose head is in a low position. Or, alternatively, the patient's head can be tilted away from the examiner in order to be able to expose the drum. If the speculum is held properly and the patient's head is at the correct angle, the examiner should be looking at the tympanum. The identification of the tympanum is made partly by the *colour*, which should be pearly-grey. It is lustrous and reflects the light. The *light reflex* takes the shape of a cone in the lower anterior part (Fig. 80).

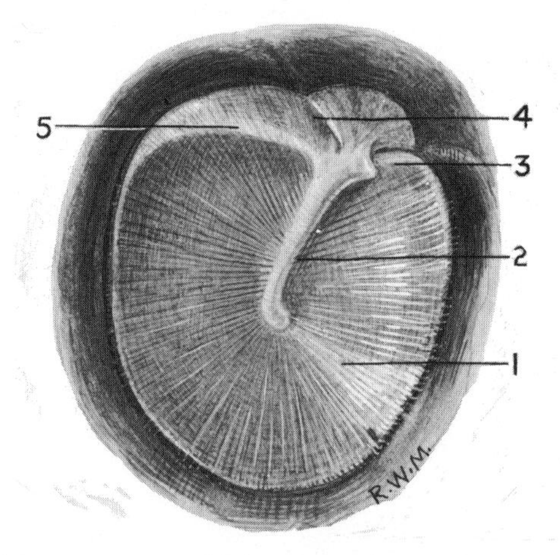

Fig. 80. Normal drum. (1) Cone of light; (2) handle of malleus surmounted by short process; (3) anterior horizontal fold; (4) attic; (5) posterior horizontal fold.

Certain landmarks must be sought in order to identify the drum. The first and most important is the *short process* of the malleus, which stands out from the drum as a small white knob about two-thirds of the way up the drum. From this a whitish streak should be seen extending downwards and backwards. This is the handle of the malleus. If these can be seen, then the drum is located. The examiner should look again at the short process of the malleus, and a fold should be seen stretching posteriorly from the process which is the *posterior horizontal fold*. Anteriorly may be seen also the *anterior fold*.

The drum lies at an angle to the observer. The upper posterior part is the nearest and the anterior inferior part is farthest away. The angle in different individuals varies considerably; but all the structures noted above are seen at an angle.

When the drum is identified any deviation from normal must be sought, *e.g.* colour, retraction or fullness, increased vascularity, scars, perforations, etc. It is also important to examine its movement by using a pneumatic speculum in order to detect underlying adhesions. Adequate magnification should be used to examine any suspected abnormality. It is also convenient to examine Eustachian tube patency at this stage by watching for drum movement when the patient autoinflates (see p. 222). Not all persons, however, can perform this manoeuvre, so failure does not necessarily indicate tubal occlusion.

If the drum cannot be seen, the examiner must not be satisfied until he has found the reason for failure. It may be that his light is not properly focussed, or it may be thrown in the wrong direction, the result of which will be that only the posterior wall of the meatus will be illuminated. Again, something may be obstructing the meatus. If this is suspected, note must be made of the colour of the obstruction, the distance of the obstruction from the speculum and its approximate consistency. Another cause of failure is narrowness of the meatus. This may be caused by inflammation of the lining membrane of the external meatus or by the presence of a boil.

The position and extent of tenderness must be ascertained, and any discharge which is present must be carefully traced to its source. If the obstruction is due to discharge or suspected wax, the ear should be syringed clean and the examination repeated. If there is a mass in the meatus which prevents an adequate view, the examiner must be prepared to identify this particular mass.

Difficulty usually arises when there is uncertainty whether the light is being directed in the correct manner or not. A good rule with regard to these obstructions is that if an ordinary-sized speculum can touch the object which is obstructing the view, then the depth of the drum has not been reached.

The obstruction may be caused by wax. This is readily identified by means of its dark brown, sometimes almost black coloration, and it can be touched without discomfort to the patient. Furuncles may also obstruct the view of the drum, but the extreme sensitiveness in such a case will readily show that acute inflammation is present. A polypus may likewise form an obstruction which is easily reached by the speculum. Polypi are, as a rule, insensitive and may be moved about by a probe.

Accumulations of debris, such as are encountered in cases of otitis externa, may require to be removed before an adequate view of the drum can be obtained. If anything of this nature obstructs the view of the drum of the ear, the obstruction should be examined carefully with the aid of a probe. If this is done with sufficient gentleness no discomfort will be caused to the patient and an accurate diagnosis is more likely to be made.

The greatest difficulties are likely to be encountered in cases in which the drum is completely absent, as, if the ear is dry, it may be very difficult for the inexperienced examiner to decide whether the drum has been reached or not. The depth of the examined object will sometimes give a clue to its nature, and the remains of the drum will usually be seen when careful examination of the periphery of the meatus is made. A history of chronic otitis will generally point to there having been some damage to the middle ear.

EXAMINATION OF THE EUSTACHIAN TUBE

Exclusion of Eustachian tube obstruction is an important part of the examination of the ear, especially if a conductive type of deafness is present.

Valsalva's method

This is conveniently done whilst the drum is kept under observation. The patient is instructed to take a breath, keep the nose tightly pinched and the lips firmly closed, and then forcibly attempt to blow the nose. The drum will be seen to move outward and a click may be audible. Not all patients however, can succeed in auto-inflation. It should never be done where there is nasal infection.

It should be emphasized that none of these methods does more than demonstrate that air can be forced up the tube. They give no indication of its functional patency. For this, various manometric methods are available, but none is entirely satisfactory.

When Valsalva's method of auto-inflation fails, inflation with Politzer bag or catheter may be successful.

Politzer's method

The simplest method of examination of the tube is by means of the Politzer bag. The olive attachment is applied to one nostril; the other nostril is closed with a finger while the olive is made to form an airtight joint in the nostril. The patient is then told to blow the cheeks out hard, or, alternatively, close off the nasopharynx by means of swallowing. At the moment of the closure of the nasopharynx the bag is compressed sharply and the intra-nasal pressure thereby raised considerably above normal. The result of this is to force air up the Eustachian tube. This is a simple procedure which can be carried out in the consulting-room. It is in many cases effective in relieving obstruction and restoring hearing.

Inflation with catheter

The catheter method of inflation is more accurate and gives greater information. The Eustachian catheter is a metal tube which can be obtained in various sizes. It is curved at one end, and at the other end has a fitting for taking the Politzer bag. A dressed probe is moistened in 10 per cent cocaine and passed through the inferior meatus before the catheter is used. This will save the patient a considerable amount of distress. The catheter is introduced through the nose, so that the end of it lies in the opening of the Eustachian tube, and, on application of the Politzer bag to the catheter, air is blown into the Eustachian tube. The method of insertion of the catheter is as follows: The curved point of the catheter is placed in the floor of the nose; it is then pushed backwards along the inferior meatus, at the same time the handle of the catheter is raised and it is pushed backwards until the posterior pharyngeal wall is reached. The point of the catheter is then turned outwards, about 30 degrees. If the catheter is drawn forwards the point will be felt to slip over the Eustachian cushion, and if it is then turned through a right angle in the same direction the point will slip into the mouth of the Eustachian tube. If the auscultation tube is placed in the patient's ear and the other end in the ear of the examiner, when air is blown through the catheter characteristic sounds should be heard by the examiner. A soft, clear, blowing sound indicates a patent tube; bubbling sounds indicate catarrh in the tube.

Difficulties of catheterization. There may be a deviation of the nasal septum or enlargement of the conchae, which renders it difficult to pass the catheter back through the nose. In such cases the bend at the end of the catheter is reduced. A small bend may enable the catheter to be passed through the nose. Sometimes it will be found possible to pass the catheter successfully by hooking the end into the inferior meatus and passing it posteriorly with the point up. On occasion it will be found useful to pass the catheter through the opposite nostril.

If deafness is due to tubal blockage then introduction of air in this way should give immediate improvement in hearing.

Formerly catherization was sometimes combined with introduction of bougies to dilate strictures, or with introduction of oils and drugs to promote decongestion. Such treatment is now seldom indicated.

29. Physiology of the Ear

The middle ear mechanism

For successful stimulation of the cochlea via the middle ear it is essential for a sound pressure differential to be present between the oval and round windows. In the normal ear this is obtained by the preferential transmission of vibration through the drum and the ossicular chain. Comparatively little sound travels direct to the round window; indeed, the presence of the drum itself provides for its *sound protection*.

Although the ossicular chain provides certain acoustic advantages and is a highly efficient part of the *sound transformer* mechanism of the middle ear, a simple columella is compatible with comparatively good hearing. This is the principle in certain types of tympanoplasty.

Good hearing can indeed be obtained without an ossicular chain as long as there are two mobile windows and sound protection for one is provided, *e.g.* by the remains of the drum. Some tympanoplasty and fenestration operations depend on this mechanism.

Interruption of the ossicular chain or total loss of the drum result in severe hearing loss largely because there is no difference in the pressure of sound reaching the two windows.

Reference has already been made to the action of the middle ear muscles (p. 213).

The cochlear mechanism

The cochlea can be stimulated directly by bone conduction as well as by sound passing through the middle ear. It is generally agreed that sound waves are analysed in the cochlea and that each frequency has its own place on the basilar membrane. There is ample evidence to support the place theories, with the higher frequencies being represented in the basal part of the cochlea and the lower frequencies in the apex. Helmholtz looked upon the basilar membrane as a simple resonator, but it has long been recognized that the mechanism is far more complicated than this.

Complex mechanical experiments as well as observation of the basilar membrane in action by the Nobel prize-winner von Bekesy resulted in his *travelling-wave* theory. He was able to show that vibration introduced into the oval window of his models resulted in a wave travelling up the basilar membrane, increasing in amplitude as it moved, and finally dying away. The point of maximum amplitude was determined by the frequency introduced, and occurred at a corresponding distance along the basilar membrane.

The means by which the complex pattern of sound energy is transformed in the organ of Corti into electrical energy suitable for transmission by the neural pathways, remains obscure in spite of increasing knowledge concerning electrolyte behaviour in the cochlea and the various electrical potentials.

EXAMINATION OF HEARING

There are two chief classes of hearing loss and the first step is to determine which is present or whether the hearing loss is of mixed type.

The terminology is somewhat confusing. The classes are:

1. **Conductive deafness** (also known as obstructive or middle ear deafness). This results from any interruption to the passage of sound up to and including the stapedo-vestibular joint.

2. **Sensori-neural deafness.** Terms, such as 'nerve deafness' and 'perceptive deafness' are out-dated. Various components of the sensori-neural system are recognised, but special tests are necessary to identify lesions of individual parts. A sensory hearing loss arises when the lesion is in the cochlea. A neural lesion is one in which a lesion affects the VIII nerve, though it is important to recognise that lesions may also affect the central neural pathways including the auditory cortex. Furthermore, one sometimes has to consider lesions of the 'perceptual' part of the central nervous system, i.e. the area of the auditory pathway close to the cortex. This has not yet been anatomically identified, but is concerned with the organisation of auditory information and when deranged may cause language impairment and communication difficulties without any hearing defect as such that can at present be recognised by audiometric testing. Non-communicating children, language-impaired children, and patients with sensori-aphasias, probably suffer from disorders of this area of the sensori-neural hearing system.

3. **Mixed deafness.** In many instances both types of deafness are present, as in people suffering from such conditions as otitis media or otosclerosis with cochlear damage. The correct assessment of hearing may be difficult but is important for prognosis and proper treatment.

Having decided whether the patient is suffering from conductive or sensori-neural deafness, which, as a rule is possible by tuning-fork tests, the second step is to determine the degree of deafness. The third is to give a prognosis concerning the disease and the results of any treatment proposed.

Tuning-fork tests

The diagnosis between the chief types of deafness is made by means of tuning-forks. These forks are of various types; the most useful type for this examination is one of about 512 double vibrations per second, and it should be clamped to eliminate the overtones as far as possible.

Rinne's test. This test indicates whether conductive deafness is present or not. The test is carried out thus: A tuning-fork is sounded and held in front of the ear with the points close to and in line with the external auditory meatus. The patient is asked frequently whether the tuning-fork is heard. As soon as the patient ceases to hear the tuning-fork it is transferred to the mastoid process. If it is not heard there, the procedure is reversed, and if the tuning-fork is heard by air conduction after it is heard by bone conduction, then Rinne's test is said to be positive – the normal state of affairs in a healthy middle ear. If the tuning-fork is heard when it is transferred to the mastoid process, after it has ceased to be heard by air, then bone conduction is said to be better than air conduction, and Rinne's test is negative.

Where the Rinne test is positive, it may be concluded that there is no marked degree of conductive deafness, but any deafness present must be of sensori-neural type.

Weber's test. This test is used for comparing the degree of deafness in two ears, both of which are affected in the same way. It depends upon the fact shown by the previous test, that in conductive deafness bone conduction is better than air conduction. The tuning-fork is sounded and placed upon the vertex, and the patient is asked in which ear the sound is best heard. In a conductive deafness of one ear the patient can be expected to point to the ear in which there is conductive deafness as the ear in which the sound is clearest. If both ears are affected by conductive deafness the tuning-fork will be heard in that which is the more affected.

In sensori-neural deafness the position is reversed. In ears which have sensori-neural deafness, presuming that the middle ear is normal, the sound being conveyed to the ear entirely by bone conduction will then be heard more loudly by the ear with the better functioning nerve and cochlea.

Schwabach's test. This test has a twofold purpose. It can detect sensori-neural deafness not only where this is the sole cause of the hearing defect, but also the underlying degree of sensori-neural deafness in those cases which are suffering from conductive deafness.

The test is carried out as follows: The tuning-fork is sounded and is placed upon the mastoid process of the patient. Whenever the patient ceases to hear the tuning-fork it is transferred to the mastoid process of the examiner, and if the examiner can hear the tuning-fork the Schwabach test on the patient is said to be shortened. This test presupposes perfect hearing on the part of the examiner, and if he has defective hearing this test, to have any value, must be done with a stop-watch and a predetermined normal. Testing should ideally be carried out under conditions free from ambient noise. If this is not possible the accuracy of the Schwabach test can be improved by closing the meatus of the patient and also that of the examiner to minimize distraction from outside noise.

There are other tests, but the foregoing are the most useful and they will serve to distinguish between the various types of deafness.

Measurement of deafness

The simplest method is to ascertain at what distance the patient can hear conversation voice or whisper in one ear, the other ear being covered. With practice an examiner who is constantly testing patients will use a voice of approximately equal loudness each time. This provides a useful clinical guide but is of course not of scientific accuracy. Alternatively a watch can be used.

The most satisfactory way of recording hearing is by audiometer, of which there are two types, pure-tone and speech.

The pure-tone audiometer gives a range of pure tones, the intensity of which can be adjusted in 5 decibel steps. The range of frequencies provided is between 64 and 8,000 cycles per second. Sound can be presented to the patient by air or by bone conduction. The latter as a rule gives a fairly accurate indication of sensori-neural function and is an essential part of the test when an operation for improvement of hearing is being considered.

A graph can be charted showing the hearing loss for a particular patient and a record kept for future reference. Such an audiogram is also valuable in the prescription of a hearing aid to meet the precise needs of the patient (Fig. 81).

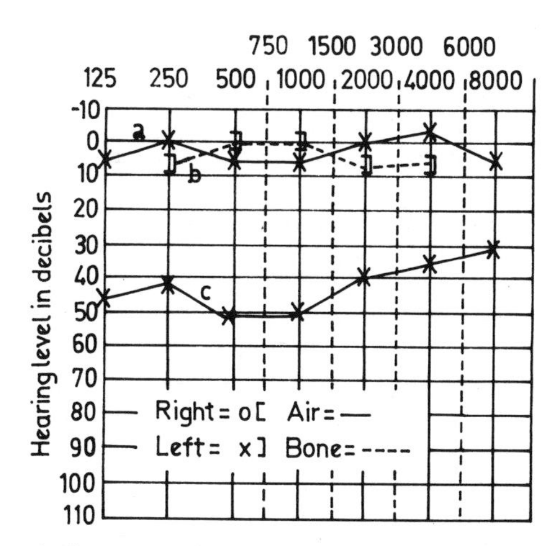

Fig. 81. Pure tone Audiogram.—Shows normal levels of hearing for (a) air conduction; (b) bone conduction, for a left ear. (c) shows air conduction curve for pure conductive type hearing loss.

When sensori-neural deafness has been diagnosed it may be necessary to test for the phenomenon of *recruitment*. There are a number of related tests which help to distinguish a sensory lesion (*e.g.* Menière's disease) from a neural one (*e.g.* acoustic neuroma). They depend upon the fact that in sensory lesions, although the hearing threshold is raised, there is increasing sensitivity at intensities above threshold. To put it simply, the deaf ear hears loud sounds abnormally loudly.

The speech audiometer consists essentially of a receiver, a high fidelity amplifier and a source of speech. This may be tape or gramophone records, or occasionally live monitored speech. Phonetically balanced lists of words are delivered in calibrated volume and the result recorded on chart as the percentage of words correctly heard and repeated for each intensity employed (Fig. 82).

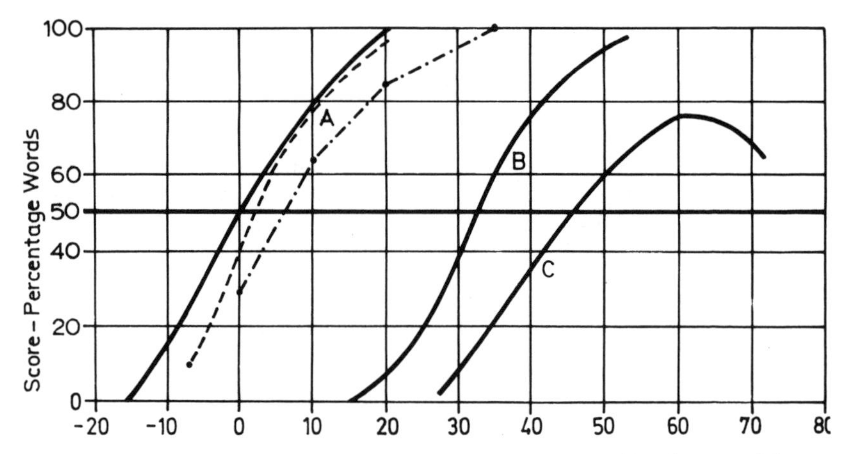

Fig. 82. Speech audiogram. – (A) Thick line shows average normal hearing, dotted lines indicate typical curves for patient with hearing within normal limits. (B) shows typical conductive hearing loss of approx. 33 db. shift. (C) shows curve of sensori-neural hearing loss of 45 db. Note that the discrimination score falls with increasing intensity.

The intensity at which 50 per cent of the words are correctly heard is known as the speech reception threshold (S.R.T.) and the subject's deviation from normal is recorded as so many decibels.

By increasing the intensity another 20 db a person with normal hearing or a pure conductive deafness will hear 100 per cent of the words correctly. But in sensori-neural deafness, and especially in neural deafness, the maximum discrimination score falls markedly and the patient becomes confused by the extra volume.

Speech audiometry is of great value not only in diagnosis, but also in assessing suitability for operation and in the evaluation of hearing aids. The test is clearly more closely related to the patient's problem than is pure tone testing.

Examination of cases of severe deafness

In examination of patients who are suffering from severe forms of deafness several difficulties are encountered. Tuning-fork tests, such as Rinne's, Weber's and Schwabach's, are comparatively simple to carry out, but are very liable to be misinterpreted owing to the fact that the patients give what they consider helpful answers, or they may actually misinterpret the sounds heard.

One of the chief sources of fallacy is that in cases of advanced conductive deafness bone conduction in the opposite ear may be interpreted as hearing in the affected ear. The same difficulty arises in estimating the amount of hearing with conversation voice, and in audiometric testing.

Masking is therefore used to minimize these fallacies. In masking, the opposite ear to that being tested is subjected to noise which can be created by various means. In clinical examination Barany's noise box is the source, in audiometry electrical methods are used. The masking noise is introduced into the external meatus of the sound ear, and the amount of noise produced is sufficient to mask the hearing ear and prevent sounds being heard by it when the deaf ear is being tested. Thus with a Barany box in the sound ear, a tuning-fork placed upon the mastoid of the deaf ear, if heard, must be heard by the deaf ear, and a loud shout into the deaf ear, with the Barany box in the opposite ear, if heard, must be heard by the ear being tested.

Tests for malingering

Careful and complete clinical examination combined with tests such as those below will usually reveal abnormalities suggestive of simulated deafness. The deafness is generally of sensori-neural type.

It must be emphasized, however, that as the experienced malingerer may have little difficulty in defeating clinical tests, complex audiometric examination is frequently necessary. Differentiation of simulated from hysterical deafness presents even greater problems.

Stethoscope test. The ordinary binaural stethoscope is placed in the patient's ears. The examiner sits behind the patient and speaks into the mouthpiece of the stethoscope. The tubes leading to the ear are clamped in succession while the patient is being made to repeat what the examiner is saying. If, with the tube leading to the good ear clamped, the patient can still repeat the words being said, the suspected ear must be functioning because the patient is unaware which ear is being tested.

The Barany box test depends upon the fact that in a noise persons usually raise their voice in order to hear themselves above the noise. A person of normal hearing, with a Barany box placed in each ear, will read or count in a much louder tone than normal. This principle is used in testing cases of suspected malingering, where complete deafness in one ear is simulated. A Barany box is placed in the sound ear, and the patient is told to count up to twenty. After a few numbers have been spoken, the noise box is set going, and if complete deafness exists the patient's voice will rise loudly in tone. If the voice does not rise, then evidently the patient can hear his own voice in the ear which is supposed to be deaf.

PHYSIOLOGY OF THE VESTIBULAR LABYRINTH

The function of the vestibular portion of the labyrinth is a subject upon which further information is still required before there is any real understanding of its mode of operation, or agreement upon the principles which govern its effects upon the body.

The vestibule is a part of the proprioceptive system to which muscle, tendon and joint sense, skin pressor receptors and the occular reflexes also make important contributions. The vestibule has three parts, the utricle, saccule and semicircular canals. The function of the saccule is still debated but it probably resembles that of the utricle, to which it has a close structural resemblance. Experimentally, however, it has been shown that the saccule can be stimulated by sound.

The reflexes produced by the utricle are due to the pressure or pull caused by lateral displacement of the otolith membrane on the macula. The utricle is accordingly concerned with identification of head position in relation to the gravitational field (whether natural or artificial) and with linear acceleration and deceleration.

The semicircular canals on the other hand are stimulated by endolymph flow occurring within the lumen during angular acceleration, the result of inertial lag of the endolymph which normally occurs at the start and finish of head movement around an axis. The three canals of one labyrinth are arranged at right angles to each other (Figs. 83 and 84) and it follows that each canal has a counterpart on the opposite side in the same plane. Movement in any plane can thus be detected. The

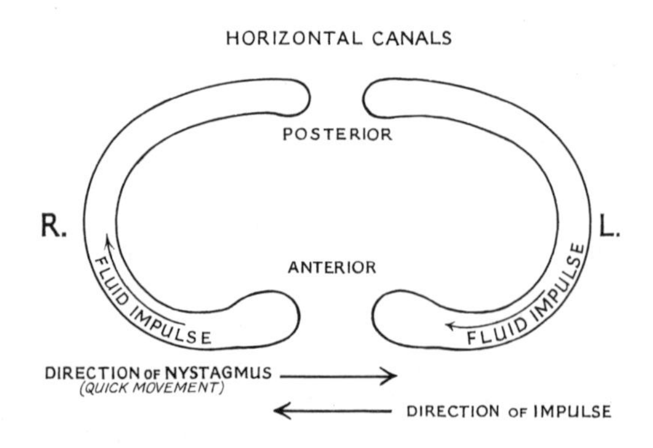

Fig. 83. Horizontal canals. (Lateral Canals).

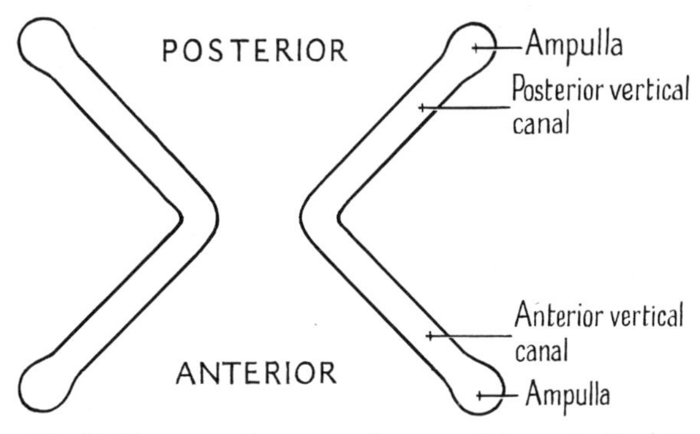

Fig. 84. Shows complementary character of the vertical canals.

endolymph movement produced in the canal acts on the crista by causing deviation of the cupola, this stimulus causes a series of reactions.

Effects produced by stimulation of the vestibular labyrinth

Vertigo is felt as a sensation of turning or, if the vertical canals are involved, of falling to one side or the other, and objects appear to move towards the affected ear.

Nausea and vomiting are visceral reflexes produced by strong stimulation of the labyrinth.

Nystagmus is a rhythmic eye movement consisting of two components, a slow labyrinthine component and a quick, correcting cerebral component. The nystagmus is named according to the direction of this more obvious quick movement.

Fistula sign

If physical examination of the patient with vertigo has shown evidence of otitis media, and especially if cholesteatoma is suspected, the fistula test should be done. If positive it is likely to make other labyrinthine tests unnecessary. Pressure is applied to the meatal entrance, or a dressed probe is used to palpate the area of the deep meatus. A positive result is indicated by the production of vertigo and the observation of a deviation of the eyes to the opposite side, with a return when the pressure is withdrawn. It indicates (1) that disease has eroded through the labyrinthine capsule, (2) that the labyrinth is still active.

Tests for vestibular function

Labyrinthine tests aim at the production of the signs described which result from labyrinthine excitation. The tests stimulate the labyrinth in a controlled manner so that the reactions may be studied. Comparison may be made between the functioning of the two sides. The test most commonly used is the caloric test; the rotation test has the disadvantage of stimulating both sides simultaneously; galvanic stimulation and the table tilting test are seldom used.

Labyrinthine stimulation results in three responses: (1) nystagmus, (2) past-pointing, (3) falling. Nystagmus has already been described.

Past-pointing is an effect due to the presence of vertigo. There is a sensation of objects moving away from the patient, who voluntarily attempts to compensate for this when trying to touch a fixed point.

Falling is similarly caused by the patient trying to correct an apparent rotation in one direction, which is produced by the vertigo. The result of this attempt to correct a movement which does not exist is that the patient falls in the opposite direction to the sense of movement produced by the vertigo.

Relationship of nystagmus and past-pointing, etc.

Where these effects are produced by stimulation of the labyrinth, the relationship of the nystagmus to the past-pointing and falling is constant. The nystagmus is always in the opposite direction to the past-pointing and the falling. This is a very important fact and should always be remembered.

The principles upon which the tests are based are demonstrated in the experiments carried out by Ewald upon the labyrinths of pigeons. Ewald introduced a cannula into the canals of a pigeon's labyrinth in such a manner that he was able to produce currents in the canals at will and was able to study their effects. By this means he discovered that the effects were as follows:

1. Movement of the endolymph produces a slow deviation of the eyes in the direction of the flow of the enodlymph.
2. In the horizontal canal the greatest effect is produced when the flow is towards the ampulla.
3. In the vertical canals the maximum effects are produced when the current travels from the ampulla to the smooth end.

As will be seen from the diagram (Figs. 83 and 84), the canals of the opposite sides are complementary, and thus interpretation depends on the understanding of the directions of the currents produced in any given case, and the effects on the canals in which they are produced.

Positional tests

If the history suggests that vertigo occurs when the head or body is moved in a particular direction, then positional tests should be carried out. With the patient sitting erect upon a couch he proceeds to lie flat with the head turned to the right, any nystagmus is then observed until it decays. The patient then resumes his original sitting-up position and a search is again made for nystagmus. The test is repeated after an interval with the patient in the head-left position and finally in the head-extended position. Any nystagmus detected is described according to its latent period, direction, duration and fatigueability. Positional nystagmus may occur as a benign peripheral disorder in which case it is fatigueable and reversible. Alternatively, it is found sometimes in certain serious lesions of the brain stem and cerebellum, though with different non-fatiguing characteristics.

Electronystagmography

This is a means by which a permanent recording of nystagmus can be made and depends on the presence of a corneo-retinal potential difference. The electrical axis of the eye corresponds to the optical axis, so movement can be accurately recorded. As well as enabling an exact analysis of speed, amplitude and frequency to be made, the test provides a means of detecting nystagmus which may not be visible to the naked eye. Fixation suppresses nystagmus, as this test is done in darkness or with the eyes closed fixation is suppressed and detection made much more likely.

The caloric test

This test depends upon the production of convection currents in the canal system by heating or cooling a portion of the labyrinth. The test may be performed in different ways. It can be done by continuous syringing with cold or hot water, by the method of Kobrak (Fig. 85), or by the differential hot and cold method of Hallpike.

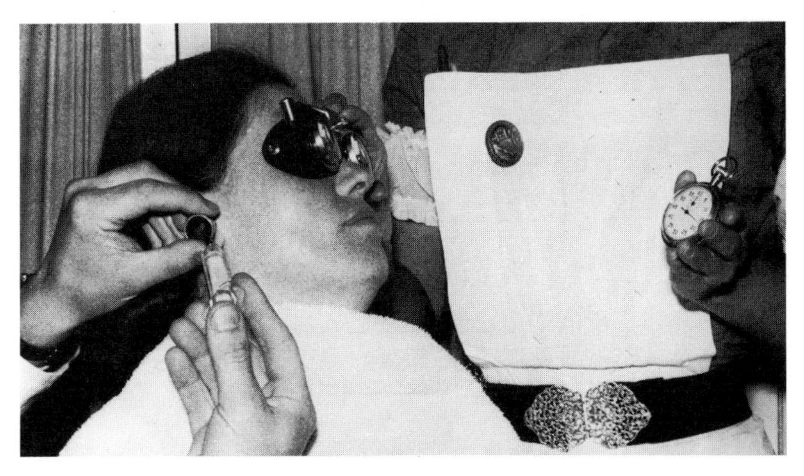

Fig. 85. Caloric test. The Kobrak test is the most convenient in ordinary practice. Frenzel spectacles are useful for observation of nystagmus, but make its end point more difficult to define.

Methods of carrying out the test.

Kobrak's method is perhaps the most convenient test and can be done rapidly during a busy clinic. With the patient seated and the head supported on the extended head rest to bring the lateral semicircular canal near to the vertical position as before, 2 ml of cold water are delivered from a syringe on to the postero-superior segment of the drum under direct vision. The nystagmus is timed, and after a short interval the test is repeated on the other side.

The differential caloric test is done according to the method described by Fitzgerald and Hallpike. With the patient recumbent and the head raised 30 degrees the ears are irrigated in turn with water at 30°F and then at 44°F, each for 40 seconds. The after-nystagmus is timed with a stop-watch and recorded on a calorigram (Fig. 86). This method of testing with water at 7°C above and below body temperature gives information not only about canal paresis but also about the function of the utricle and the temporal lobe of the brain. If an ear under test gives no response with the stimuli mentioned above, then continuous stimulation with water at 20°C. Up to four minutes may be necessary before deciding that the labyrinth is functionless.

Past-pointing and falling are not generally tested for during the caloric test. In performing these it is useful nevertheless to recall that

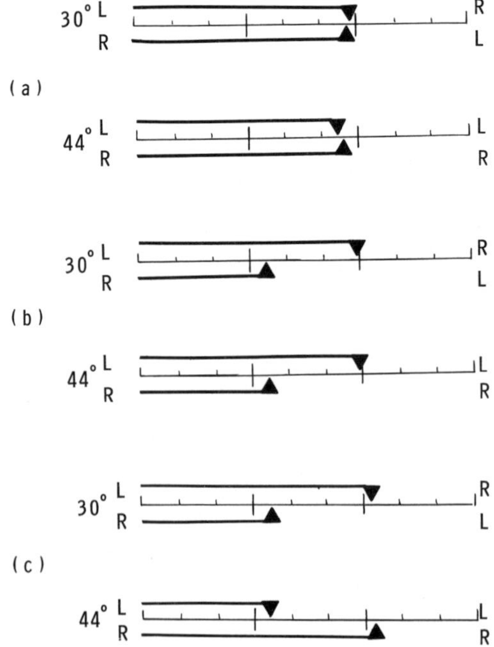

Fig. 86. Differential caloric test. (a) Normal response. (b) right canal paresis. (c) directional preponderance to the right. Timing interval – 20 secs.

the direction of the endolymph flow, past-pointing, falling and the slow component of the nystagmus are all in the same direction, *i.e.* opposite to the direction of the quick element of the nystagmus.

The rotation test

The patient is seated in a chair which can be rotated horizontally and has provision for support of both the head and the feet. A special chair, known as the Barany chair, is usually employed for this test. The patient is seated upright with the head tilted forwards 30 degrees. This brings the horizontal canals into the plane of rotation. Rotation is then carried out, with the patient's eyes closed, for ten complete turns in twenty seconds. At the end of this rotation the chair is stopped abruptly and the patient is directed to look at the examiner's finger, which is held in front of the patient and towards the side of the ear being tested. In this test the duration of the after-nystagmus is timed in seconds, and, in the normal, should last from about 25 seconds to 35 or 40 seconds.

Explanation of the test. The patient is rotated the number of turns which is known to be the smallest number sufficient to overcome the initial lag or inertia of the endolymph within the canal. Therefore at the time the chair is stopped the canal and the endolymph are rotating at the same speed. With the sudden stoppage of rotation the fluid tends, by its mass, to continue its movement and so sets up a current within the canals. This current produces effects in accordance with Ewald's laws.

In practice the horizontal canals only are tested, though it is possible to test the other canals by placing the head in different positions.

Comparison of the tests

The advantage of the caloric tests is that one ear only is tested at a time. One disadvantage is that if a perforation of the drum exists it is inadvisable to use water. This difficulty can be overcome by using cold air.

The rotation test gives information as to the degree of compensation which has taken place in the sound labyrinth. This may be of importance where operations for ablation of one labyrinth are under consideration.

SCHEME OF FUNCTIONAL EXAMINATION OF THE EAR

Otoscopy always precedes functional examination.

Examination of the cochlea

1. Tuning-fork tests:
   (*a*) Rinne's test.
   (*b*) Weber's test.
   (*c*) Schwabach's test.

2. Hearing test: conversational voice and whisper.
3. Audiometry, with special tests if necessary.
4. Repeat hearing tests and audiometry after Eustachian inflation if appropriate.

N.B.—In cases of severe deafness use the Barany noise box to confirm the results of tests (1) and (2).

Examination of vestibule

1. Observation of spontaneous signs: Nystagmus. Past-pointing. Falling.
2. Fistula test where appropriate.
3. Positional tests.
4. Simple caloric test.
5. Differential caloric test if indicated.
6. Rotation test: if indicated.
7. Electronystagmography in special cases.

30. Diseases of the External Ear

CONGENITAL ABNORMALITIES

The external ear, the middle ear and the inner ear differ not only in their embryological origins but also in their times of development. This accounts for the wide variation in the types of abnormality, for it is not unusual to see patients with an absent auricle and external auditory canal who are found to have only a moderately severe deformity of the middle ear and its contents and who have normal internal ears. On the other hand, children may be encountered who have a normal or almost normal external ear, and at the same time congenital malformation of the middle ear or internal ear. Abnormalities may be unilateral or bilateral and may be associated with other congenital malformations (Fig. 87).

These deformities may arise from genetic defects or from a virus or from toxic drugs acting during early pregnancy. In many cases, however, the cause of the abnormality cannot be determined.

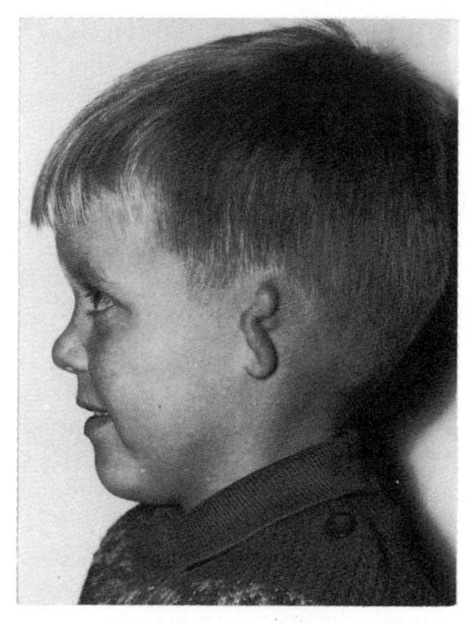

Fig. 87. Congenital atresia of the ear. In spite of the severe deformity of the pinna and total bony occlusion of the external meatus, the middle ear and ossicles were relatively normal and the internal ear was entirely normal.

The pinna may be absent; it may be small and deformed, or consist of a few skin tags only. The position of the deformed pinna is also frequently abnormal.

The management of these patients is always difficult. It is essential that hearing should be accurately assessed, even in apparently unilateral cases. Surgical reconstruction of the pinna involves elaborate multi-stage plastic procedures. The alternative is some kind of prosthesis worn for cosmetic purposes. The reconstruction of the external canal and middle ear is likewise complex. It is generally agreed that operation should be carried out in bilateral cases so that a hearing aid can be fitted and speech can be acquired, but not all otologists agree that reconstruction is justifiable in the case of unilateral atresia.

THE AURICLE: INJURIES

One result of injury to the auricle is the formation of a haematoma. The haematoma is an extravasation of blood and serum beneath the perichondrium. The appearance of the auricle is that of a large, bluish swelling, the outline of the conchal folds is lost, and the ear itself may be slightly tender with a feeling of heat and discomfort. If left alone the result of this haematoma may be distortion of the auricle and the eventual thickening which is known as 'cauliflower' ear, so frequently seen in boxers who have suffered repeated trauma.

The treatment of such a condition is aspiration of the contents of the swelling. This is most easily done with a 5-ml syringe and a needle of fairly large bore, by inserting the needle into the swelling and aspirating until no more fluid can be withdrawn. This should be repeated daily until the auricle returns to normal. Antibiotic cover should be given to prevent infection and consequent necrosis of cartilage.

INFECTIONS OF THE AURICLE

Perichondritis

Perichondritis is inflammation of the immediate covering of the cartilage, the perichondrium. This infection may obtain entry in various ways. It may follow the infection of a haematoma or other injury, and is a rare complication of a mastoid operation when the cartilage is cut in presence of an obvious infection. In perichondritis the auricle is found to be uniformly enlarged and thickened. Its surface is red and shiny. There is great pain, and frequently considerable constitutional disturbance.

The treatment of perichondritis is tedious. A broad spectrum antibiotic is essential because the infecting organism is generally penicillin resistant. Ampicillin may be given orally until the organisms and their sensitivities are known. Local treatment consists of the application of soothing soaks, such as glycerine and ichthyol or magnesium sulphate.

If sub-perichondrial abscesses form they need incision and drainage, but incision should only be carried out when definite fluctuation can be elicited. Premature incision may result in a further spread of infection and more extensive necrosis of the cartilage.

Furunculosis

Furunculosis is the infection of a hair follicle and so is usually staphylococcal. It differs from the foregoing by being localized to one particular part of the ear, though by deep extension it may give rise to perichondritis.

Furunculosis is treated on general lines. Heat and soothing soaks are applied until the boil is localized, and surgical measures are postponed until pus has formed.

Dermatitis

Dermatitis of the auricle is an infection, usually of a streptococcal type, of the skin covering the auricle. It is characterized by a weeping, scaly condition, with the formation of yellow crusts on the skin, which may spread from the auricle to the neck or face. It differs from perichondritis in that it is not necessarily confined to the auricle itself.

The origin of dermatitis is usually in an infection of an abrasion. It may readily be transferred from ear to ear, or one person to another by contact, or by towels. In children one of the most frequent causes of this disease is neglect of a discharging ear. Treatment of dermatitis consists of the application of soaks such as glycerine and ichthyol or magnesium sulphate, creams consisting of steroids and antibiotics can be used when the skin condition is improving.

Erysipelas

Erysipelas is sometimes seen following operation, and is the spread in the sub-epithelial tissues of an infection by streptococci. It also is characterized by a reddened swollen auricle, but the spread to other parts of the face or the head, and the formation of the typical blisters, will very quickly make the diagnosis clear.

Treatment of erysipelas is usually straightforward; being a streptococcal infection it usually responds rapidly to penicillin.

Diagnosis. All these diseases in the earlier stages resemble each other closely and may give considerable difficulty in differential diagnosis. There is in each a reddening of the skin, heat, pain and a feeling of thickness of the auricle. As the condition progresses, however, it becomes easier to make the diagnosis. Perichondritis, as has been already mentioned, is confined to the cartilaginous auricle. Furunculosis rapidly becomes manifest in its local character. Dermatitis and erysipelas spread beyond the limit of the auricle readily, erysipelas being accompanied by the typical constitutional reaction, that is, by a high temperature, sickness and a feeling of extreme illness. Locally the typical advancing raised edge is found and blisters may form. In dermatitis constitutional disturbance is less, the condition is more diffuse and the surface is scaly and weeping.

Treatment. Treatment of the early stages is similar, and consists in soothing the part. Soaks of magnesium sulphate and glycerin, or ichthyol and glycerin, are the chief aids. As the condition advances treatment diverges in each particular condition. If a perichondritis proceeds to suppuration and pus is formed, then multiple incisions should be made down to the cartilage. Necrosis of cartilage in these cases will almost certainly follow, and deformity of the external ear may be considerable. In dermatitis the crust should be removed by poultices – for example, starch poultices – and the surface dressed with some ointment, such as an ichthyol-zinc-oxide paste, and as the condition dries, and the crust formation becomes less, painting with gentian violet 2 per cent is one of the most valuable remedies. Another method of applying these remedies is to paint the part with gentian violet first and then apply the starch poultice. Erysipelas is treated by the application of magnesium sulphate soaks, and by dealing with the general constitutional disturbances with antibiotics as usual.

Herpes

Herpes may occur around the auricle as part of herpes zoster oticus (p. 332) sometimes known as Ramsey-Hunt syndrome. This will be described more fully later. The vesicles quickly heal spontaneously if the part is kept dry. A painful neuralgia may precede or follow the eruption of the vesicles.

Tuberculosis (lupus)

Lupus of the auricle is always accompanied by lesions on the face or mucous membrane (p. 52). The appearances are those of lupus in other situations – the usual apple-jelly nodules and the scarring, with a tendency to resolution in one part and extension in another; but on the ear, besides these appearances, there is a distinct tendency to ulceration and destruction of the cartilage.

Tumours of the auricle

Epitheliomata present as indurated ulcers with everted margins and require surgical treatment, possibly also radio-therapy, depending upon their site and extent. Basal cell carcinomas also occur, adequate excision or radio-therapy are usually curative.

DISEASES OF THE EXTERNAL MEATUS

FURUNCULOSIS

This is an infection of the hair follicle and so can occur only in the skin of the outer part of the meatus.

Symptoms. Acute pain is the outstanding symptom of furunculosis. The pain may spread up the side of the head into the jaw, or down the neck as far as the shoulder. It may be so severe as to deprive the patient of any hope of rest. There is swelling of the parts round the ear, corresponding to the location of the boil within the meatus. If it is in the anterior wall the tissue in front of the tragus is swollen, if behind, the oedema may spread over the mastoid process, or above to the temporal region, superficially simulating acute mastoiditis. Tenderness on pressure is marked, but the tenderness is found more in front of the ear and below the ear than on any other part. The acute pain produced by movement of any part of the cartilaginous meatal structure is typical of this condition, for any movement of the cartilage naturally puts tension upon the already extremely painful tissues lining the ear. Deafness may be present, but is not typical of furunculosis, because it will occur only when the furuncle is of sufficient size to occlude the external auditory canal completely.

Appearances on examining the meatus. It is frequently difficult to obtain an adequate view of the deeper part of the external meatus. The walls appear to be in apposition, and on attempting to introduce the speculum within the external canal extreme pain is caused to the patient. If examination is carefully pursued it will be seen that the swelling is confined to one or other wall, and if the condition has advanced a discharging point may be seen when the furuncle has burst, and it may be possible to express pus from this opening. The most difficult types of furuncle to diagnose are the deep-seated, early types, in which there is little to be seen on superficial examination. The canal appears to be wide open, the drum membrane may be normal, but if examination is carried out carefully a small swelling or fullness will usually be found in the floor or other aspect of the external auditory canal, and if probed there is usually a definite spot of tenderness. In this type of infection there is a deep tenderness in front of and below the tragus. The treatment of furunculosis will be considered later in conjunction with otitis externa.

OTITIS EXTERNA

This is a generalized infection involving, as a rule, the whole of the skin of the external canal, including the surface of the drum membrane. It varies widely in the severity of the infection, from a slight itching to an acute crippling disease.

Aetiology. Certain conditions predispose to the affection such as moist humid atmosphere. Dust and other irritants predispose by reason of the irritation which induces scratching of the ear. This is undoubtedly the common factor in the initiation of an attack. An allergic diathesis is present in many cases and in such circumstances psychological factors play a part in its origin.

Organisms. A wide variety of organisms is concerned, such as haemolytic streptococcus, staphylococcus aureus, pseudomonas pyocyaneus. These organisms commonly gain entrance to the skin after abrasion of the protecting surface layers of the epidermis. Fungi are often present as secondary invaders and often unsuspected. They may predispose to recurrence or chronicity.

Diagnosis. In the acute infective condition the diagnosis is simple. The meatus is acutely inflamed, tender and weeping freely. It is extremely painful to handle and nothing can be seen of the interior of the canal without causing the patient acute pain. At this stage no conclusions can be formed as to possible causes and treatment is directed towards soothing the inflamed tissues.

In less acute forms there is swelling and redness of the skin of the external meatus and the canal may be filled with debris. The ear is tender to touch and the glands in front of the tragus may be enlarged. The drum membrane may or may not be visible, but as a rule deafness is not marked. This observation is of prime importance because otitis media may be present and may be the cause of the maceration and infection of the skin of the canal. As the treatment for external otitis may on occasion be incorrect in the case of otitis media this distinction should be made at the earliest opportunity. In very slight cases the meatus may be open and the only sign of disease is a little dry crusting and scaling of the epithelium.

In allergic affections the external canal becomes moist quite suddenly, and a thin watery secretion is seen coming from the ear. Many of the less acute forms of otitis externa appear to be exacerbated by warm confined conditions as when in bed, or where the occupation demands the wearing of ear phones or protective ear muffs. In cases of long standing there may be chronic thickening of the skin of the external canal which makes observation and treatment extremely difficult. When irreversible by conservative treatment, this may require surgical intervention and skin-grafting to correct the stenosis of the canal.

Treatment

As the treatment of external otitis and furunculosis in the acute phase is similar they will be considered together.

Acute pain is one of the outstanding characteristics and the use of heat in the form of fomentations is soothing. Hot pads and other applications can be used if preferred. The meatus should be packed as far as possible with soothing lotion such as ichthyol in glycerin on strip gauze. Aluminium acetate solution 8 per cent is an extremely useful lotion also. Gauze 1 cm broad is required, a good reflected light and a suitable pair of forceps such as Politzer's angled forceps, to pack the gauze sufficiently deeply into the ear. If a furuncle should become very large it is necessary to incise it, but incision of small early furuncles is more likely to spread the infection than to cure it.

A very large number of drugs, both for systemic and for local use, have been recommended, but none have been specially successful, and complete and careful treatment is the best insurance against recurrence.

The affected canal should be packed with one of the recommended remedies, *e.g.* aluminium acetate or ichthyol in glycerin, till the acute stage has passed, and some view of the meatus can be obtained. Twice or thrice weekly treatment is not sufficient in the early stages, treatment must be given daily by a competent person who can use a head mirror or headlamp.

Few antibiotics are of value in otitis externa, and some of the most severe cases seen are the result of ill-judged treatment with these drugs. Neomycin and soframycin are the most valuable and should always be combined with hydrocortisone. While cortisone is an anti-inflammatory agent it should not be used by itself as it has no effect on the bacterial infection where this is present; it is better combined with one of the antibiotics. These drugs can be obtained as a cream or in a water-soluble base.

Chronic disease. These form the bulk of the cases seen, the condition is equally demanding for both the patient and the doctor. For adequate control frequent and prolonged treatment is necessary. It is essential that all discharge and debris should be cleaned from the ear at each visit, especially from the deep part of the meatus and the anterior recess. This may be best accomplished by syringing the ear provided the meatus is carefully dried afterwards. It is also essential to avoid repeated trauma, whether it be caused by matchsticks, hair grips or long fingernails. Many of these patients have allergic skins and have become sensitised to repeated courses of ear drops containing antibiotic.

After cleaning out the meatus completely a dressing is inserted. This should consist of ribbon gauze impregnated with glycerine and ichthyol, alternatively a wick of Ototrane can be used. In the initial stages treatment must be carried out twice or thrice weekly. As the condition is gradually brought under control steroid-antibiotic drops may again be tried, but with great caution. When the meatus has been brought to the best possible condition the situation may be kept under control by the very sparing use of hydrocortisone cream or an ointment containing 2.5% ammoniated mercury in order to promote the development of a resistant epithelium. For a long period after the condition has been brought under control it is important that the patient should keep the ear dry and to use discretion, especially in respect of bathing and swimming.

Very occasionally the otologist sees patients in whom gross stenosis of the canal prevents any possibility of access for treatment. In such cases total excision of the thickened, unhealthy skin, together with meatoplasty, widening the bony meatus, and skin grafting can sometimes be curative.

OTOMYCOSIS

Fungoid infection is found in the external meatus either as a primary disease or complicating otitis externa. The usual organisms are aspergillus albicans or aspergillus niger. The presence of masses of material like wet blotting paper in the meatus upon which the mycelia can be seen is characteristic, the colour of the mass may be white, through brown to black. The condition responds to repeated and careful cleaning out of all debris and powdering with a fungicide such as nystatin or amphotericin. When the condition is under control then powdering with hydrargaphan or the use of 2% salicylic acid in spirit can be useful. Local treatment must be continued for at least three weeks after apparent cure otherwise recurrence is inevitable. In persistent cases of external otitis the presence of a fungus should always be considered.

WAX IN THE EAR

Wax in the ear is the result of a discharge from glands situated in the skin of the ear. Wax is nature's provision for the removal of dust and other foreign material from the canal of the ear. The accumulation of wax varies greatly in different people, but is more commonly found in those engaged in dusty occupations, such as miners, firemen, dust-men, etc.

Wax may cause a variety of symptoms, the chief of which is deafness. There may be irritation in the ear amounting to actual pain, and noises are not infrequently the chief symptom owing to pressure upon the drum.

The sudden onset of deafness is explained by the fact that where only a small aperture exists in the wax, a sudden movement of the wax may completely occlude the passage. Another common occurrence is the onset of deafness after bathing or washing, due to water entering the external meatus. The water causes the wax to swell and the passage is completely blocked.

Treatment consists of the removal of the wax. This is not difficult, provided care and gentleness are exercised. Wax can be removed safely by picking it out or by the more usual method of syringing. If the wax is hard it should be softened to begin with by the instillation of a saturated solution of bicarbonate of soda, or olive oil three times daily for two or three days before removal. If a patient is unlikely to carry out these instructions, it may be of advantage to instil some oil into the ear. If there is no time to soften the wax, some drops of peroxide of hydrogen are put in and allowed to remain for a few minutes. This will help in the removal. Syringing wax from the ear is not necessarily a simple operation, and there is a right way and a wrong way to do it. The syringe used for removal of the wax should be of a sufficient capacity to enable a fair pressure of water to be obtained. Unless the user is competent the nozzle should not be a fine one, otherwise harm may be done to the external canal. The stream of water should be directed upwards and backwards along the posterior wall of the meatus. If this syringing has little effect upon wax, a wax curette or probe should be used to make a small opening along the posterior wall behind the wax, so that the water may enter behind the mass and force it off the posterior wall. It must be emphasized that it is possible to rupture a drum membrane if a jet of water is driven directly on it from a syringe, therefore the syringing should be indirect. After the wax has been removed, careful examination of the external meatus must be made, as occasionally part of the epithelial lining is removed with the wax, or abrasions may have been caused by the syringe. If these are found it is wise to dry out the ear gently and then insufflate a small amount of dusting powder. In practically all cases examination of the drum membrane after syringing will show a degree of injection. This is found chiefly round the short process of the malleus and along the handle. This must not be confused with an early otitis media, particularly as the deafness caused by a large accumulation of wax may not recover completely for a day or two after the removal of the wax.

KERATOSIS OBTURANS

In this condition wax accumulates in the inner part of the external meatus, and with continual desquamation of the epithelium a mass is formed of wax and epithelium which contains cholesterol, and which exerts pressure on surrounding tissues.

By continued enlargement the keratotic mass causes progressive erosion and expansion of the bony meatus and may go on to invade the middle ear. The mass may be fairly silent until an external otitis supervenes and gives severe pain. The ring of granulation tissue which forms superficial to the expanding keratotic mass is almost diagnostic. Removal may be accomplished by careful softening of the mass, but in many cases a general anaesthetic is required. The condition may occur alone or as part of a syndrome with sinuso-bronchiectasis.

FOREIGN BODIES IN THE EAR

Foreign bodies in the ear are almost invariably confined to children, and for the purposes of removal may be divided into two classes – those which are vegetable and those which are not. The importance of this is that while in the non-vegetable forms of foreign body the syringe is one of the most useful instruments for removal, in the case of the vegetable foreign body a syringe may be a very dangerous instrument. For example a pea, which is quite a common article for a child to insert in the ear, will, if a syringe is used, immediately swell and become wedged in the bony canal in such a way as to cause excruciating pain to the patient. Removal will be exceedingly difficult, as the foreign body may have to be cut out piecemeal. Such foreign bodies as beads, pieces of indiarubber, stones, etc., can be removed by syringing or by the use of a small hook. Alligator forceps are particularly to be avoided on smooth, round objects which may escape and shoot still deeper into the meatus. In small children, however, if they are refractory, it will be very much wiser to take the precaution of administering an anaesthetic. It is impossible safely to remove a deeply embedded foreign body from the ear of a wriggling, struggling child. It is unwise to attempt to remove such a foreign body without adequate preparation, particularly if an anaesthetic is to be given. In this way accidents happen. Proper instruments also are essential, and if the foreign body is found in circumstances where proper equipment is not available, it is wiser to wait until instruments which can do the work are obtained, or to transfer the patient to a hospital more fully equipped. The use of a large, clumsy pair of forceps to remove a small bead from an ear will in many cases result in the bead being pushed through the drum into the middle ear, and a tympanotomy may be required to remove it.

EXOSTOSIS

An exostosis is a bony outgrowth from the wall of the external auditory meatus. It may be composed of cancellous bone or of ivory bone. Exostoses are usually multiple and bilateral, affecting chiefly the anterior and posterior walls. The condition is frequently found in swimmers. The patient may be completely unaware of their existence, or, on the other hand, he may come for advice regarding deafness, and when examined the meatus may be found to be completely blocked by the growth. Otitis externa may be present, and may be responsible for the final closure of the meatus. The treatment of otitis externa in these circumstances is of the greatest difficulty. Removal of an exostosis is not an operation to be lightly undertaken and, unless essential, it is better avoided. As the exostosis is usually attached to the posterior meatal wall, removal endangers important structures, such as the facial nerve. As an exostotis is usually of very much more dense bone than the wall of the meatal canal, an attempt to chip or break off the exostosis may result in a fracture of the wall of the meatus. The motor-driven burr is the best instrument for the removal.

MALIGNANT DISEASE

Cancer of the auditory meatus

Mention has already been made of growths which affect the pinna. Tumours of the meatus itself are much rarer, but malignant polyps may present which have their origin in the middle ear or in a mastoid cavity. They are nearly always the result of prolonged suppuration. Malignancy is to be suspected, especially in older patients in whom a fleshy-looking polyp is present which bleeds easily.

Treatment of these patients is always difficult and often disappointing. Radio-therapy alone rarely controls the condition, an extended radical mastoidectomy may be considered. Extensive or recurrent growths can sometimes be best controlled by total excision of the petrous bone.

31. The Tympanic Membrane

The tympanic membrane may be involved in many conditions affecting the external ear, the middle ear and the Eustachian tube. Although the colour of the normal drum is pearl grey and the surface smooth and shining, some variation is possible without the presence of any pathological change. The drum is concave and tense and it moves freely with the pneumatic speculum.

INFECTIONS OF THE DRUM

Otitis externa

In this condition the drum membrane rapidly loses its lustre, becomes thickened and sometimes pink. The surface begins to desquamate, the epithelium covering the drum comes off in flakes, giving the drum a rough, whitish appearance, and there may be a certain degree of oedema. This can be so marked as to obscure the landmarks. In less severe degrees the otitis externa may spread on to the posterior part of the drum from the adjacent external meatus and may cause suspicion of attic disease.

The condition of the drum will improve when the infection of the external meatus is brought under control. After repeated or prolonged attacks, however, the drum may be permanently thickened and fail to regain its normal healthy lustre.

Myringitis bullosa

This is probably due to virus infection, and may have serious intracranial accompaniments. Often it is seen during influenza epidemics. Haemorrhagic bullae are formed on the drum, and may spread on to the wall of the meatus. They are usually seen under these circumstances on the postero-superior aspect of the canal. They appear as dark bluish or red swellings, which may be the size of a split pea, or large enough to obscure the drum completely. At first the hearing may be unaffected, and the chief complaint is that of acute pain. The pain is extremely severe, prevents sleep or work, and may completely incapacitate the patient. Bullae may occur on a small portion of an otherwise normal membrane or they may include the whole drum and part of the meatal wall. They either burst, discharging sero-sanguineous fluid, or they dry up into blackish crusts. The condition frequently proceeds to acute otitis media. Viral labyrinthitis and meningo-encephalitis sometimes occur.

Treatment. Energetic antibiotic treatment should be given to prevent secondary infection leading to acute otitis media if not already present.

Herpes

True herpes of the drum is seen in the condition known as herpes zoster oticus. This condition will be described more fully in dealing with the internal ear (p. 332).

RETRACTION POCKETS

The normal drum is tense and devoid of any retained epithelial debris. These two features result from firstly the presence of the middle elastic layer in the pars tensa, and secondly the normal migration of the epithelial layer from the drum along the meatal walls to the exterior.

One or both of these conditions may become disturbed by mechanisms which are still not fully understood. Damage to the middle layer of the drum may follow from middle ear infections, and impairment of middle ear aeration from Eustachian tube insufficiency may cause part of the drum to collapse and form a pocket. This is seen most often in the postero-superior segment. As long as these pockets remain small and there is no retention of epithelial debris it is safe to keep them under observation.

In deeper retraction pockets, however, the self-cleansing mechanism may fail and there will be accumulation of epithelial debris with subsequent infection. These epithelial accumulations must be recognized and removed, so that the self-cleansing mechanism may recover. Failure to do so may result in the development of a true cholesteatoma (see Attico-antral Disease, p. 271).

INJURIES OF THE DRUM

Injuries of the drum may be due to violence from without or from within. Thus, perforations may be caused by foreign bodies of various kinds, such as hairpins or other instruments being forced through the drum from the external meatus. Foreign bodies may be pushed through the drum in misguided attempts at removal. Matches are a cause of injury, and this may occur if a patient receives a jog in the elbow while scraping the ear with a match. A blow on the ear or compression of air in the external meatus may be sufficient to rupture the drum. A blast from shot-firing or gun-fire may cause sufficient displacement of air to rupture the drum, either inwards by direct blast or outwards by blast suction. In the latter case the edges of the rupture are seen to be everted. From within, traumatic perforation occurs by fracture of the petrous bone running along the roof of the middle ear and involving the tympanic ring with rupture of the upper part of the drum.

Treatment of injuries in all cases. The minimum is done. A plug of sterile material should be put into the ear and the patient made to rest. On no account should the ear be syringed but it may if necessary be mopped, with strict aseptic precautions. If the perforation results in otitis media, as it may, then the usual regime for the treatment of discharging ear is instituted. Chemotherapy is employed prophylactically. If the drum fails to heal, repair of the drum and ossicular chain may be considered later.

PERFORATION OF THE DRUM

Three main types of perforation of the tympanic membrane are found. They are central, marginal and attic. Perforations are usually single but may be multiple, in which case they suggest tuberculosis.

Central perforations

In this type of perforation a margin of drum membrane is left all round, and the annulus remains intact. Frequently the handle of the malleus can be seen projecting into the perforation which is described as anterior, inferior or posterior, according to its relationship to the handle of the malleus. A 'kidney' perforation is larger and the term is self-descriptive. Sometimes the defect in the pars tensa is so great as to merit the description of sub-total perforation. Any of these various types of perforations may be seen in chronic otitis media of tubo-tympanic type whether active or quiescent. Perforations associated with acute otitis media are always central.

Marginal perforations

These are perforations in which the tympanic ring is involved. This means that disease of the bone is present, and such perforations frequently indicate long-standing and advanced middle ear disease, very often with cholesteatoma formation. Cholesteatoma can be recognized by its white wax-like appearance and its foul sickly smell. Marginal perforations are usually seen posteriorly and many of them probably have had their origin in retraction pockets. In some cases destruction of the drum margin allows squamous epithelium to grow from the meatus into the middle ear cavity.

Attic perforations

An attic perforation is one situated in the membrana flaccida. Perforations of this kind are associated with the most serious variety of destructive middle ear disease because of their invariable association with an invading cholesteatoma. These perforations are characterized by lack of symptoms, and are frequently unsuspected. The attic perforation should be looked for above the short process of the malleus. It may be pin-hole in size, but it may, by spread of the disease, involve the whole of the membrana flaccida, and possibly the posterior horizontal fold also. Sometimes an attic perforation is characterized in its chronic form by the presence of a small brown crust, closely resembling a piece of wax, on the superior wall of the external meatus. If, on examination of an ear, the only wax to be seen is located in the roof near the drum, the removal of this wax will, in the majority of cases, reveal an attic defect. Although small such a defect may be associated with a large cholesteatoma. Like marginal perforations these attic defects probably originate by the part of the drum concerned collapsing or being dragged inwards. Although infection and discharge may be minimal both types of perforation are always associated with chronic progressive destructive middle ear disease.

GENERAL POINTS TO OBSERVE IN EXAMINATION OF PERFORATIONS

If an ear discharges and there are no signs of external otitis, there must be a perforation, and the examiner should be able to find it. More erroneous diagnoses are made because the ear has not been adequately cleaned than for any other reason. The drum must, therefore, be cleaned carefully before attempting to make a diagnosis.

If a perforation does not become obvious after this, the patient should be told to inflate the ear by Valsalva's method (p. 222). This may be sufficient to cause secretions to exude from the perforation. An aspirating speculum may be used to draw fluid from the middle ear through the perforation. When the perforation has been found, the malleus must be identified, and its relation to the perforation noted. The edges should be examined for thickening, which is a sign of chronicity. Whether the perforation is moist or dry, and the character of the secretion, if any, must be ascertained. If the perforation is moist, the surgeon should decide whether it is adequate for drainage. Especially is this important in the case of pin-hole perforations. When a large perforation is moist, the condition of the lining of the middle ear should be determined. If it is polypoid or shows signs of granulation tissue formation, this has an influence on the prognosis. In chronic perforations, especially of the upper part of the ear, cholesteatoma should be looked for. Its presence will frequently determine the nature of the treatment (p. 271).

THE EUSTACHIAN TUBE

The Eustachian tube plays an important part in the physiology of the middle ear, and is frequently of primary importance in the course of diseases of the ear.

Acute insufficiency of the Eustachian tube

This is a frequent cause of deafness. It is a concomitant of almost every acute coryza, and the precursor of acute otitis media. If temporarily superimposed on another type of hearing loss (especially sensorineural hearing loss in the elderly) as in a cold, a moderate degree of deafness can become severe until the Eustachian tube is re-opened. In children and occasionally in adults it causes considerable pain. Eustachian insufficiency may become chronic, and give rise to recurring attacks of deafness of middle ear type.

Treatment. This consists of inflation with a Politzer bag or, if necessary, with a Eustachian catheter. Adenoids or nasopharyngeal disease should be dealt with.

Sometimes self-inflation by Valsalva's method is useful (see p. 222).

In otitis media, infection of the Eustachian tube is frequently responsible for keeping up the discharge from a perforation. The discharge is of a mucoid character, and the perforation is in the anterior part of the drum.

Chronic Eustachian insufficiency

This may be the result of a mass in the nasopharynx (commonly adenoids), or chronic infection in the nose or sinuses, or sometimes of allergy. It may also be associated with a chronic infection in the ear and in such instances does much to militate against a successful tympanoplasty.

In those cases not associated with chronic ear disease it is important to control nasal and sinus infection and allergy. Eustachian catheterization is generally successful in reopening the Eustachian tube and aerat-

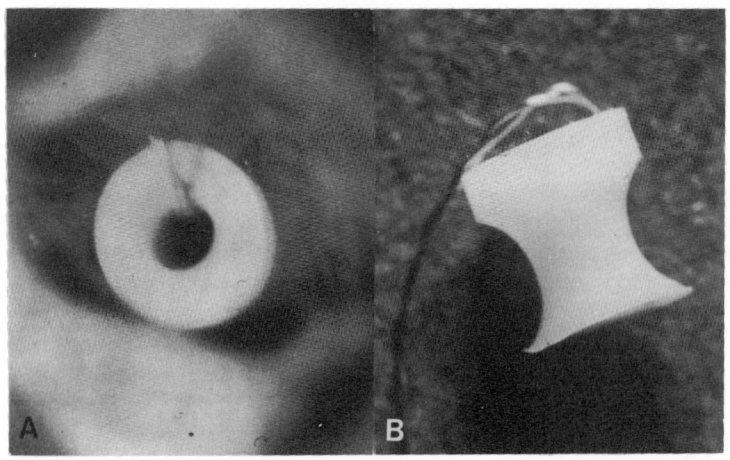

Fig. 88. Mucous otitis. (A) the tube in situ in the tympanic membrane, (B) pressure equalising grommet prior to insertion. (The outside diameter is about 2 mm.)

ing the ear. This should restore hearing, but in some cases fibrous stenosis of the tube may be present. For these patients there is no entirely satisfactory treatment though passage of bougies is still sometimes recommended.

Following a radical mastoid operation persistent discharge of tubal origin may render an otherwise successful operation a failure from the patient's point of view. This unfortunate sequel poses difficult problems of treatment; one of the modern tympanoplastic procedures offers the greatest promise of success.

Eustachian tube insufficiency, which may be persistent or recurrent, is frequently seen in children and probably plays an important part in mucous otitis ('glue ear'). Adequate middle ear aeration must be maintained by inserting a plastic tube or 'grommet' through the anterior part of the drum. This will equalize the pressure within and without the middle ear. This procedure is especially valuable in children, but must always be associated with whatever treatment is necessary for adenoids, nose or sinuses. The grommet is eventually extruded after several months, but during this time the Eustachian tube in most cases has recovered sufficiently to function normally. Maintenance of middle ear aeration by these grommets is essential not only for a satisfactory level of hearing, but also for the prevention of severe damage to the drum and middle ear structures which could be permanent. Accordingly there should be no hesitation in re-inserting a grommet a second or even a third time if necessary (Fig. 88).

This is necessary in a substantial minority of children and in a few of these the problem may extend over a period of two or three years or even more. In these particularly difficult cases middle ear ventilation may be encouraged by Valsalva type exercises. It is important not to overlook a masked mastoiditis.

32 Acute Otitis Media

Acute otitis media is the name given to inflammation of the lining membrane in the middle ear cleft. This condition includes all grades of infection from the least degree of catarrh up to the formation of frank pus, with all the accompanying changes in the lining membrane. The reader is reminded that in these cases the whole middle ear cleft must be considered as one. The membrane lining in the middle ear is continuous with that which passes through the aditus into the mastoid antrum (tympanic antrum) and the mastoid cells. As in the nose, when the mucous lining of the nasal cavity is infected, the lining of the nasal sinuses, being in continuity with that of the nose, shares in the inflammatory reaction, so in the ear there is some reaction in the mastoid antrum and cells in most cases of middle ear infection. Possibly the inflammation may stop short at the aditus or in the mastoid antrum, but it is essential in all cases to look upon the inflammation of the various parts as one disease, and not as a disease which involves the middle ear and then afterwards may involve other parts or structures.

Sources of infection in otitis media

The Eustachian tube is the chief route by which infection reaches the middle ear. The cause of infection in such cases is nasopharyngeal disease and in children this usually means adenoids. Occasionally the infection may be diffuse, as in a coryza, or alternatively the causative infection may be in the nose or sinuses or in the oropharynx and tonsils. In all of these conditions an ascending infection of the Eustachian tube occurs. In the earlier stages the lower end of the tube is involved, but as the salpingitis spreads farther the tube becomes blocked, the air within the middle ear is absorbed and is replaced by exudate which may later become purulent.

Although extension along the Eustachian tube is nearly always an extension of inflammation in the lining membrane, occasionally otitis media may result from infected secretions being forced up the tube by pressure changes associated with excessive nose-blowing, diving, underwater swimming or flying.

Occasionally, infection may enter the middle ear from the external auditory meatus if there is a pre-existing perforation of the drum. It is not unusual to see patients who have had a dry perforation for a long period of time who re-infect their ears by swimming. Very occasionally infection may enter from the external meatus if the drum has been ruptured by trauma.

The great frequency of otitis media in children calls for special comment. The most common cause in children is undoubtedly adenoids. The shortness, patency and the position of the Eustachian tube in the child makes it a particularly easy journey for the organisms to pass from the nasopharynx into the middle ear. In exanthemata, otitis media is frequently encountered in those cases in which purulent nasal complications are prominent. The acute degree of the rhinitis and accumulation of pus in the nasopharynx, combined with the inability on the part of a debilitated child to cleanse the nose properly, is frequently responsible for the infection.

Bacteriology

The use of antibiotics has not greatly influenced the variety of organisms causing acute otitis media. *Streptococci*, *staphylococci* and *haemophilus* are those frequently found. Pneumococcal otitis is not unusual, and while apparently less severe it has a higher risk of complications.

Symptoms of acute otitis media

Pain is the most prominent symptom. In most cases the presence or absence of pain appears to depend to a large extent on the speed of the accumulation of fluid, just as in other parts of the body the rapid production of tension is responsible for pain. In the middle ear the degree of tension of the drum and the production of that tension in a short space of time cause the acute pain which is so frequently experienced in otitis media. There is also in these cases an added source of irritation from the inflammation in the drum structure or in the formation of bullae, which may form the first stage of the infection. The pain is usually described as being of a sharp, lancinating character located in the ear itself, and does not as a rule seem to radiate in the early stages.

Deafness is also a constant sign in cases in which accumulation of fluid has taken place in the middle ear. Deafness in the earliest stages of middle ear inflammation may be almost absent. This is the stage of inflammation without any outpouring of secretions. When, however, fluid commences to accumulate, the hearing tends to become impaired, and with the accumulation of fluid, the normal movement of the ossicles, their ligaments, and the membranes covering the ligaments is prevented, and the hearing steadily deteriorates. This is one of the most reliable guides in estimating the progress of acute otitis media. If we assume the normal to be the hearing of a whisper at 25 to 30 feet, moderate impairment may be said to have occurred when hearing is reduced to 5 to 10 feet; great when a whisper can only just be heard, and severe when a conversation voice is audible at only a few feet. The deafness is of conductive type.

Discharge is the other cardinal symptom. It occurs only in the more severe cases, however, that is in those cases in which spontaneous resolution has failed to occur in the earlier stages of the disease, or in those cases in which the disease has not been arrested by treatment. Discharge indicates that necrosis of the drum with consequent perforation has occurred. The appearance of discharge is usually associated with substantial lessening of pain due to the decrease in tension in the drum membrane. The purulent discharge may be initially bloodstained, and later become mucopurulent.

Other symptoms. These may include tinnitus and voice resonance. Giddiness and sickness occasionally occur from irritation of the inner ear. There is always some general disturbance shown by elevation of the temperature and pulse rate, and a dry, furred tongue.

Signs of acute otitis media

Appearances of the drum membrane. The diagnosis of acute otitis media in the early stages rests largely upon the appearance of the drum membrane. Therefore, if the membrane cannot be seen clearly, either from the lack of skill on the examiner's part or from the presence of some condition in the external canal, such as wax, furunculosis, etc., the diagnosis of otitis media will be by inference only, and complete reliance should not be placed upon this diagnosis. The earliest appearance of infection will be found around the malleus, and consists of the injection of the vessels around the short process and the handle. Care must be taken not to confuse this injection with that which may follow clearance of the external meatus by syringing or other means. The inflammation spreads until it involves the whole drum. The drum loses its lustre, changes from grey to greyish pink, and from pink to bright red. Gradually the outline of the drum itself is lost, and when the fluid at first accumulates the drum bulges in its posterior aspect. The swelling gradually spreads until it involves the anterior portion of the drum, and finally a condition is found in which the drum appears as a doubled roll, the dimple in the centre representing the point of attachment of the handle of the malleus. The colour by this time may be dark red, and all the landmarks will have vanished.

The appearance of the drum membrane in advanced suppuration differs from that in the early forms. A yellowish tinge frequently may be seen instead of the acute red appearance. A hair line may appear to be stretched across the drum, which is the level of the fluid within the middle ear. If a drum is examined when on the point of bursting, a yellow nipple at the point of a projecting red bulge indicates the part of the drum which is in process of sloughing.

Tuning-fork tests. Tuning-fork tests are a very valuable guide to the presence or absence of middle ear involvement. For the purpose of carrying out tuning-fork tests, it must be assumed that the external meatus is to a great extent clear of obstruction. It is useless to lay any stress upon tuning-fork tests in cases in which the external meatus is obstructed by furunculosis or by wax, but when the drum can be seen they are a valuable assistance in deciding upon the presence or absence of disease. The tests have been described fully, and Rinne's test is the most useful. In the earliest stages of inflammation Rinne's test may still be positive, but if the involvement has reached any degree of gravity, the test will be negative. In bilateral infections Weber's test is used to differentiate between the two ears, the one in which the tuning-fork is heard best being that in which the infection is the more advanced.

Tenderness of bone. As already observed, the lining of the middle ear is continuous with that of the mastoid antrum and the mastoid cells. It is, therefore, obvious that the inflammation inside these cells may give acute tenderness over the bone of the mastoid process, and the more acute the infection in the ear the more probable is tenderness in the bone behind the ear. This is due to the simultaneous inflammatory reaction inside the mastoid antrum and cells.

If recovery takes place and pus or serum is released from the middle ear then, as a rule, the tenderness behind the ear subsides, but if not, and if the catarrhal condition of the ear becomes manifestly purulent, then the infection within the bone becomes more advanced and passes into the stage which is called 'mastoiditis'. This will be gone into more fully when we come to deal with complications of middle ear disease (p. 278).

OTITIS MEDIA IN CHILDREN

Diagnosis presents special difficulties in infants and young children because they are unable to co-operate. In infants there is often remarkably little to draw attention to the ear. The infant is simply unwell and has a temperature. Accordingly, any infant with an undiagnosed illness or pyrexia must have the ears examined. Sometimes in the infant, restlessness, crying or screaming (at night time in particular), putting up the hand to the head, rolling the head on the pillow, are signs which should suggest examination of the ears. In older children, apparent disobedience, which is in reality due to deafness, may call attention to the ear condition. It may be very difficult to estimate hearing, and tuning-fork tests are of little use until the child is of an age to co-operate intelligently. Discharge from the ear will solve the problem in some cases and cause relief of pain, if the condition has not been identified and treated by myringotomy. In some cases the appearance of discharge is the first sign of the disease. In these cases, in all probability there is an accumulation of fluid owing to Eustachian obstruction from the presence of adenoids. This fluid may be almost sterile in character, but the gradual accumulation has caused stretching of the drum to such an extent that eventually part of the membrane has sloughed away, and there is present the typical running ear of childhood, causing little or no discomfort to the child.

In the case of a child who proves refractory under examination, it is advisable to give an anaesthetic in order to clean the ear out at leisure and under a good light. Where an accurate diagnosis is important this will be found to be the most satisfactory method.

Diagnosis after perforation

When perforation of the drum has taken place, diagnosis is usually simplified. The history is of considerable importance and will typically include the statement that the acute pain ceased when something burst, and the discharge appeared.

Clinical signs. The meatus is full of discharge, which may be thin sero-sanguineous fluid or yellow pus. When this is mopped out the discharge may be seen to be coming from a perforation. In many cases the exact location of the perforation may be difficult to determine, owing to the oedema of the drum and the free flow of discharge.

Pulsation, however, may be made out. This is movement of the discharge, synchronous with the pulse. The degree of inflammation present causes this movement, and the sign is indicative that an acute process is present. The pulsation is detected by watching a light reflex, or point of reflected light on the discharge, and the point of light is seen to have a small regular movement.

Hearing is still impaired, but is probably showing signs of improvement. Increase in deafness from this time is to be regarded as a sign that the otitis is not clearing up, or that complications may be expected.

Tuning-fork tests indicate conductive deafness. This may persist for a considerable period.

Constitutional disturbance should settle down and any temperature abate. If temperature and pulse remain elevated, danger of extension of disease is still present, and the patient must be confined to bed under close observation.

Differential diagnosis. The differential diagnosis and the exclusion of other conditions form an important part of the diagnosis, and it will be considered fully when the condition of mastoiditis has been dealt with on page 278.

Recovery from acute otitis media

Recovery takes place in one of three ways:

1. There may be spontaneous recovery *without perforation.*
2. There may be spontaneous recovery *after perforation.*
3. There may be recovery *after myringotomy.*

1. Recovery without perforation. The landmarks gradually begin to reappear. One of the first signs is the cracking of the overstretched epithelium of the drum head causing a patchy appearance of desquamation on the surface of the drum. As resolution proceeds, the vessels in the drum begin to stand out, and what is known as the 'cart-wheel' injection develops. Surrounding the drum there is a large vessel like the rim of a wheel, and running to it radially, like the spokes of the wheel, are other vessels. This appearance is typical of the recovering drum. If it has been severely stretched it may take a long time to recover tension completely, and a myringotomy may be of value to release fluid lying behind the drum, and allow a quicker recovery. At the same time, if the inflammation has passed its peak, and the cart-wheel injection referred to is appearing, myringotomy should not be performed, as the time for it is past. The reopening of the Eustachian tube may relieve the tension within the middle ear at any time and initiate improvement in the condition. Full recovery has been obtained only when hearing is again normal.

2. Recovery after perforation. The extreme stretching of the drum membrane gradually produces a devitalization of the tissue, with the result that a portion of the drum sloughs, and the contents of the middle ear are released. The condition of the typical discharging ear with perforated drum membrane follows. Recovery from the infection may leave a permanent perforation or a flimsy scar. In more favourable cases a good firm scar may result, or even a scar which is hardly visible with magnification.

3. Recovery after myringotomy. The third method of releasing the contents of the ear is by means of myringotomy. This consists in making a small cut in the drum, and in presence of an infection a clean surgical cut offers a very much better chance of good healing than when the release of fluid follows the sloughing of part of the membrane. The object of carrying out a myringotomy therefore is not only to relieve pain and release fluid, but to facilitate healing with a good, firm surgical scar instead of risking a large perforation closed with a thin delicate membrane.

Treatment

The chief aim in the treatment of acute otitis media is the preservation of normal hearing. Since the introduction of chemotherapy the danger to life is so reduced that the whole attention can be given to the problem of restoring and safe-guarding function. It cannot be too strongly emphasized that mere recovery from acute symptoms is not sufficient. Misuse of chemotherapy and antibiotics may give apparently good immediate results, only to cause loss of hearing in the future. How far treatment has proved successful is gauged by the degree to which the ear-drum, tuning-fork tests and hearing have returned to normal.

Treatment before myringotomy or perforation. General treatment consists of confining the patient to bed in a warm but adequately ventilated room. Relief from pain, caused by the irritation of nerve endings in the inflamed ear-drum, is important and at times essential.

Pain can be relieved by the application of local heat and the administration of analgesics aided where necessary by the use of ear drops (see Appendix).

Re-establishment of drainage of the Eustachian tube is important. This can be encouraged by the use of nasal drops and inhalations. Suitable decongestant drops are ephedrine in saline; they are given four-hourly in the head-hanging position and followed by an inhalation of medicated steam. Either Friar's Balsam or menthol is appropriate. (Fig. 26).

Chemotherapy

Chemotherapy has greatly reduced the incidence of suppurative conditions of the ear, and the surgery of acute suppuration now forms a very small part of otology. It must be stressed, however, that the descriptions of acute disease are not unnecessary, because without some knowledge of the classical course of the disease the variations produced by chemotherapy cannot be understood. Organisms insensitive to drug treatment are increasing in numbers, and therefore it is essential to understand the management of otitis media without the aid of chemotherapy.

Administration of antibiotics

These drugs, when used, should always be given in adequate dosage. To give small doses of sulphonamides or antibiotics is to invite trouble, and most of the difficulties in hospital work arise from the uncertainties created by half-hearted treatment. Masked mastoiditis (see p. 281) may result from such inadequate treatment.

Inadequate dosage may succeed in sterilizing, wholly or partially, the contents of the ear, which remains full of pus. The infection, therefore, may only be damped down and will soon recur. Organization and formation of adhesions may be encouraged. Alternatively discharge may become chronic. Although parenteral administration of antibiotics may be considered preferable and is the most certain way of obtaining adequate blood levels there are certain objections to this method in practice. It has to be accepted that the great majority of acute infections respond satisfactorily to suitable antibiotics by mouth. Moreover, most practitioners are reluctant to give repeated injections to children unless they are absolutely essential. They are almost inevitably associated with some emotional trauma with consequent loss of confidence and loss of co-operation during any future illness. With so many effective antibiotics now available injection can be reserved for those ear infections which prove resistant to treatment.

Identification of organisms

Wherever possible, bacteriological studies should form the basis of administration, and sensitivity tests should always be carried out. In the majority of cases the organisms are penicillin sensitive, but if practicable a swab should be taken from the nose and throat, and from the ear if myringotomy has been done or discharge has occurred. Only by these means can satisfactory bacteriological control be achieved. Sometimes in difficult cases aspiration of the middle ear contents, or myringotomy, is indicated purely for the purpose of identifying the organisms and their sensitivities.

The choice of antibiotic and dosage

Ampicillin is the drug of first choice and it should be given in full dosage and continued for not less than five days. In rare cases injection may be judged the best method of obtaining a high blood level of the drug quickly.

If examination of the ear after an interval of about twelve hours shows that the infection is responding, the treatment is continued.

If examination at the second visit shows no response, then a switch to a wide spectrum antibiotic can be made. If possible swabs should be taken for bacteriological investigation.

It is also worth remembering (*a*) that other effective oral preparations include the sulphonamides and erythromycin; (*b*) although oral preparations may be prescribed the patient may not take the full dosage.

Whatever drug is chosen, treatment must always extend from five to seven days if emergence of insensitive strains of organisms is to be prevented.

When the condition is not arrested by these measures, and the drum membrane becomes obviously full and bulging, and the patient's symptoms are not improving, it becomes necessary to consider the operation of myringotomy to permit free drainage.

MYRINGOTOMY

Extreme pain is the most usual indication for myringotomy. Where a perforation appears almost certain, or where symptoms suggest an extension of the inflammatory reaction throughout the mastoid cells, then drainage by the quickest surgical method becomes good practice. Healing of a perforation caused by spontaneous rupture usually occurs by regeneration of the outer and inner epithelial layers only, the middle elastic layer often does not regenerate. Accordingly, the scar is often flimsy and fragile and may readily break down at some future time. A myringotomy results in a much more satisfactory scar, and the probability of good hearing after the operation is very much greater than if the drum is allowed to slough. When carrying out the operation of myringotomy it is frequently good practice to remove any adenoids in the nasopharynx at the same time. Sometimes the discharge persists for a long period unless the adenoids are removed, and a further operation may be avoided if the adenoids are removed at the time the drum is incised.

Summary of indications for myringotomy

1. Excessive pain demanding relief.
2. Presence of increasing hearing defect caused by accumulation of fluid in the middle ear.
3. Pus in the middle ear which is causing toxic symptoms.
4. Severe bulging of the drum which is not quickly lessened by chemotherapy.

Technique of myringotomy

A good light is essential for carrying out this operation. If possible a properly equipped operating theatre should be used, but it is quite permissible to carry out the treatment in a patient's home. Under such circumstances the greatest difficulty is that of illumination, and some form of focussing headlight or operating otoscope is advisable.

Anaesthesia by means of gas-oxygen or pentothal sodium will be adequate for the experienced surgeon, but those without experience are advised to use some form of anaesthesia which will give ample time to carry out the operation with deliberation and care. If myringotomy is urgently needed and facilities for general anaesthesia are not available, it is possible to operate after using Blegvad's drops (see Appendix). Analgesia, however, may be incomplete and an accurate incision therefore more difficult to make.

The outer ear is painted with antiseptic, the speculum is inserted, and any wax or debris is removed from the meatus. The knife used is of special design for the operation, and it is essential that the handle should be angled to give a clear view of the point during the operation. The incision is 'J' shaped, and should commence in the posterior part of the drum about the level of a line dividing the drum horizontally into upper and middle thirds (Fig. 89). The incision is then brought down vertically, and curved round well below the tip of the handle of the malleus. The point of the knife should be passed through the drum only far enough to cut the drum itself, as if passed far through the membrane there is danger of injury to the structures in the middle ear. Some operators prefer to incise the drum from below upwards, believing that this method avoids danger to the ossicles and inner ear. This objection, however, appears to be theoretical. In most cases pus immediately follows the knife. A specimen is taken for bacteriological purposes, and a strip of ribbon gauze can be inserted to absorb any blood or pus, and by capillary attraction to help to drain the middle ear. This wick can be removed in a few hours' time, and the drum inspected to make sure that the opening made is adequate, and that drainage is free. Thereafter the treatment should be that of a case of acute otitis media with a discharging ear. If the method of mopping under direct observation is adopted skilled supervision will be required.

Although diagrammatically it appears simple to divide the drum at the proper place, the beginner must be warned that the incision should be farther forward on the bulge of the drum than would appear to be correct. The chief fault in carrying out this operation is to make the cut too far posteriorly, and when the drum collapses the incision lies so close to the posterior wall that the drainage is seriously impeded. It should be noted that the operation of myringotomy consists of making a full-length incision. In paracentesis, by contrast, only a small stab is made. This is often done for diagnostic purposes, or for aspiration of watery fluid in serous otitis. In 'glue ear' (p. 267) the stab is usually made in the anterior segment and in a radial direction when a grommet is to be inserted.

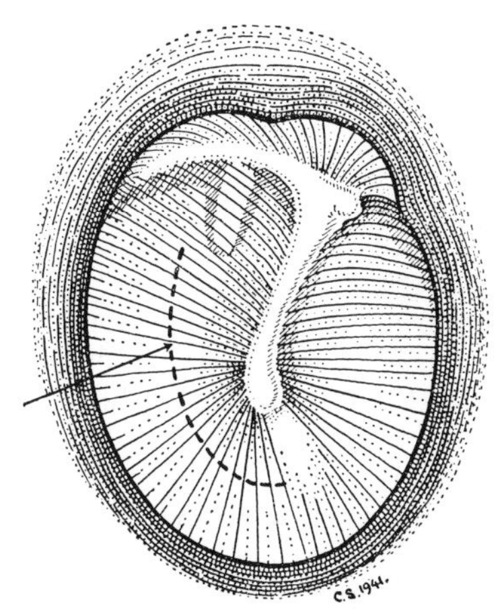

Fig. 89. Myringotomy. In acute suppurative otitis media the incision is as shown. For a diagnostic paracentesis a small stab is usually made anteriorly in a radial direction.

Following myringotomy an immediate fall in temperature and improvement of general condition is to be expected. Failing this, further complications must be anticipated, in particular advancing mastoid infection. The discharge, passing gradually from a purulent condition to a serous one, should clear up within a few days. Before passing a patient as recovered, careful examination of the hearing must be made, and, if necessary, the Eustachian tube must be inflated. This is a part of the treatment which must on no account be omitted. Failure to do this small examination after treatment may mean partial deafness for life to the patient.

A bacteriological examination should be made of the discharge following myringotomy. The organisms most commonly found are *streptococci*, *staphylococci*, and *haemophilus*. The *pneumococcus* may also be found. Information on this particular point is a valuable help in planning further treatment. Antibiotics can be given accurately, and complications prevented.

Treatment after myringotomy or perforation

The object of treatment is primarily adequate drainage, and the drying-up of discharge. Pain does not enter into consideration in these cases in which myringotomy or perforation has occurred. Should pain be present at such a stage in the disease, treatment does not consist of soothing the pain, but of treating the cause, for subsequent pain, when adequate drainage has been established, is a symptom which indicates extension of disease, and must be looked upon as a danger sign. In certain cases, however, a slight recurrence of pain may occur after the perforation. In those cases in which the perforation has been inadequate to release the whole of the purulent contents of the middle ear the perforation tends to close, and may by oedema seal off completely. It may be necessary to enlarge the opening in the drum to drain the pus. Premature closure by healing of the perforation may also occur and may necessitate another myringotomy.

The perforation or opening in the drum may become obstructed if the discharge in the external meatus is allowed to collect. Drainage is inadequate and the movement of the secretion in the various parts of the ear is prevented. The discharge should, therefore, be removed. This may be done by two methods – the dry method or the wet method. In the dry method the canal is cleansed by mopping. This is done by dressed probes and by small wicks of cotton wool. A good light and a certain degree of skill and previous training are necessary. This treatment is followed by leaving a small wick in the meatus. Capillary attraction draws the secretions out of the middle ear. It is essential in employing this method to change the wick at very frequent intervals.

This treatment, while theoretically sound, presupposes a considerable degree of skill on the part of those attending the patient, and is hardly one which can be entrusted to the hands of an untrained nurse or friend. It is, therefore, the experience of those working in hospital clinics that where the patient has to be sent home a considerable distance, and has to be attended by those who have little skill or knowledge of ear diseases, that the treatment by wet methods will achieve more than the dry method inefficiently carried out.

The wet treatment consists of the instillation of hydrogen peroxide drops. These are allowed to remain in the ear for half a minute to a minute in order to loosen the accumulated discharge. The discharge is then syringed out gently with warm boric lotion and the ear is mopped dry. This treatment is carried out daily, or if discharge is very copious and thick, twice daily.

In the normal process of resolution the discharge gradually becomes thicker and more mucoid, then it slowly assumes a more serous appearance and finally dries up. The condition may pass normally through these stages in the course of a week or so, or it can take two to three weeks. On the other hand, it may enter a subacute stage, which may last weeks or months. The longer discharge continues, the greater is the danger of some permanent damage to hearing. If syringing has been instituted for some days, and the acute stage is passing off, spirit drops may be instilled. About six drops of boric acid in rectified spirit are poured into the ear morning and night. (See Appendix.)

Boric and iodine powder (0.75 per cent iodine in boric acid powder) is a more popular remedy for achieving the same object. The boric acid dissolves in the discharge of the ear and liberates nascent iodine which exercises a bactericidal effect. This powder is introduced by means of an insufflator.

Antibiotics. These should be continued until the full course has been completed. The antibiotic used may have to be altered, depending upon the bacteriological report. Ear drops consisting of antibiotics and steroids have no significant place in treatment, but are occasionally helpful in drying up the last trace of discharge. Drops should always be used with care because of the risk of local reaction.

If the discharge from the ear continues, search should be made for the condition responsible for its chronicity. This may be found to be nasopharyngeal disease which, in children, may be caused by adenoids. Sinusitis, also is responsible sometimes for the condition, and inadequate nasal airway with poor aeration of the post-nasal spaces may be found to be at the root of the trouble. These conditions may require to be corrected before recovery can take place.

It is also important to exclude the possibility of a masked mastoiditis, especially if chemotherapy may have been given in inadequate dosage or the organisms are only partially sensitive (p. 281).

RECURRING OTITIS MEDIA

Patients are occasionally seen in whom repeated attacks of acute otitis media cause great problems. A most careful search should be made for any focus of infection in the nose, sinuses, mouth or pharynx. Swabs for bacteriological examination may be taken from other members of the family if there is reason to suspect outside sources of infection. In children who have already had an adenoidectomy the possibility of a recurrence of adenoids should be considered. Similarly, in children, the possibility of hypogammaglobulinaemia should be borne in mind. Occasionally in both adults and in children the focus which is responsible for recurrent attacks of an apparently acute otitis media lies in the mastoid. Such patients have often received repeated courses of antibiotics which have produced a latent mastoiditis. There is often no clinical evidence of mastoiditis as such, although good X-ray studies are invaluable. The final diagnosis may be made only by exploring the mastoid.

33. Chronic Otitis Media

Chronic otitis media may be defined as 'infection of long standing in which there are no signs of acute inflammation'. It may be caused by the failure of an acute infection to resolve completely or by the infection of a cholesteatoma or of a serous effusion into the middle ear.

Types of disease

Chronic otitis may be classified as follows:

1. Non-suppurative.
   (*a*) Serous otitis.
   (*b*) Mucous otitis or 'glue ear'.
2. Suppurative.
   (*a*) Tubo-tympanic suppuration.
   (*b*) Attico-antral disease.
3. Tuberculous.

MUCOUS OTITIS AND SEROUS OTITIS

The accumulation of fluid in the middle ear occurring in the absence of acute inflammation appears to be increasingly common. It may vary from a thin serous fluid to thick viscid material, hence the label 'glue ear' is often used clinically. These collections of fluid are encountered at all ages and some observers believe that the affection in the child is a different condition from that found in the adult. There is much to support this view.

Mucous otitis

This is the form of the disorder usually seen in children. It is almost invariably bilateral and the fluid is in most cases thick and mucoid. It may even be semi-solid. The condition is very common about the age of five or six and is probably the result of upper respiratory tract viral infections occurring in association with inadequate Eustachian tube function. Insufficient dosage of antibiotics in otitis media has sometimes been blamed, but a history of true acute otitis is rare. It is possible that administration of antibiotics early in an attack of otitis media may sterilize the contents of the middle ear, and a blocked Eustachian tube and unhealthy adenoids may prevent evacuation of fluid and re-aeration.

The only symptom is impaired hearing, but the onset of this is insidious so that the child is frequently accused by the parents of being awkward or inattentive. In some children the deafness is first noticed by the schoolteacher or a visiting relative, others are only discovered during routine audiometric screening at school. Pain is absent, though a mild aching may occur if infection supervenes. There is no discharge unless an acute otitis media should develop.

On examination the drum may appear normal, even when a magnifying speculum is used. Typically, however, the drum is lustreless and often has a yellow or orange tint: fine blood vessels are often seen coursing inwards from the drum margin. The most important and obvious signs are the lack of mobility of the drum when using the pneumatic speculum and the discovery of a negative Rinne. When these two clinical signs are present the child in most cases has a 'glue ear'. In cases of long standing, the drum often becomes thinned, atrophic and collapsed.

Treatment is surgical. This usually consists of an anterior myringotomy, the aspiration of the thick mucoid material, and the insertion of a plastic tube or 'grommet' (Fig. 88). The 'grommet' provides for adequate ventilation of the middle ear space and is essentially an artificial Eustachian tube. Adenoids are removed and any other infection of the nose, sinuses or pharynx must also be dealt with. As long as the grommets remain *in situ* the disorder rarely recurs and hearing remains at a normal level. After several months, however, the grommets are slowly extruded and if the Eustachian tube function has not meantime returned to normal a recurrence of the fluid is frequent. Accordingly, these children must be kept under careful observation and, if necessary, the grommets must be re-inserted. It is extremely important that these children should be identified and treated adequately, not only to restore their hearing but perhaps even more important to prevent eventual damage to the drum and to the middle ear. Neglect may result in the formation of adhesions, collapse of the drum with formation of retraction pockets, and possibly cholesteatoma.

Serous otitis

This name is more applicable in the case of adults. Although the disorder just described can occur in adults it is not common. Usually the fluid is thin and watery and probably is a transudate. It is nearly always unilateral and the aetiology is uncertain, although upper respiratory infections and allergy are probably predisposing factors. Occasionally a lesion in the nasopharynx, such as carcinoma, may present in this way. The onset is usually acute; the ear feels blocked and hearing is impaired. The patient may be aware of a splashing sensation inside the ear when moving the head and may also notice that hearing varies in different head positions as the fluid moves around the ear cavity.

On examination of the drum the line of the fluid level is often visible and this remains horizontal as the head is moved. Occasionally bubbles may be seen behind the drum. In contrast to the findings in children the hearing loss is often slight and may not be sufficient to produce a negative Rinne. A search should always be made for any disease in the nose, sinuses, pharynx and especially in the nasopharynx.

Treatment is straightforward; indeed certain cases resolve without treatment, as for example when an acute cold settles. Frequently the fluid will clear on a short course of an antihistamine. If the fluid persists then inflation of air through a Eustachian catheter will usually disperse it. Occasionally the fluid must be removed through a myringotomy incision. Obstinate cases are rarely seen, but may call for the insertion of a grommet as described above.

TUBO-TYMPANIC SUPPURATION

Aetiology. This type is very common in children but is found also in adults, and may follow acute otitis media. Not infrequently it is accompanied by disease in the nose or the sinuses or in the pharynx.

Clinical features. The discharge is mucoid or muco-purulent. It may be constant, but it may dry up at times to reappear with the onset of upper respiratory infection. The perforation of the drum is anterior or central, and does not involve the drum margin. In acute exacerbations the middle ear mucosa may be swollen and oedematous and may on occasion produce polypi. There is usually a conductive deafness present, but hearing can remain good; in untreated disease there is danger to the hearing though there is rarely any threat to life.

There is no evidence of cholesteatoma or disease of bone, which is usually indicated by granulation tissue or necrotic bone. X-rays may show some clouding of the mastoid cells due to preceding acute disease. The ossicles are often intact, though they may undergo ischaemic necrosis.

Treatment

If the surgeon is satisfied that there is no complication and that no deep-seated disease exists, conservative treatment is started, and perseverance with this treatment is essential. The type of case suitable is one in which there is a clean central perforation without complication.

Any concurrent disease in nose, sinuses or pharynx should be cleared up. In children particular attention should be paid to adenoids if present. Local treatment is directed towards strict cleansing of the ear and the adoption of measures designed to dry up the discharge.

If discharge is profuse the best way of cleansing the ear is by gentle syringing. First, a few drops of peroxide of hydrogen are instilled into the ear and left for one minute. The ear is then syringed with warm boracic lotion and mopped dry. Boric acid and spirit drops (see Appendix) or antibiotic-steroid drops are instilled thrice daily. This will assist the ear to dry up and prevent stagnation of discharge. If the spirit causes pain it may be omitted. Where skill is available the ear is mopped under direct vision, or the discharge may be aspirated.

Instillation of chemotherapeutic drugs. Antibiotic drops must be used with caution as sensitization may occur. The use of antibiotics involves careful bacteriological studies, otherwise more harm than good may be done by permitting free growth of antibiotic-resistant organisms. The addition of steroids is an advantage if combined with an antibiotic, *e.g.* neomycin, by reason of their anti-inflammatory properties.

Insufflation of powder. Boric and iodine powder (0.75 per cent of iodine in boracic acid powder) is still one of the most useful. It is appropriate when discharge is not copious, or in the recovery stages where cleansing treatment has caused a marked diminution of discharge. A light dusting of powder is sufficient.

Polypi

In some cases of tubo-tympanic disease there may be oedema of the mucous membrane of the middle ear which may appear through a perforation as a polypus. In such cases removal of the polypus should be the first step in treatment, as the obstruction caused by the polypus prevents proper drainage of the ear. In more advanced instances clearance of the middle ear by suction is undoubtedly the quickest method of obtaining good results.

Healing

When the ear becomes dry and the perforation remains it is said to be quiescent. To obtain complete healing, repair of the drum defect is necessary. While the perforation exists, pressure caused by nose blowing, diving, etc., can re-introduce infection into the middle ear by driving nasopharyngeal secretions through the middle ear. Also infection can enter the middle ear from the external auditory meatus and cause recurrence of the otitis.

In such circumstances closure of the perforation should be considered.

This may be accomplished in several different ways, depending upon the size and position of the perforation. Touching the edges with trichloracetic acid, or similar substance, may stimulate granulations and lead to healing of small perforations. Blood clot, oil silk, or polythene film can be used as a scaffold for the epithelium and will hasten healing. This method is useful but after many treatments may still end in failure or a weak scar, but as it is an out-patient procedure it is convenient in some instances.

Surgical repair is indicated in larger perforations and in patients in whom there is the possibility of discontinuity of the ossicular chain. Temporalis fascia is generally used for closure of the perforation; such a repair is known as myringoplasty. If the ossicular chain is broken then an ossiculoplasty is indicated. Sometimes the patient's own tissues can be used. If not, preserved homograft materials can be employed for reconstructive purposes (see below, General Considerations in Tympanoplasty, p. 276). All these operations are of advanced technical difficulty. In tubo-tympanic disease, there being no mastoid infection, operation on the mastoid is not indicated. Sometimes an inspection window is made into the antrum to confirm the diagnosis.

ATTICO-ANTRAL DISEASE

This differs radically from tubo-tympanic disease in that it is dangerous to life and may be so silent in onset that it may give little indication of its presence until complications make their appearance. There are two forms of the disease: (1) suppurative disease, (2) cholesteatomatous disease. These forms may be combined. In both types there is destruction of bone and usually some damage to the contents of the middle ear.

Suppurative

This may occur at any age and may follow an acute process as a sequel to otitis media. At the present time because of the prompt administration of antibiotics the widespread suppurative type of disease is rare, but it may follow inadequate treatment of acute disease with antibiotics, where there is some mastoid involvement. In such circumstances there is destruction of the mastoid cells, and possibly some exposure of the dura or the lateral sinus. In the absence of symptoms due to complications X-rays will, as a rule, enable a diagnosis to be made. Discharge, which may be yellow, copious and foul, is a common feature, and deafness is marked. Occasionally, however, the discharge is scanty. Perforations of the drum are as a rule posterior, but do not necessarily follow any particular pattern when the disease follows an acute otitis media.

Granulations. These are typical of disease of bone and grow on dead or dying bone. In certain cases, however, especially in the earlier stages of disease, swollen mucous membrane may produce polypi as well.

Cholesteatomatous disease

Discharge may be scanty, foul and creamy where secondary infection is present, and comes from a perforation which is typically marginal, *i.e.* it involves the bony rim of the drum, or it may be in the attic and may extend downwards to involve the posterior part of the drum.

If there is little infection the discharge may consist of a flaky, waxy deposit which is found adhering to the roof of the external meatus near the drum membrane. This may obscure the attic perforation which may be difficult to identify.

Cholesterol granuloma has no relationship to cholesteatoma, though the names are confusing and the two conditions may co-exist in the middle ear or mastoid. Cholesterol granuloma is caused by the presence of cholesterol crystals from a previous sero-sanguineous exudate. The crystals lead to a foreign body type of reaction and so become embedded in granulomatous tissue.

Cholesteatoma is the result of accumulation of squamous epithelium and its products in the middle ear and mastoid. It not infrequently forms an encysted putty-like mass. The suffix '-oma' may suggest that it is a tumour. This is not the case, though as it expands it is destructive.

Cholesteatoma is classified as (1) congenital cholesteatoma, (2) acquired cholesteatoma, which may be primary or secondary. Debate continues concerning the exact pathogenesis.

Congenital cholesteatoma

Primary inclusions occur within the petrous bone, but are rare. They produce extensive destruction and are usually diagnosed when interference with VII and VIII nerve function occurs. They are often closely related to the internal carotid artery and the jugular bulb and their removal calls for the most advanced otological techniques. These usually give better access than a neuro-surgical middle fossa approach.

Acquired cholesteatoma

It is believed at present that the most frequent cause of acquired cholesteatoma is collapse and invagination of various parts of the drum leading to the formation of retraction pockets. These have been discussed on page 249. Such pockets develop consequent upon Eustachian tube insufficiency. They do not recover when middle ear ventilation has been re-established, but remain as collapsed areas in the attic or, alternatively, in the posterior segment of a damaged pars tensa. Keratinising squamous epithelium normally throws off its dead layer and no accumulation of debris occurs, but when a pocket forms and the normal self-cleansing process fails, debris builds up and eventually becomes a true cholesteatoma. Extrusion of the epithelium through the narrow neck of the sac becomes increasingly difficult and expansion of the lesion occurs. The drum is not 'perforated' in the true sense of the word. The hole one sees is really the small, narrow opening of what can be a very large flask-like retraction, the flask itself being full of wax-like epithelial debris.

Other theories of cholesteatoma formation postulate that squamous metaplasia of the middle ear mucosa may occur in response to a chronic infection or that ingrowth of squamous epithelium around the edges of a perforation may take place, especially in the case of marginal perforations. It has also been suggested that ingrowth of basal cells from the outer layer of the attic part of the drum into persisting sub-mucous tissue within the attic spaces may occur. It is possible that each of these three mechanisms can play a part, but present opinion is that they are not of great significance.

Secondary acquired cholesteatoma

This form does not differ basically from the primary form. By reason of infection, progress is more rapid and the suppurative element introduces further risks to the patient. The primary cholesteatoma may be silent and unsuspected for years, whereas the secondary has overt symptoms of discharge. This may be profuse or scanty, but it is always foul.

Destruction of bone is a feature of both primary and secondary acquired cholesteatomas; this is probably the result of a chemical process rather than pressure alone.

Investigation

As this disease is frequently silent yet invasive in character, investigation of a suspected case of attico-antral disease must include tests to confirm or eliminate signs of involvement of important structures.

Hearing

The level of hearing must be ascertained and in instances of marked hearing loss care must be taken to ensure that such results as are obtained are a true reflection of the hearing in the ear under examination. This implies the use of adequate masking.

The tuning-fork tests will indicate a conductive type of hearing loss, but it is always wise to repeat these tests using a noise box. Otherwise it is possible to miss a 'false negative Rinne' and the fact that the patient has a 'dead ear', *i.e.* a total sensori-neural deafness. This is a complication indicating internal ear destruction.

The fistula sign

In certain cases, especially in those in which there is cholesteatoma formation, the disease causes erosion of the bony capsule of the labyrinth. The most frequent site for such a fistula is in the lateral semicircular canal, where it lies in the floor of the aditus. Where such a fistula is present any sudden change of pressure in the middle ear will immediately be transmitted to the labyrinth, and will produce strong labyrinthine reaction.

The sign may be elicited by sudden pressure on the tragus, or the nozzle of a Politzer bag may be inserted into the external auditory meatus and pressure or suction applied. This will cause a momentary oscillation of the patient's eyes, and a sensation of giddiness. The direction of the nystagmus is not constant and may be to one side or the other.

The interpretation of this sign is firstly that there is a fistula in the bony covering of the labyrinth, and, secondly, that the labyrinth is functioning.

Radiological examination

This is occasionally useful and may show the extent of the disease, such as erosion of the attic region, destruction of the ossicular chain, enlargement of the Eustachian Tube, and encroachment on other structures. (Fig. 90).

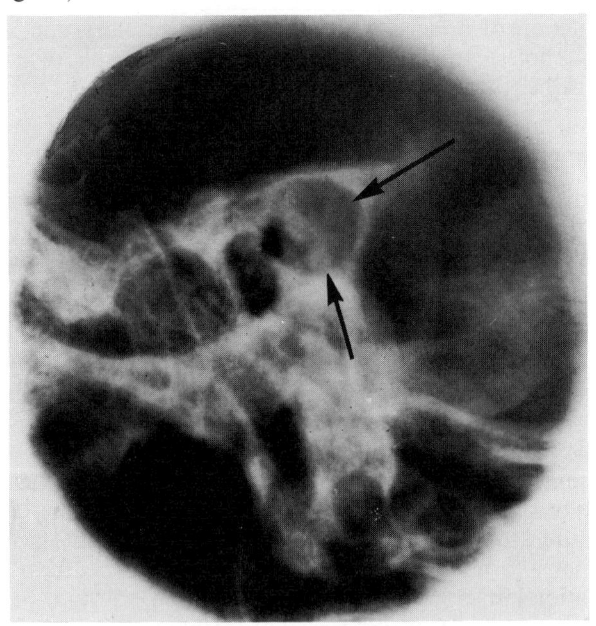

Fig. 90 Cholesteatoma mass arrowed.

It must be emphasised, however, that diagnosis is essentially clinical, by recognizing the site of the perforation and character of the discharge. And though X-rays and tomograms are helpful, only surgical exploration can accurately define the extent of the disease.

Treatment

Conservative treatment has only a limited part to play. Careful use of suction under magnification occasionally results in removal of all diseased tissue and healing may result if the disease happens to be very limited. As already emphasized, however, the extent of disease is difficult to diagnose and such management carries a high risk of leaving trouble behind. Nevertheless such 'suction-clearance' can provide a valuable preliminary to definitive surgery in that it allows for more accurate estimation of the condition in the ear and occasionally it will control very early disease.

Instillation of antibiotic drops has no place in treatment, except for a few days prior to operation when it is useful to suppress infection. The antibiotic should be selected according to bacteriological studies of sensitivity and should be combined with a steroid.

Treatment is surgical and is aimed at the elimination of a dangerous disease. The majority of serious complications occur during acute exacerbations of chronic disease, and if this is realized it becomes obvious that a patient with attico-antral disease leads a precarious existence. The second consideration is the preservation or improvement of hearing. Uncontrolled disease will, over the years, produce a severe degree of deafness, or even total destruction of hearing in the affected ear. The use of chemotherapy, however, has so changed the prognosis of the dangerous complications of chronic suppurative otitis media that the preservation of hearing may now be said to be the chief preoccupation of the surgeon, and success is often judged by the level of hearing it is possible to save or restore. The third aim in treatment is the elimination of discharge from the ear, so providing a symptom-free ear. Hearing improvement and a dry, stable ear are to a great extent dependent upon avoidance of an open mastoid cavity, which nowadays constitutes an important part of the technique of mastoid surgery.

Before proceeding to any reconstruction of the hearing mechanism all disease, whether of bone or other tissue, must be eradicated. There is much to be said for doing the necessary reconstruction as a separate operation after a substantial interval.

Excision of the disease may require a relatively limited operation on the attic (the operation of atticotomy). Frequently the antrum must also be opened (attico-antrotomy), or if disease extends into the mastoid, some kind of mastoidectomy will be required. In radical mastoidectomy the middle ear and mastoid cavities are thrown into one space by removing the bony posterior wall of the auditory meatus as far down as the facial nerve allows. The increasing emphasis, however, on preservation or restoration of function makes it necessary for the patient to be left with an intact posterior meatal wall whenever possible. Intact posterior wall procedures demand a high degree of surgical skill and are by no means suitable for all patients. The major risk of operations in which the approach is partly permeatal, partly trans-mastoid (combined approach tympanoplasty) is that disease may be left in the posterior part of the mesotympanum. The creation of a window from the mastoid into the posterior meso-tympanum (posterior tympanotomy) does much to overcome this difficulty, but is not without danger to the facial nerve.

GENERAL CONSIDERATIONS IN TYMPANOPLASTY

Certain basic materials are essential for any reconstruction. The poorer the quality of these, the poorer the result will be. Ear operations are no exception and sometimes the situation will be such that any attempt at reconstruction is contra-indicated. A brief note of the types of operation to excise diseased bone has been given above, together with some account of the terminology used. Such operations are needed only in attico-antral disease and are sometimes done as a preliminary and separate operation so that swollen, oedematous mucosa can recover and regenerate, infection can settle and vascular engorgement can diminish. The middle ear reconstruction can then be done under more favourable conditions.

Apart from adequate skill and experience in micro-surgical techniques the following factors influence the functional result obtained after reconstructive operations for either tubo-tympanic or attico-antral disease.

(*a*) The level of the sensori-neural reserve. This is a factor beyond the surgeon's control, but if the reserve is inadequate the functional result will be affected accordingly. Sometimes the sensori-neural reserve is so poor that reconstruction is contraindicated.

(*b*) The adequacy of Eustachian tube function. This, too, is largely beyond the surgeon's control; steps to improve it pre-operatively are of doubtful value as are elaborate pre-operative methods of testing Eustachian tube function.

(*c*) The quality of the middle ear mucosa. The condition of the mucosa can be greatly improved when the associated infection has been controlled by appropriate preliminary medical and surgical measures. During tympanoplasty formation of adhesions can often be diminished by the implantation of suitably tailored sheets of plastic film.

(*d*) The presence of an intact tympanic ring to support the new drum. This is not affected in any case by tubo-tympanic disease; after operations to eradicate attico-antral disease it is retained intact only if the techniques of combined approach tympanoplasty are utilized.

(*e*) The feasibility of providing for adequate sound transmission. This implies the passage of vibrations from drum to oval window across the closed air-containing, mucosa-lined middle ear, and the provision of adequate sound protection of the round window in order to produce a differential between the two windows. For sound transmission some kind of ossicular chain must be slung across the middle ear. Sometimes the patient's own damaged incus can be interposed between the malleus and the stapes. With increasing frequency preserved homograft materials are being used, either homograft ossicles, or homograft cartilage which can be carved to suitable shape and size. The drum is usually reconstructed from the patient's own temporalis fascia, but homograft drums are not infrequently used to repair sub-total perforations. In patients with total loss of drum and ossicular chain a complete tympano-ossicular homograft can be used. These methods are still under development and it will readily be appreciated that all these complex micro-procedures demand much time and skill. It can be said that the results are constantly improving and that much more can be offered to patients than was possible a decade ago.

Details of micro-surgery of the ear are beyond the scope of this book, but it is hoped that this brief account will help to explain some of the procedures and help familiarize the reader with some aspects of the various problems and their solution.

TUBERCULOSIS OF THE EAR

This disease occurs mainly in children and is insidious in onset; widespread disease of bone may be present with little outward evidence. Infection is secondary to disease elsewhere and usually reaches the ear via the Eustachian tube by infiltration of its mucosa. In adults infected material may pass up the lumen. Haematogenous spread also occurs.

Diagnosis is seldom made pre-operatively, except in countries where tuberculosis is still common. Multiple perforations of the drum and rapidly recurring pale granulations may draw attention to the possibility, but most cases are seen at a late stage when the ear is already disorganised. Associated secondary infection usually makes bacteriological diagnosis difficult, but biopsy of granulations shows the typical appearances.

Occasionally complications such as facial palsy and labyrinthitis may first draw attention to the disease. Mastoid surgery is necessary, it consists of the removal of granulations and necrotic bone with conservation of whatever is considered possible. Intensive anti-tuberculous chemo-therapy and a sanatorium regime are essential for the healing of what is usually a more generalised disease.

34. Complications of Otitis Media

ACUTE MASTOIDITIS

Now a rare disease in this country, acute mastoiditis is still common elsewhere. It is a complication of acute otitis media and is seen more frequently in children than in adults. It can occur also as a complication of chronic otitis media which may have been present for some time without signs of mastoid involvement. Acute mastoiditis occurring under such circumstances is as a rule more extensive and requires more radical treatment than in a hitherto normal ear, and symptoms may be confused by the pre-existing disease.

Inflammatory reaction within the mastoid area frequently accompanies acute otitis media. Its extent is decided by several factors, among them the cellularity or otherwise of the mastoid, the anatomy of the aditus and the virulence of the infection. Swelling of the lining of the aditus may prevent proper drainage of infection in the mastoid area and accelerate destruction of the bone cells. Continuous hyperaemia in presence of infection causes decalcification of the bone trabeculae so that in advanced cases the whole area becomes one large cavity filled with pus and granulations. If the disease continues uncontrolled the infection may break through towards the middle cranial fossa, the posterior fossa or the sigmoid sinus; in more fortunate cases the pus may break through the superficial cortex and form an abscess under the periosteum.

Signs and symptoms

Mastoiditis is invariably preceded by acute otitis media. This may not have been observed, but evidence of it can always be found.

Pain. One of the outstanding signs of the onset of mastoiditis is pain. As already stated, pain often accompanies otitis media. After myringotomy, or the spontaneous perforation of the drum, pain disappears in a few hours, or at most after three or four days. Should pain recur, or, not having completely disappeared, increase in severity, it is an indication of advancing mastoid infection. In these circumstances the pain may be in the ear, but it is more often located behind the ear in the mastoid bone. The pain may remain localized in one spot, but it may on occasion radiate all over the side of the head in severe spasms.

Discharge. With the onset of mastoiditis, as a rule, the discharge ceases or it becomes more profuse. Cessation of the discharge means that the membrane lining the aditus has become so swollen that the discharge is being dammed up in the mastoid cells. In these cases relief by mastoid operation will almost certainly be required. Increase of discharge suggests the further involvement of mastoid cells by infection.

Temperature. Rise of temperature usually accompanies the spread of infection, but in uncomplicated mastoiditis the temperature seldom rises above 38.5°C. Sharp rises above this suggest further complications, in particular, blood infection. Generally speaking, temperature is an unreliable guide to the condition in the mastoid cells, since many a case of advanced suppuration is afebrile.

Pulse rate. A more reliable indication of the course of an infection can be obtained by careful observation of the pulse rate. Especially is this true in the case of children. A slowly rising pulse rate is always a danger sign, and of itself may constitute sufficient reason for operation. Conversely, sudden and unexplained fall, without corresponding fall of temperature, must always arouse suspicion of intracranial complication. Where mastoid involvement is suspected, a patient must never be considered out of danger until the pulse rate has fallen to normal.

Deafness. In the majority of cases the onset of mastoiditis is accompanied by increase of deafness.

General appearance. The general appearance of the patient must always be taken into account. With the rise of temperature the patient appears flushed and has an anxious look. The tongue, in most cases, is heavily coated.

Local signs

Tenderness. There is increasing tenderness over the mastoid area. This is most marked in front of and behind the mastoid tip, but may spread all over the bone. In children the tenderness is frequently found over the mastoid antrum as the mastoid process itself may not be developed.

Oedema. If careful search is made over the mastoid area thickening of the periosteum will be detected. This is most easily found by standing behind the patient with one hand on each mastoid, comparing carefully the sensation when palpating the bone. On the sound side the bony outline is clear and the root of the zygoma and the meatal spine are distinct. On the affected side there is a feeling that a thin sheet of rubber overlies the bone. The progress of the condition is an extension of these signs. There is increasing oedema of the overlying skin and tissues, which is found initially over the mastoid antrum and the posterior wall of the external meatus. When fully developed the swelling produces a characteristic appearance. The auricle is pushed outwards and downwards by the oedema and the sub-periosteal accumulation of pus, while the skin fold behind the auricle is preserved. There is still tenderness over the bone on deep pressure. If the external meatus is examined, the condition will be seen to differ from normal in that there appears to be a narrowing of the meatus. If this is examined closely, the narrowing will be found to be caused by depression of the roof of the meatus. The sagging appears to commence at the drum membrane, giving the passage a funnel shape.

Drum membrane. In the majority of cases a perforation is seen in the drum membrane through which pus is flowing or pulsating. It must be borne in mind, however, that mastoiditis may occur where the drum membrane appears to be intact. In some cases the pus may burrow along the posterior meatal wall under the periosteum and finally perforate the posterior wall of the auditory canal. At first the symptoms closely resemble furunculosis. A swelling is seen on the posterior wall from which pus is oozing, but owing to the oedema no view can be obtained of the drum. Before a diagnosis can be made other points such as the position of pain and tenderness, and pain on movement of the auricle must be considered. The state of the hearing, the tuning-fork tests and X-rays also are important.

Differential diagnosis

The differential diagnosis between mastoiditis and those conditions closely simulating it should be considered. Confusion may arise with a number of conditions, but of these the chief are furunculosis, otitis externa and erysipelas. The points of similarity are pain and discharge from the ear and oedema of the tissues surrounding the auricle. In a certain number of cases deafness is present.

The difference between mastoiditis and one of these other conditions may be so slight as to give even an experienced clinician great difficulty in diagnosis.

It must constantly be remembered that an otitis externa or furunculosis may co-exist with an acute or subacute otitis media. The presence of discharge in the external meatus may have set up the external irritation which was responsible for the otitis externa and it is in this class of case that the greatest difficulties arise. The most certain method of making a diagnosis is by examining the drum membrane. If this is normal there can be no otitis media or mastoiditis. Sometimes it is impossible to see the drum and experience shows that it is in such cases that mistakes are most common. To these the following observations particularly apply.

Comparison of symptoms

Pain. The pain of acute otitis media and mastoiditis is as a rule of a different type from that of furunculosis. Furunculosis and otitis externa cause a dull aching pain, differing considerably from the sharp, lancinating spasms of the otitis media and mastoiditis. In the external conditions the pain is usually localized in front of and below the ear. In mastoiditis or acute otitis the pain is described as being in the ear itself or behind it.

Tenderness. The position of the tenderness is one of the best guides. This has already been described in connection with the disease of the external meatus (p. 241). The position of the tenderness and the pain on movement of the auricle are characteristic of otitis externa. If these are found otitis externa may be diagnosed. Tenderness characteristic of mastoid infection must not be overlooked since both conditions may be present.

Discharge. The character of the discharge gives little or no help, except in certain cases of very early discharge, when the sero-sanguineous fluid is released from the haemorrhagic bullae which have formed.

Hearing. When it can be tested adequately hearing is a reliable guide. It is very rare that a patient with otitis media has good hearing. If, therefore, a case is seen in which the drum cannot be made out owing to swelling of the meatus, but a whisper is heard at, say, 12 feet (3.6 m.), established acute otitis media is unlikely to be present. Should it be found it is not sufficiently advanced to give any real anxiety.

Tuning-fork tests. Tuning-fork tests may help. If Rinne's test is undoubtedly positive the diagnosis of otitis externa can be made confidently.

Radiology in mastoiditis

X-ray photographs of the mastoid region can be of value, especially now that widespread use of antibiotics and consequent masking of typical symptoms is common. X-rays are by no means essential in every case, but on occasion indispensable information can be obtained through them.

In the majority of skulls the mastoid bones are symmetrical, therefore in the first instance the examination is based upon comparison of the two sides.

As already pointed out, the degree of cellularity of bone may have some influence on the symptoms, for example, where the bone is acellular an early symptom is tenderness accompanied by some oedema. In such cases the X-ray will give the surgeon information as to the type of mastoid being examined. In the cellular type of mastoid the X-ray will be of value in estimating the amount of absorption of bone which has taken place (Figs. 91 and 92), and may demonstrate the presence of abscess formation. Occasionally X-rays repeated at intervals of a few days will be a useful aid in watching developments.

VARIETIES OF MASTOIDITIS

Masked mastoiditis

In most western countries classical acute mastoiditis is rare. Its place is taken by masked or 'silent' mastoiditis. The disease is seen mainly in

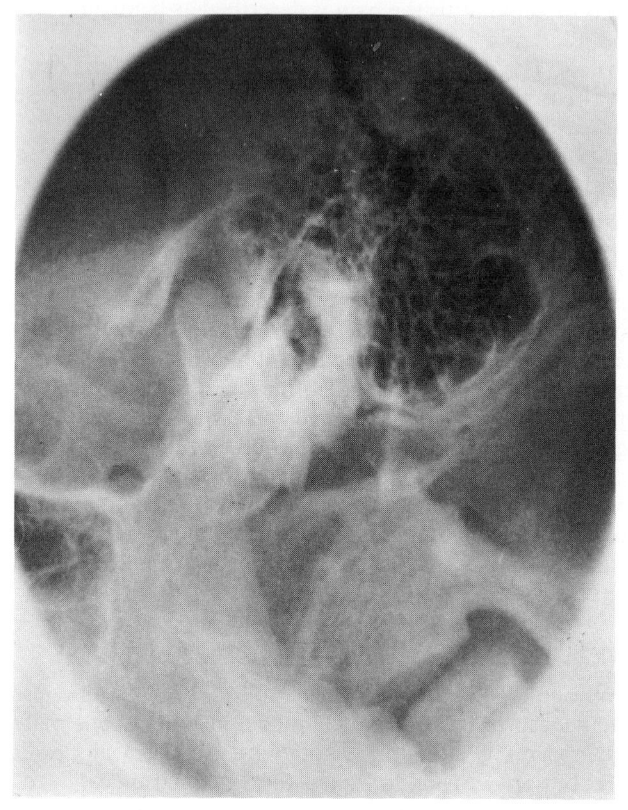

Fig. 91. Normal pneumatized mastoid. Left side. Normal mastoid cells.

children who have had repeated short courses of oral antibiotics for recurring ear symptoms such as earache and hearing loss, with or without otorrhoea.

During an attack, aching pain is felt in or behind the ear, there may be a temporary increase in hearing loss, and there may be transient discharge. The picture differs in small degree from that of otitis media though there may be more mastoid tenderness. The main difference is that the ear and hearing do not return to normal and mild exacerbations continue to occur.

Between attacks a degree of conductive deafness persists, the drum remains dull, immobile and featureless. Tenderness and periosteal oedema over the mastoid are usually absent.

The condition is diagnosed partly by ability to recognize these unusual signs and partly by X-ray, and is confirmed by surgical exploration. X-rays show clouding of the mastoid cells and decalcification

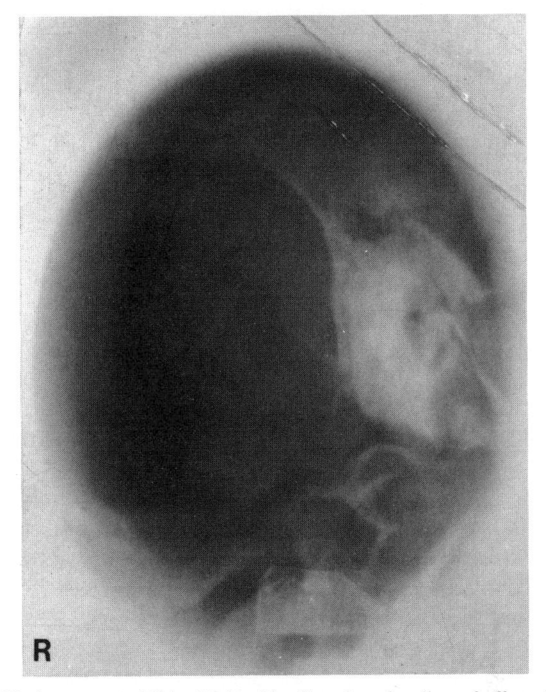

Fig. 92. Acute mastoiditis. Right side. Showing clouding of affected cells.

compared to the opposite side. Actual breakdown of the cellular outline is seen only in the more advanced case.

Treatment is drainage by a Schwartze mastoidectomy (p. 294). The bone is abnormally soft, and the mastoid cells full of thickened ulcerated mucosa and exudate.

Zygomatic mastoiditis

The zygoma may be so extensively pneumatized that the infection may extend forwards and thus appear to cause swelling and tenderness in front of, and above, the auditory meatus. This pneumatization may be so extensive that the pus extends practically to the back of the orbit. The appearances in this type of case may resemble furunculosis closely, since the swelling and tenderness may be entirely above and in front of the auricle.

Bezold's mastoiditis

Another form of extension, which is known as Bezold's mastoiditis, is the condition in which a large tip cell gives way and the pus extends downwards into the muscles of the neck. The sterno-mastoid muscle being attached around the tip of the mastoid, the downward extension of the pus will proceed along the muscle within its sheath giving the so-called 'sinking abscess' of the neck. This form of abscess is characterized by a brawny swelling in the neck below the mastoid tip and sometimes closely resembles a gland infection.

Mastoiditis in children

Mastoiditis in children presents so many difficulties in diagnosis that attention must be drawn to some of the more important facts.

The presence of mastoiditis in a child is frequently unsuspected and in a great many cases a swelling behind the ear is the first sign of the complication. Owing to the thinness of the bone overlying the mastoid antrum, pus readily finds its way to the surface of the bone and in a great many cases has an easy means of exit in the petro-squamous suture. Because of this fact complications are comparatively rare and treatment may be simplified. The operation sometimes consists only of the curettage of some small cells in the line of the mastoid antrum. Wilde's incision was designed for this purpose.

In all cases of unexplained pyrexia in a child, where there is any suspicion of middle ear infection, the possibility of mastoiditis must be kept in mind. X-rays give considerable help in these cases.

TREATMENT OF MASTOIDITIS

The treatment of mastoiditis is a matter of considerable controversy and the introduction of antibiotics has rendered the decision for or against operation even more difficult. Each case must be judged on its merits and the optimum time for interference must be chosen within the experience of the surgeon in charge of the case. Should the case occur during an epidemic, the locality, the prevalent type of infection and the organism responsible must all be taken into consideration.

To those who have worked through successive waves of respiratory infection, it would appear that every epidemic differs from the last in some characteristic or other. The wide variations in severity, speed of onset and incidence of complications may render a method of treatment suitable at one time, inapplicable at another. Different localities may be found to present their own problems. The lack of unanimity of opinion regarding the treatment of this disease may be accounted for in this way, and statistical accounts should be studied keeping these points in mind.

The operation used for treating acute otitis media with acute mastoiditis is the *Schwartze operation*. The object of the operation is threefold. It provides drainage of a septic focus, prevents extension of the sepsis into neighbouring structures and preserves hearing.

The first duty of the surgeon is to ensure the safety of the patient and this is best done through timely and adequate surgical drainage.

It must be realized also that once hearing is lost over a period the patient will remain deaf, and the longer an infected area is allowed to drain through the middle ear the less likely becomes return to full function. Thus increasing deafness in presence of a mastoid infection becomes an adequate reason for drainage by the most direct route.

The results of operation carried out on conservative lines are excellent. Barring accidents and neglect, results should approach 100 per cent recovery. In children the results are naturally superior to those obtained in adults, but this is only to be expected in the rapidly growing tissues of children with the reparative powers which they normally possess. The poorest results functionally are those obtained in adults in whom deafness either of middle ear or of sensori-neural type has previously been present.

Bearing these facts in mind, the indications for mastoid operation may be summarized as follows:

1. Cases showing manifest subperiosteal abscess formation, Bezold's abscess, or sagging of the roof of the external meatus.
2. Recurrence of pain and constitutional disturbance following apparent recovery after myringotomy or perforation. This is most important when associated with cessation of discharge.
3. Increase of profuse creamy discharge when associated with rising pulse rate, and increasing oedema over the mastoid area.
4. Persistent or increasing deafness associated with thick copious discharge lasting for a period of several weeks.
5. Persistent throbbing and headache on the affected side when associated with thick creamy discharge.
6. Evidence of extension of disease beyond the limits of the mastoid and middle ear, such as rigors, giddiness or papilloedema or other intracranial signs.
7. Suspected masked mastoiditis. Increasing deafness with radiological evidence of advancing bone disease.

Chemotherapy and antibiotics (p. 334)

Schwartze mastoidectomy. For details of the operation see page 294.

35. Complications of Otitis Media (Cont.)

In some cases mastoiditis tends to erode the cortex of the mastoid bone and becomes evident by outward extension. Instead of this, owing to various factors such as density of the cortex, position and direction of previous bone disease, the suppuration sometimes takes the line of least resistance, and travels inwards and invades the structures within the skull.

These complications are found more frequently in adults than in children, owing to the relative thickness of the cortex in the adult and the firm union of the sutures. These complications are—perisinus abscess, lateral sinus thrombosis, cavernous sinus thrombosis, extra-dural abscess, otogenous brain abscess and meningitis, and in some cases labyrinthitis and petrositis.

PERISINUS ABSCESS

In cases of prolonged suppuration the plate of bone covering the lateral sinus becomes eroded by disease and the sinus wall is exposed. This condition is found frequently where the cortex of the mastoid bone is dense, preventing the easy escape of the pus outwards. The abscess may be found also where there is extensive necrosis of bone. Any portion of the sinus in contact with the mastoid bone may be involved, and the abscess may not be limited exclusively to the wall of the lateral sinus but it may extend as part of an extra-dural abscess of the middle or of the posterior fossa.

The perisinus abscess causes no characteristic symptoms, but it is important because it is the precursor of lateral sinus thrombosis. On exposure the sinus will be found covered with granulations and it may be difficult in certain instances to exclude sinus thrombosis.

Treatment of perisinus abscess consists in the free drainage of the affected area by appropriate mastoid surgery. The removal of bone should be sufficiently extensive to uncover healthy dura in every direction round the area of granulations. These cases must be watched with great care for some days owing to the possibility of the infection having extended into the lateral sinus.

LATERAL SINUS THROMBOSIS

The granulations which normally form upon the wall of the lateral sinus when it is exposed offer considerable resistance to the passage inwards of infection. This reaches the interior of the blood channel either by direct extension, or sometimes by the retrograde thrombosis of veins passing into the lateral sinus. At first this infection may take the form of a mural clot. This is a thin ring of thrombus which may extend round the whole lumen of the vessel. Gradually the clot is built up until the vessel becomes occluded and then the condition of lateral sinus thrombosis is established.

In position and extent the thrombosis is subject to wide variations. The thrombus may extend upwards to the torcular or may invade the superior sagittal or other sinuses. Downwards the infection frequently extends into the jugular bulb, and through it into the internal jugular vein. The jugular bulb is sometimes infected by direct extension through the floor of the middle ear and in these cases diagnosis may present great difficulty. Formation of a healthy thrombus is essentially a defence mechanism, but the thrombus may become infected, soften and break up. The result will be pyaemia and septicaemia.

Symptoms of lateral sinus thrombosis. The classical symptom of a lateral sinus thrombosis in the presence of disease of the ear is a sharp and high rise of temperature. This may be accompanied by a rigor followed by an equally sharp fall. A rise of this type occurring two or three days after a mastoid operation is almost pathognomonic of a sinus infection. On the other hand, thrombosis of the lateral sinus, if present before the patient is first seen, may be difficult to diagnose with certainty.

The attack is ushered in with a rigor. The patient feels chilly and then commences to shiver. The shivering may last a few minutes only or may continue for half an hour or longer, and then the temperature rises sharply to 39°C. These attacks come on usually in the evening and next morning the temperature has again fallen to normal or sub-normal. It is to be noted, however, that the pulse rate remains fast. During the rigor the patient looks anxious, grey and ill, but between attacks is well and feels fit. This is a deceptive stage, and may delude the inexperienced into fatal delay.

The clinical picture of sinus thrombosis may be confused because many patients have been given antibiotics. Rigors are frequently absent and the temperature is only moderately elevated. The ear condition may appear to respond to treatment, but in spite of this the patient fails to show commensurate general improvement, he may be anxious and toxic. The suspicion remains that all is not well, but at the same time nothing definite can be pin-pointed. The Tobey-Ayer test (below) may be helpful, but a definite diagnosis is often only possible by exploring the mastoid and aspirating the exposed sinus.

If untreated, the rigors recur daily and the patient steadily loses strength, becoming emaciated, flushed and hollow-eyed. The tongue is furred and constipation may be marked. If recovery takes place the rigors become less severe and more infrequent and the temperature gradually settles. Pyaemic abscesses may make their appearance and they may signal the commencement of improvement, but, on the other hand if multiple, they may so exhaust the patient that death follows.

Blood culture. This must always be carried out in suspected thrombosis, as a positive result is a strong argument for active interference. The converse does not hold good, for a negative result is an indication for repeating the test.

Blood count. The white cell count is high, with a large percentage of polymorph cells. This examination may be of very great value, especially in those cases in which the original ear suppuration has largely cleared up.

Inflammation in the neck. Occasionally a thickening will be felt in the neck over the affected vein. This may be accompanied by some tenderness and is due chiefly to inflammation and enlargement of glands overlying the jugular vein.

Retinoscopy. Papilloedema and swelling of the veins of the retina indicate stasis in the cerebral circulation and are frequently found in lateral sinus thrombosis. In many cases it will be more marked on the side of the lesion.

Headache. This is not a common symptom of sinus thrombosis, but may be found in conjunction with papilloedema, and indicates hydrocephalus, due to the accumulation of cerebro-spinal fluid.

Temperature and pulse rate. Unless modified by previous chemotherapy there is a swinging pyrexia, as already indicated. The morning temperature is often subnormal. As the condition progresses the regular character may change, and with the appearance of a pyaemic stage, rigors and rises of temperature may become irregular. Although emphasis has been laid on the typical character of such symptoms, the inexperienced observer is warned never to lose sight of the fact that some other condition such as brain abscess may co-exist. The relationship of the pulse to the temperature is of great importance.

Cerebro-spinal fluid test (Tobey-Ayer). This is a useful test in cases of bilateral otitis media, and may help to make a diagnosis before operating. In bilateral cases it should be clearly realized that if an error is made and the patent sinus is opened instead of the thrombosed, the risks are greatly increased. The test consists in introducing a needle into the lumbar spinal canal. The needle is attached to a manometer, and the effect of compression of the jugular veins on each side is compared. When one vein is thrombosed the compression of the other causes a much greater comparative rise. Compression on the thrombosed side may produce no increase at all. A test based on similar principles is used for observing the veins of the retina, but it is less reliable.

Operative findings. If sinus thrombosis is suspected clinically, or if there is any evidence of disease in the bone overlying the sinus, the surgeon must examine and expose the sinus. Even then it is not always easy to decide on the nature of the contents. These may vary between a firm healthy aseptic thrombus, which is really a defence response, and a suppurating thrombophlebitis which is softening and breaking up and producing septicaemia and pyaemia. To determine with certainty the condition within the sinus it should be aspirated with a wide-bore needle inserted a short distance. If there is still doubt the sinus must be opened as described below.

Differential diagnosis

Occurring in the course of a manifest mastoiditis the diagnosis does not as a rule present serious difficulty. There are certain other complications, however, which must be taken into consideration.

Meningitis may commence with a rigor, and its onset may be comparatively abrupt. The temperature rarely shows the high swing of thrombosis, and when it has risen, though it may fall slightly, it does not have the plunging character shown by sinus infection. Neck rigidity and Kernig's sign are early in evidence and serve to clarify the situation. Lumbar puncture will be decisive.

Acute brain abscess. This condition also occasionally commences with a rigor, but the initial rise of temperature is not high and it quickly settles to an irregular low level. Localizing signs may be present and the mental state of the patient contrasts unfavourably with the alert condition of the patient with sinus thrombosis.

Labyrinthitis is easily distinguished by the typical labyrinthine disturbance.

Fevers, such as typhoid or malaria, occurring during the course of an acute otitis may give rise to considerable anxiety. History and blood examination will help in making a diagnosis, though in some of these instances a conservative attitude will have to be adopted.

Treatment

The treatment of sinus thrombosis, when diagnosed, consists in opening the sinus and the removal of the infected clot. Superiorly bone is removed until healthy-looking sinus has been exposed for about a centimetre. The sinus is then opened longitudinally. Using a soft rubber catheter for suction, the septic clot is then removed until free bleeding occurs from the upper end. Bleeding is readily controlled by inserting a pack of medicated ribbon gauze between the bone and the sinus wall, and so compressing the lumen. Packing preferably should not be placed in the lumen, otherwise at the first dressing bleeding will restart when the pack is removed.

The lower end of the sinus is dealt with in a similar manner as far as is practicable. If healthy sinus cannot be exposed, septic clot is aspirated with the sucker as far as possible and free bleeding encouraged before packing the area as before.

Ligation of the jugular vein, with drainage of septic thrombosis in its lumen, is now rarely needed; and only if signs of pyaemia or septicaema continue.

Anticoagulants are not normally given. Chemotherapy is continued in full dosage, the choice being dictated by bacteriological studies.

MASKED THROMBOPHLEBITIS

The preceding account is based on the natural course of the disease uncomplicated by chemotherapy. Antibiotics have caused a virtual disappearance of the classical picture, and diagnosis must be made by combining knowledge of the basic character of the disease with that of the probable effect of the drugs employed.

Masked disease may be seen both in the child and in the adult, but is probably more common in the child where it is likely to follow acute mastoid disease. In the adult it is more likely to be the result of infection of cholesteatoma which has eroded the bony covering of the lateral sinus or of the dura mater. The features which are suppressed in most cases are the occurrence of fever and rigors, and infection of the blood stream. In cases following cholesteatoma formation a rigor or sharp rise of temperature may occur but is likely to be suppressed immediately by antibiotic administration.

In children on the other hand, as antibiotics have in all probability been given for some time, it is unlikely that any definite symptoms will appear. Malaise and listlessness on the part of the child are probable, and there may be some local tenderness over the mastoid area. Diagnosis is not difficult when X-ray signs are obvious or when the Tobey-Ayer test is positive, but in the absence of information of this kind, diagnosis may depend on exploration of the mastoid and examination of the sinus itself.

CAVERNOUS SINUS THROMBOSIS

This is now a very rare complication.

It is characterized by oedema of the inferior fornix of the eye, proptosis, swelling of the upper eyelid, and fixation of the eyeball. Owing to stasis in the retinal veins papilloedema is an early sign. Reliance should be placed upon antibiotic and anticoagulant therapy.

OTITIC INTRACRANIAL HYPERTENSION

Obstruction to venous outflow may result in this serious condition, which causes papilloedema, and sometimes sixth nerve paralysis. Papilloedema demands immediate relief by reduction of cerebrospinal pressure, otherwise optic atrophy may follow, together with loss of power of concentration and memory. Reduction of C.S.F. pressure by frequently repeated lumbar puncture is essential. If this fails a sub-temporal decompression is advisable to prevent blindness.

OTITIC SEPTICAEMIA

This is seen typically as a sequel to sinus thrombosis in which softening of an infected thrombus has permitted blood infection.

The temperature is high, swinging and irregular, and the patient obviously extremely ill. Blood examination will usually show a high leucocytosis and blood culture may be positive. It should be noted, however, that a negative result means little, whereas a positive one merely confirms the diagnosis. In severe overwhelming infections there may be little or no increase in the white blood count due to the patient's inability to resist, so that even with modern chemotherapy and prompt surgical eradication of the primary infection the outlook is poor.

Otitic septicaemia is also associated occasionally with an acute otitis or fulminating acute mastoiditis. In young children this may occur during epidemics of gastro-enteritis. The infecting organisms may be streptococci, staphylococci, bacterium coli or pneumococci. Owing to debilitation and malnutrition this disease is extremely dangerous and, while antibiotics and chemotherapy must be used, measures to counteract dehydration and the use of blood transfusion will save many lives.

LABYRINTHITIS

Labyrinthitis is a rare but serious complication of otitis media. Early recognition and treatment will aid the preservation of function in the affected ear and help to prevent dangerous spread of infection.

The chief routes of infection into the labyrinth are–

(1) Direct infection of the labyrinth after erosion of the bony capsule by middle ear disease.
(2) By extension of acute middle ear infection through vascular channels, or directly through bone.
(3) By trauma during operation, or directly through the drum membrane, or as part of a fracture injury of the temporal bone.
(4) Rarely by infection from the meninges.

Clinical types of Labyrinthitis

Erosion of the bone of the labyrinth may expose the membranous labyrinth to infection from the middle ear. This is caused most frequently by cholesteatoma, usually in the horizontal or lateral semicircular canal. This may result in repeated attacks of localised serous inflammation known as 'circumscribed' labyrinthitis. Infection by this route or by any other, may be widespread throughout the labyrinth and in the very early stages is known as 'diffuse serous' inflammation. If this inflammation becomes purulent the labyrinthitis is said to be 'diffuse purulent'. When this infection settles down one of two things happens, either the pus becomes organised and the labyrinth fills with bone or pus becomes locked up within the labyrinth. This stage is called 'latent labyrinthitis'.

Signs and Symptoms

In addition to symptoms already present due to middle ear disease, symptoms and signs due to labyrinthine irritation and failure become evident. These consist of giddiness, loss of balance, vomiting and nystagmus, as well as increased hearing loss. This further hearing impairment is of sensori-neural type. As always past-pointing and falling are in the opposite direction to the fast component of the nystagmus.

When giddiness is intense the patient often takes up a characteristic attitude in bed. He lies on the sound side and looks to the affected ear as in that position the giddiness and nystagmus are greatly lessened.

The level of hearing depends upon the stage of the infection. The primary disease in the ear may already have produced considerable deafness which is of middle ear type. Any deafness caused by the labyrinthitis will be of sensori-neural type but in older patients the possibility that sensori-neural deafness was present previously must be remembered. The fistula sign should be sought and if it is present it means that the labyrinth is exposed and also that it is functioning. The cold caloric tests should not be used in the diagnosis of acute labyrinthitis as they may initiate extension of infection to the meninges.

When the disease advances all signs of function may be lost and tuning forks and noise box indicate a dead ear.

In latent labyrinthitis however, full compensation may have taken place when the patient is first seen, and all tests may be required to identify a dead ear.

Management of Labyrinthitis

Antibiotics should be given in full dosage when this disease is suspected. Labyrinthitis may be arrested at any stage with energetic and appropriate treatment, and operation should not be contemplated until it is evident that control has not been established. Return of function depends upon the speed and efficiency of treatment, provided that inflammation has not already caused severe damage within the labyrinth.

In the early stages of serous labyrinthitis if the patient is kept in bed with the head immobilised between pillows, the nystagmus may be expected to subside within a few days. Where a fistula has been identified as the cause of infection the problem of operation on the primary disease and its timing must be decided. This may be undertaken whenever the labyrinth has settled down as shown by the disappearance of the nystagmus. The form of the operation selected should permit careful examination of the area of the semicircular canals, particularly the horizontal canal as that is the most frequently eroded.

When a fistula has been identified the surgeon must decide to what extent he should clean the area of the fistula. There is no unanimity on this point but opinion seems to be that the thin layer of cholesteatomatous membrane covering the fistula may be left provided the fistula is exteriorised, but if the tissues are to be closed over the fistula the membrane is better removed. Any middle ear reconstruction necessary can be undertaken at a later date.

Another problem of management occurs when the latent stage is reached. Here the surgeon must decide when doing an operation to eradicate the chronic otitis media whether to leave alone a labyrinth which may still contain pus or to explore it. In latent labyrinthitis the labyrinth spaces may have become obliterated with fibrous tissue or bone, or may be filled with pus, infected or sterile. To leave a potentially infective condition in the ear is dangerous and it is recommended that the labyrinth should be explored. (see Hinsberg's operation p. 302).

The outstanding danger when control is not achieved with antibiotics is meningitis. This can be anticipated if watch is kept on the cerebrospinal fluid. A rise to 10 cells per cmm. means danger and if the rise continues drainage of the labyrinth should be undertaken. (See Hinsberg's operation p. 302).

Loss of one labyrinth may cause difficulties in balance especially in older people and rehabilitation exercises under a competent physiotherapist will do much to hasten recovery.

36. Operations for Mastoiditis and its Complications

THE SCHWARTZE OPERATION (SIMPLE MASTOID OPERATION)

Descriptions of these operations are included because they may have to be undertaken on occasion by those lacking special skill or training, in order to save life.

Detailed descriptions of reconstructive procedures, involving modern microsurgical techniques, are considered too advanced for a book of this kind.

Preparation. Preparation for this operation is the same as for any surgical operation. If necessary the bowel should be properly cleared, and the patient brought to the operating table in a fasting condition.

Local preparation. The hair should be shaved up to 3 inches at least from the ear. The skin should be cleansed with fluid soap and spirit. This is followed by the application of chlorhexidine or a similar preparation.

Anaesthesia. The farther the anaesthetist can be kept from the patient the easier it is for the operator. Therefore, although an open anaesthetic is quite efficient when administered with a mask, intra-tracheal insufflation of the anaesthetic of choice is very much better, and gives the operator considerably more facility and freedom.

Pre-operative medication. This should always include atropine, with or without an hypnotic such as morphia, as the circumstances of the case require.

The position of the patient. The patient should be lying on the back with the head turned to the side on a fairly firm pillow. It is frequently of assistance if the shoulder on the side to be operated on is also raised slightly on the pillow.

The arrangement of the towels. Two sterile squares are placed on top of a sterile mackintosh. They are all three slipped under the head, and the upper towel is folded round the head. A pad of cotton wool is placed in the shoulder angle to absorb blood or pus, and sterile mackintoshes and towels are spread over the patient from the shoulders down. Finally a towel with an oval opening is placed over the operation field and clipped in position.

The operation

As the incision is to be a curved one, it is wise to mark the skin with

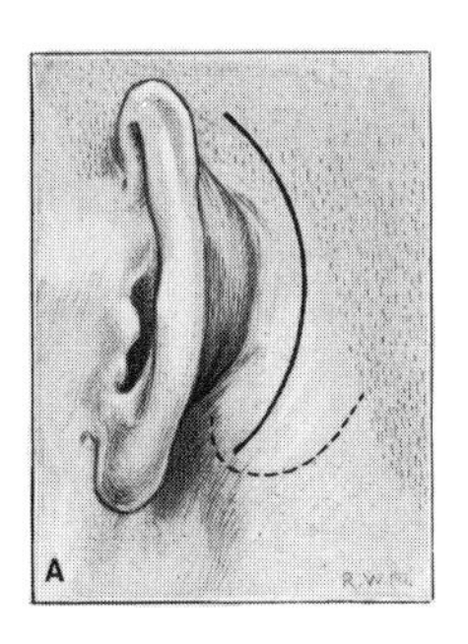

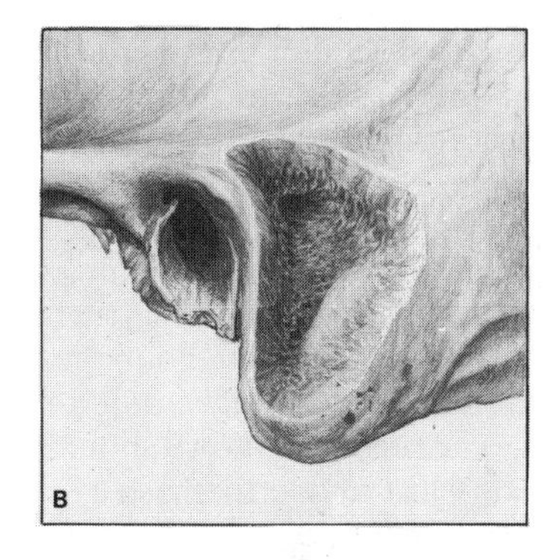

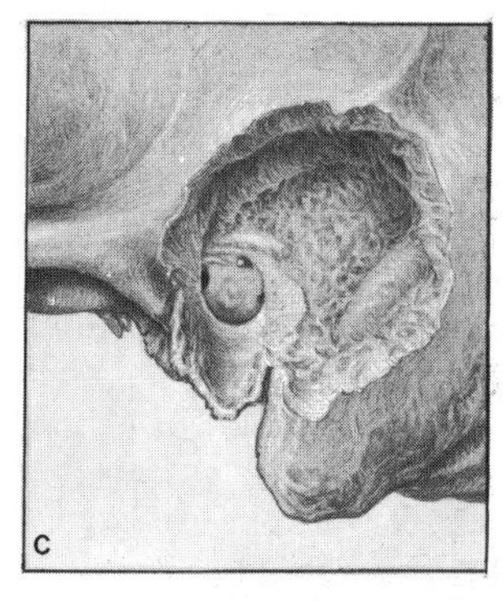

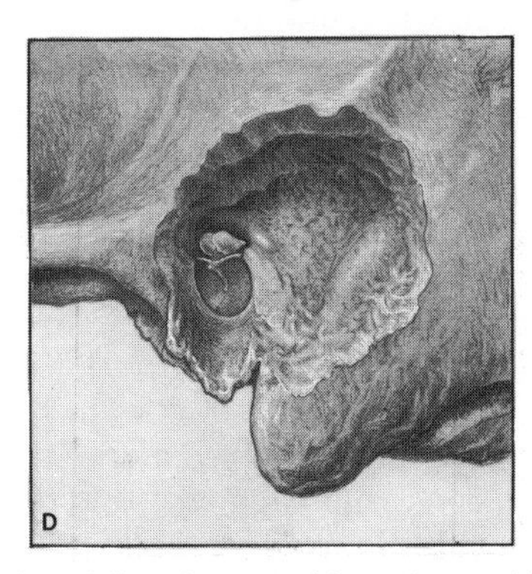

Fig. 93. (A) Incision for mastoid operation (dotted line shows position of mastoid process). (B) Completed Schwartze operation. (C) Completed radical operation. (D) Completed modified radical operation.

scratches to facilitate accurate stitching. This done, the skin incision is made at a distance of half an inch from the skin fold, following the curve of the auricle. The incision should extend from a point vertically above the centre of the external meatus to the level of the lower border of the cartilaginous meatus below. It is a great mistake to make too small an incision, especially where there is considerable oedema of the tissues.

The incision is quickly deepened through the skin, superficial fascia and muscle to the periosteum in the lower part of the wound; to the sheath of the temporal muscle in the upper part. The sheath only is incised and the muscle elevated with the periosteum. This is carried forward till the suprameatal spine is exposed and the external bony meatal wall.

The muscular fibres of the sternomastoid, which take origin from the mastoid process, are exposed in the lower end of the wound. These may have to be cut with scissors, or they may, if not powerful, be scraped off with the periosteal elevator.

A self-retaining retractor is then inserted in order to leave the field of operation clear. A high-speed rotating drill or a gouge and hammer, according to the preference of the surgeon, may be used to remove the cortex. The drill is much more commonly used today than the gouge. If a gouge is used a large size of gouge should be selected to begin with, and the operator should always remember the principle that the safest gouge to use is the largest which can comfortably approach the work to be done. Throughout the mastoid operation this principle holds good. In the average adult a number 15 or 16 gouge is used first.

The cortical removal should be begun in the lower part of the exposed bone just above the base of the mastoid process and well behind the meatal ridge using a fast cutting burr. As soon as the surface of the cortex is removed an idea will be obtained as to the type of mastoid with which the operator is dealing.

Whenever the cortex is opened pus may flow in quantity, and after the pus is mopped away a large cavity may be found filled with necrotic debris, granulations and pus. When such is the case the cavity should be carefully examined, as the lateral sinus may be exposed at some point within this cavity, and so is readily damaged. The cortical removal is then continued, and the beginner should avoid the mistake of attempting to do a mastoid operation through a small cortical opening.

If the mastoid appears to be cellular – a point which can be determined almost immediately – the cortex is removed widely; it will have to come off in any case, and the sooner it is removed the greater is the facility of access for the operator. In the removal of bone if the gouge is being used the gouge stroke should always be directed upwards and into the position of the antrum. In handling the gouge and shoulder of the gouge must never be permitted to bite into the bone; the centre must be invariably at the deepest portion of the cut. This fact will be appreciated when working round curves.

From time to time after the opening has been deepened, search should be made for the antrum. This is found with a bent probe or a spoon which slips into the antrum and through the aditus into the upper part of the middle ear with a characteristic sensation. When the antrum has been found the remainder of the operation is, as a rule, perfectly simple and straightforward, for it consists in the removal of all diseased bone and the opening of all diseased cells which are found.

The removal of diseased bone may be carried out with the gouge, with a bone scraper or with a spoon. Care must be taken in curetting the floor of the aditus, for here lie the delicate structures of the horizontal semicircular canal and the facial nerve. As far as possible overhang must be avoided in the removal of bone and the upper part of the antrum and the aditus should be opened up. The dura may be exposed, but this is of small moment provided it is uninjured. The lateral sinus also may be exposed, and this too is a safe procedure, provided the sinus is not damaged. Indeed, in certain circumstances, such as with a high swinging temperature or long-standing disease, it is advisable to expose the lateral sinus and sometimes also the dura for the purposes of inspection in order to ascertain if they are healthy.

In all cases the tip of the mastoid should be carefully examined and frequently it will be found to contain a large cell. The outer wall of this cell should be removed so that the tissues can fall in. There is frequently a deep gallery of cells behind the posterior meatal wall; but it must be remembered that in this region lies the facial nerve. Extra care must be exercised here. The sinus plate and dural plate must be cleaned of cells and also the angle between sinus and dural plates. When the operator concludes that no more infected bone or cells remain, the cavity may be irrigated and the wound is closed with interrupted silkworm gut stitches and a small drain is inserted at the lower end of the wound. The soft tissues will fall into and obliterate the dead space. Finally, the external ear is cleared of pus and debris and a light pack inserted. As far as possible, interference with the posterior meatal wall is avoided. This wall is required for the support of the meatus, and if it is damaged or removed there may be a narrowing of the external auditory meatus which will be very difficult to correct.

A dry dressing and a bandage are then applied. Many variations of the method of closing the wound have been proposed and practised.

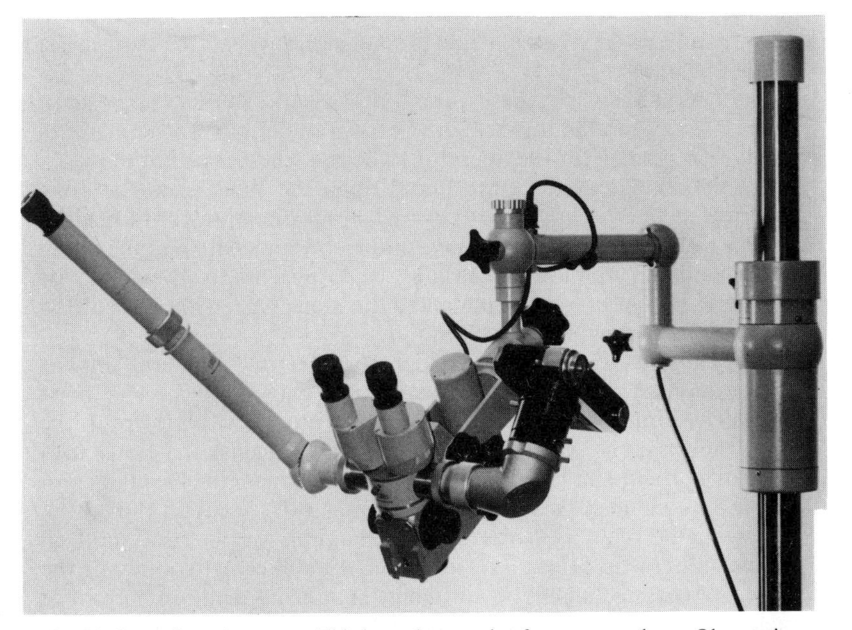

Fig. 94. Operating microscope. This is used as routine for ear procedures. Observation tube and camera can be fitted as illustrated. With a longer objective lens the microscope is also used for micro-procedures on the larynx as well as for operations on the pituitary using the trans-sphenoid route.

Simple closure with drainage is probably the best for the occasional operator, with antibiotics used in the usual way when required.

Difficulties and dangers

Necrosis of tissue. In certain cases of advanced sub-periosteal abscess there will be found such a widespread necrosis of the soft tissues and also of bone, that primary union is not to be expected. In such cases a more rapid and satisfactory convalescence will be obtained after operation if the wound is not stitched at operation. It is wiser to pack the wound with gauze soaked in liquid paraffin and B.I.P.P. mixed to the consistency of thin cream or with an antiseptic cream. Antibiotics should be given in high dosage systemically, depending on the bacteriological sensitivity reports. It will be found possible in most cases to suture the wound on the fifth day. Thus the minimum of time is lost and healing is rapid.

Density of bone. Density of bone may render the mastoid hard and acellular, and this in turn may render the location of the mastoid antrum of considerable difficulty. In such cases the removal of bone must be kept about the level of the suprameatal spine and deepened with care forwards and backwards. In case of doubt it is quite good practice to expose the dura mater of the middle fossa and work forward along it to the middle ear. There is no real danger above, all the danger lies below the aditus.

The **lateral sinus** may be exposed in cases of extensive necrosis of bone. It may be found to be covered with granulations, and sometimes it will be necessary for the operator to decide whether or not the sinus is healthy. If granulations are found upon the sinus, then the bone covering the sinus should be removed in all directions until healthy sinus is reached. By pressure above and below and watching the filling of the sinus an opinion can usually be formed as to its patency or otherwise. Some operators puncture the sinus wall with a needle to find if blood is flowing freely within it.

Injury to the lateral sinus. Accidental injury to the lateral sinus is not uncommon, and this is very frequently caused by chips of bone being driven into the wall, or the sinus being nipped with forceps. If the injury is slight, it may be sufficient to pack against the sinus with paraffin gauze or similar material in order to control the bleeding, or a graft of muscle may be applied to the sinus wall to seal off the injury. If these methods are unsuccessful, then the sinus may be packed off. In cases of injury where there is no infection, it is sufficient to obliterate the sinus by packing outside; no attempt should be made to introduce packing within the sinus cavity.

Injury to the dura. The dura mater may be exposed by disease, and if granulations are found upon it the same principles apply as for exposure of the lateral sinus. Excessive bleeding from the dura mater may be stopped by small muscle grafts taken from the temporal muscle.

Injury to the facial nerve. In this operation the facial nerve may be injured, and this sometimes occurs in misguided attempts to locate the antrum while the operator is working at too low a level and is below the aditus. Damage to the facial nerve should be identified before the patient is removed from the operating table, and the operator will save a great deal of worry if a practice is made of examining the face on each occasion and verifying normal facial movement, before the patient leaves the operating table.

Post-operative treatment. In the normal course of events the wound is left undisturbed for five days. On the fifth day the bandages and dressings are removed. The stitches are cut and the packing or drain inserted into the lower end of the wound is removed. The packing of the meatus of the ear is also removed. The wound is cleaned with peroxide and spirit and a small wick drain is inserted in the lower end of the wound. This treatment is continued daily. Usually the ear is mopped dry at each dressing, but if there is copious discharge it is good practice to cleanse the ear by syringing when the dressing is being carried out.

Points to be observed in dressing a mastoid wound. The less handling there is of the wound the better. The wound should be expressed gently from above downwards and the excess of secretion mopped away. Excessive probing and swabbing of the cavity is not desirable. Stitch abscesses sometimes occur, and when found they should be evacuated. Non-adherent absorptive dressings should be renewed as necessary and antibiotics given systemically as required; the choice of antibiotic will depend on the bacteriological sensitivity reports. Gentleness and care are advisable, since it is possible for the wound to open and subsequently require restitching.

COMPLICATIONS DURING THE CONVALESCENT PERIOD

Pain. If a patient complains of excessive pain before the first dressing has been carried out, the dressing should immediately be taken down and the wound inspected. If normal, no attempt should be made to move the packing or otherwise disturb it. On the other hand, pain at this time frequently means infection of the wound. This may be either a deep infection or a skin infection. In some cases, particularly in patients with a dry scalp, the use of antiseptic may set up a dermatitis, which may be the cause of distressing symptoms to the patient. If unchecked, this condition may go on to complete infection of the wound and the breaking-down of the whole area. When this happens a considerable period of treatment is required before it can be restitched.

Where inflammation of the wound or surrounding skin is found, suitable chemotherapy is continued and it may be wise to remove a stitch or two from the lower end of the wound in order to aid drainage.

Rise of temperature. Rise of temperature may have a similar significance. A very acute rise of temperature, accompanied by sickness, is not an uncommon symptom, and it may indicate a superficial infection such as erysipelas. On the other hand, it may be the first sign of sinus thrombosis or other intracranial complication.

Wound infection. When infection of the wound has occurred and is not controlled by antibiotics, it will hasten recovery if the wound is completely reopened and packed with a moist dressing, or some sulphonamide paste, the dressing being changed at frequent intervals until the inflammation of the soft tissues has completely subsided.

THE RADICAL MASTOID OPERATION

Only a very brief description need be given as this operation is not primarily an emergency operation. The approach can be post-aural or endaural. Occasionally a Schwartze operation is embarked upon in cases of disease which can only be satisfactorily dealt with by radical procedures, therefore anyone undertaking the former ought to have some knowledge of how to proceed in such circumstances.

When the Schwartze operation has been completed the surgeon continues by lowering the posterior meatal wall. This is cut away until the bridge, which separates the attic portion of the middle ear from the aditus and antrum, has been removed.

For the inexperienced operator who is required to carry out this procedure without thorough training, it will be found that, if a straight line is drawn from the horizontal semicircular canal to the outer edge of the floor of the bony meatus, all bone above this line can be removed with safety and without fear of damage to any important structures.

The experienced operator may remove considerably more than this, but such refinements of technique need not be described in detail.

Curettage of the Eustachian tube may be called for in cases in which granulations are found filling the mouth of the tube.

Access is provided through the meatus by making two horizontal cuts in the posterior meatal wall to include most of the wall. Redundant skin, muscle and cartilage are removed from the flap so formed and the flap is stitched to the skin just behind the ear. This ensures a large opening. The wound behind the ear is closed completely and all after-treatment is carried out through the enlarged meatus.

After-treatment. The wound should be dressed on the fifth day. If the patient's condition is satisfactory and if the ear itself is comfortable then only the outer part of the pack need be loosened. The deep packing can often be left for a total of three weeks, especially if it consists of gauze ribbon which has been well soaked in liquid paraffin to which B.I.P.P. has been added. Further treatment in such cases consists of regularly cleaning out any discharge and debris, cauterizing any granulations, and powdering with either an antibiotic powder, or simply with boric and iodine powder until epithelialization is completed. Sometimes the cavity can be skin-grafted in order to expedite healing, but this should only be carried out when the cavity is sufficiently clean and healthy to enable the grafts to take.

Occasionally, infection may have been so gross that daily syringing of the cavity may be required, but even the dirtiest cavities usually respond satisfactorily to repeated cleaning and the use locally of antiseptic packs and drops.

Difficulties and complications of the radical mastoid operation. The difficulties which may be met with in carrying out the radical mastoid operation are many, and so varied that it is impossible to describe all the points which may arise. It will readily be appreciated that as the radical mastoid operation is carried out primarily for the relief of chronic suppuration, the varying degrees of destruction of bone which may have been produced by the suppuration will give rise to problems which differ in almost every case.

The radical mastoid operation should not be undertaken by the inexperienced except when demanded by complications of an acute infection. The outstanding dangers are two in number: firstly, danger of injury to the facial nerve; and secondly, injury to or infection of the labyrinth.

Injury to the facial nerve. This may be due to the fact that disease of the bone has caused erosion around the facial nerve, or it may be that when the ear is being scraped to clear away granulations, etc., the facial nerve is damaged. It is also liable to be injured when the posterior bony wall of the meatus is being lowered with gouge or burr. The face should be examined at the end of every operation, especially if there is the least suspicion that the facial nerve has been exposed.

Where complete paralysis is discovered skilled assistance should be sought immediately. The nerve should be exposed and the cut ends brought into apposition. If paralysis does not appear for some time after the operation then it is probably due to oedema of the nerve sheath and can be expected to recover without treatment, though recovery may be delayed for a considerable time, especially if degeneration is found on electrical testing.

Damage to the labyrinth. Damage to the labyrinth may take place either by direct injury to the horizontal canal or by injury or displacement of the stapes. The treatment and conduct of these cases are detailed in the section on labyrinthitis.

THE MODIFIED RADICAL MASTOID OPERATION WITH TYMPANOPLASTY

As this operation is rarely, if ever, performed as an emergency operation, no detailed description is called for here.

OPERATION ON THE LATERAL SINUS

When it is decided to open the lateral sinus, a portion of about 5 cm of sinus should be exposed. Packing is then introduced between the sinus and the bone, at both upper and lower ends, in order to shut off the sinus and prevent excessive bleeding.

The sinus sheath is then slit with a knife and the clot is picked out. The lower pack may be gently removed, and if no bleeding follows, the clot should be extracted with a pair of forceps until free bleeding is obtained from the lower end, whereupon it is packed firmly. The upper end is then inspected in a similar fashion. The sinus wall is slit upwards and the clot removed, the overlying bone being removed where necessary. This process is continued until free bleeding is obtained. It is packed chiefly outside the lumen to control the bleeding. Paraffin gauze, or gauze impregnated with iodoform forms a very useful packing. The diseased sinus walls should be clipped away.

The last step is the ligation of the jugular vein if this is required. This is done through an incision in the skin fold of the neck, below the jaw. The common facial vein should be ligatured at the same time. If a clot is found or pus is suspected, the vein may be divided between ligatures and dissected upwards till the whole of the septic tube is removed. Some surgeons advocate opening the upper end of the vein and syringing through from the mastoid area. In most cases, however, adequate drainage will be provided if the upper end is stitched into the upper part of the neck wound.

OPERATION ON THE LABYRINTH

The simplest operation on the labyrinth is that named after Hinsberg, and the steps of the operation are as follows: the convex portion of the horizontal semicircular canal is planed down with a fine gouge until the lumen of the canal is exposed. This is then followed forwards along the canal until the roof of the vestibule is reached. Care should be taken to keep rather to the inner side of the canal, as a facture of the anterior or outer wall will involve the facial nerve which lies immediately below it, and will almost inevitably cause a facial paralysis.

When the vestibule is reached the opening in the roof is enlarged so that a probe can be passed straight down into the cavity. The stapes is now removed from the oval window. The next step is the removal of the promontory. This is done with a drill or with a gouge which will comfortably fit the curve between the oval window and the round window, thus outlining part of the promontory. A short tap on the gouge will enable the promontory to be levered up, exposing the whorls within the cochlea. Milligan's spoon should now be passed from the roof of the vestibule into the opening in the cochlea. When it is possible to do this it is evident that there is free drainage from the more important parts of the labyrinth.

The wound can be packed with a suitable dressing, such as bismuth, iodoform and paraffin paste (B.I.P.P.) with paraffin to make a cream, and the operation is complete.

There are other more elaborate modes of opening the labyrinth, but they are longer and are technically more difficult, and do not provide any very outstanding advantages as far as clinical results are concerned.

BRAIN ABSCESS

The diagnosis and the management of a discrete brain abscess are described in the following chapter. Occasionally, however, during the course of a mastoidectomy it becomes evident that infection has passed through the meninges into the brain and that an abscess has formed in contiguity with the disease in the mastoid. In other words, part of the abscess wall is in the mastoid and part is provided by cerebral tissue, the intra-cranial part being effectively sealed-off by meningeal adhesions and a fibrotic abscess wall. The principles in treatment under such conditions are to use great gentleness and to do as little damage to the brain as possible. The mastoid disease is dealt with as necessary, great care is taken to avoid disturbing the surrounding adhesions. The abscess is emptied and the mastoid operation completed in the ordinary way. The resulting cavity is gently packed with gauze, well soaked in idioform and liquid paraffin. It is again emphasised that the utmost gentleness should be used to avoid breaking down the surrounding protective adhesions. Healing usually occurs without any problems, though a repair of the dura at a later operation through a craniotomy is advised by most neuro-surgeons.

37. Intracranial Complications of Otitis Media

EXTRA-DURAL ABSCESS

By the direct extension of infection, disease may reach the middle or the posterior fossa. There an abscess may be formed which may be extra-dural. This may be part of a mastoid abscess. The extension of inflammation and the absorption of bone in the mastoid areas can cause an infection and necrosis of the dural plate. The dural plate having given way, the dura mater is exposed to the infection. A reaction in the dura mater takes place. There is a thickening of the membrane, granulations are formed upon the surface and the condition is then known as an extra-dural abscess. This type is frequently found in the middle fossa and may track back until it comes into contact with the lateral sinus. The posterior fossa also may be the site of the abscess. Such cases are usually an extension of a perisinus infection which burrows forwards into Trautman's triangle beneath the labyrinth.

This may be suspected in cases suffering from headache with signs of early meningeal irritation, but it is rarely diagnosed prior to operation. The extra-dural abscess, beyond the usual signs of mastoid infection, gives no special symptom.

TEMPORAL LOBE ABSCESS

Otogenic brain abscess usually arises by direct extension through thrombophlebitis or via peri-vascular sheaths and therefore is adjacent to the temporal bone into which a track often exists. Diagnosis may be obscured by co-existent complication, *e.g.* meningitis, caused by the traverse of the infection across several tissue planes on its way into the brain.

Most abscesses arise from chronic otitis, particularly from the type with cholesteatoma. Initially the lesion is a poorly defined encephalitis which gradually localizes and encapsulates; treatment is accordingly planned to encourage encapsulation.

Metastatic abscesses from embolism are rare, often multiple, and often at a distance from the primary focus. Traumatic abscess can complicate a penetrating wound or a skull fracture in the presence of a chronic ear infection.

The abscess enlarges mainly at the expense of the white matter, spread is thus towards the ventricle into which fatal rupture can occur.

Brain abscess passes through the following stages: (1) initial invasion, encephalitis; (2) a latent period; (3) stage of increasing intracranial pressure; (4) terminal stage.

Symptoms. A long standing otorrhoea may have diminished or ceased prior to the onset of symptoms, which can be considered under the following headings:

1. Symptoms of cerebral infection and suppuration.
2. Symptoms of intracranial pressure.
3. Focal symptoms.

Cerebral infection. Chills or rigor may occur, with initial rise in pulse rate and temperature and sometimes with vomiting and headaches. Many of these symptoms are common to various febrile diseases and may be overlooked. When the suppuration is established it may pass into the latent stage, in which it can remain for several weeks. During this period the patient may go on working and appear normal. It is common, however, for the patient to have some feeling of malaise, occasional headache and vomiting. The temperature usually becomes subnormal and the pulse rate shows periodic slowing to perhaps forty to fifty beats per minute. Convulsions or fits have been noted during this stage.

Intracranial pressure. As the abscess absorbs more brain tissue, the surrounding oedema causes signs of cerebral compression. These are: headache of great severity, occasional vomiting, periodic drop in pulse rate and indefinite signs of meningeal irritation.

Ocular changes may be found but are not constant. These are papilloedema and indefinite nystagmus. Paresis of ocular muscles occurs but normally only in the terminal stages.

Focal symptoms. These are of interest, but to await their appearance may be courting disaster.

The main focal findings are as follows:

Aphasia. This sign is pathognomonic of an abscess in the left temporal lobe provided the patient is right-handed. The type of aphasia is that in which the patient cannot name common objects such as a key, or a coin, although he can describe them and explain their use.

Paralysis. Contra-lateral paralysis is a comparatively common symptom and is due to pressure on the internal capsule, or on the cortical motor area. In the latter the face is affected first and the paralysis spreads down the body. In the case of the internal capsule the paralysis may vary and is usually greater in extent. Paralysis of the sixth nerve can occur in any case of raised intracranial pressure.

Visual field changes. When the abscess is large it may involve the optic radiation and cause homonymous hemianopia.

Special investigations

Carotid arteriography is now standard practice in the diagnosis of the presence, and exact site, of a space-occupying cerebral lesion such as an abscess. Electroencephalography is sometimes helpful. Air encephalography and ventriculography can be hazardous.

Lumbar puncture is best avoided, but if essential must be done with the utmost care. The cerebro-spinal fluid is under pressure and fatal 'coning' may occur. Characteristically the fluid is clear, the protein raised and there is an increased cell count. The cells are mainly lymphocytes. Sugar and chlorides are reduced only if meningitis is present.

CEREBELLAR ABSCESS

An abscess in the posterior fossa is due chiefly to extension of an infection from either labyrinth or the lateral sinus. Also it may occur by direct extension of a perisinus abscess extending through the dura to the posterior fossa. Symptoms, again, may be divided into the same groups as for otitic temporal lobe abscess. Those due to intracranial tension, such as headache, vomiting, drowsiness and papilloedema, may occur. General symptoms are as previously described. It should be noted that as in all subtentorial tumour formation, papilloedema in posterior fossa abscess occurs early.

Localizing symptoms. Localizing symptoms are those of the cerebellar syndrome and are homolateral. Nystagmus is of an irregular character and may change its direction from day to day; spontaneous pointing error is to the side of the lesion. There may be found also ataxia, rhombergism, dysdiadochokinesia, indistinct speech, atony of muscles, incoordination, skew position of the head, increased reflexes on the affected side and clonus.

TREATMENT OF ABSCESS OF THE BRAIN

Cerebral and cerebellar abscesses should be approached in the most conservative attitude it is possible to adopt to permit maximum localization and encapsulation. Penicillin remains the antibiotic of choice; this may be altered later, depending upon bacteriological studies. The use of antibiotics makes it possible to wait for the optimum moment to undertake surgical treatment. After the meningitis, septicaemia or other condition has settled, the closest watch is kept upon any localizing symptoms to determine the precise locality of the abscess.

Intensive chemotherapy and control of the ear infection during the invasive stage can sometimes abort abscess formation.

The time to operate requires experienced judgment and is deferred until the abscess is believed to have been walled off. This is determined largely by the patient's general state and the degree of intracranial pressure. It has also to be decided whether to approach the abscess via the infected mastoid or by a suitably placed burr-hole.

As a rule, aspiration via a burr-hole is advisable, but transmastoid aspiration can be life-saving if the surgeon is unacquainted with neuro-surgical techniques. Exploration is made with a special blunt brain cannula; the pus is aspirated, and penicillin and thorotrast are injected. The latter enables the size of the abscess to be watched radiologically. Aspiration is repeated as necessary until only a scar remains. Occasionally repeated aspiration fails to produce a cure and the abscess must be excised. The ear infection is treated as is appropriate, and as soon as the patient is sufficiently fit a mastoid operation is indicated.

MENINGITIS

Meningitis is inflammation of the covering membranes of the brain.

Pachymeningitis is inflammation of the dura mater alone, and can vary in extent between a small abscess and a large subdural collection of pus.

Leptomeningitis is inflammation of the pia-arachnoid.

Routes of infection

1. Through the labyrinth by the internal auditory meatus, or the perilymphatic duct.
2. From lateral sinus thrombosis usually through the blood-stream.
3. Along the vessels passing through the subarcuate fossa.
4. Rupture of an abscess into the lateral ventricle or into the subarachnoid space over the surface of the brain.
5. By direct extension of disease from the middle ear cleft or the apex of the petrous bone.

Types of meningitis

Serous leptomeningitis is simply the prodromal stage of diffuse purulent meningitis. Therefore no object is served in describing the conditions separately.

Localized and cystic meningitis are rare results of adhesion formation.

Symptoms. The onset may be gradual or it may be rapid as is found in fulminating infections. The earliest sign is moderate elevation of temperature accompanied by slight transient headache which is easily controlled by such drugs as salicylates. The patient may show some anxiety but is otherwise mentally normal. The tongue is dry and heavily furred and constipation may be marked. Extensor spasm is frequently found, being most marked in the toes.

As the disease becomes established, headache is severe and spasmodic, the temperature climbs and the patient becomes confused and irritable. Later, neck stiffness and rigidity occur and inability to extend the knee when the thigh is flexed on the abdomen. This is called Kernig's sign.

The attitude may be characteristic. The patient lies curled up on the side, but with the neck extended, frequently with the face buried in

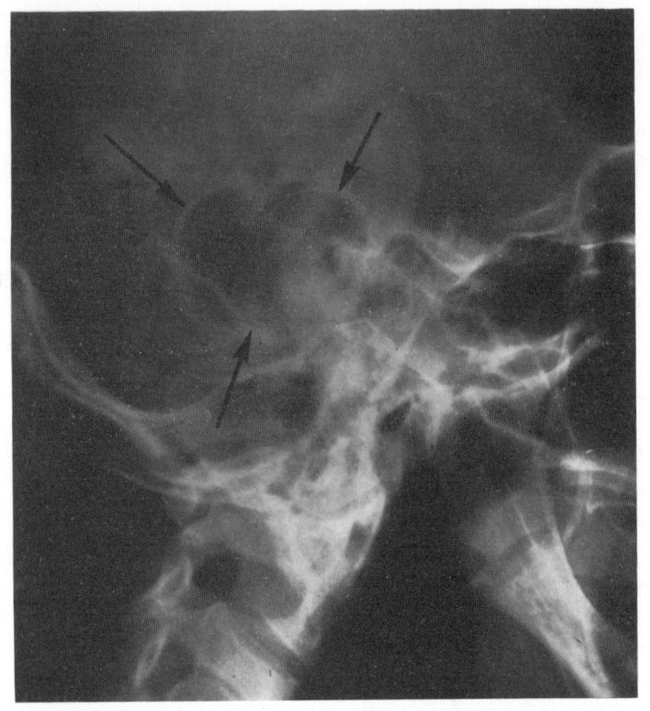

Fig. 95. Extensive erosion of bone by cholesteatoma. This led to invasion of meninges and meningitis. The patient was seen only when meningitis developed.

the bedclothes owing to photophobia, and he resents being moved or touched.

Diagnosis. Meningitis may complicate an attack of acute otitis media or may follow a chronic infection of many years' duration. Temperature characteristically climbs without the periodic fall which occurs in lateral sinus thrombosis. The pulse rate shows a steady increase. Blood examination reveals a leucocytosis of possibly 15–20,000. Increasing papilloedema may be found on examination of the optic discs, but this is usually a late change. In the final stages hyperpyrexia leads to increasing confusion, coma and death.

The cerebro-spinal fluid examination. Fluid may be withdrawn by lumbar or cistern puncture and its examination is the most valuable guide to diagnosis.

Normal cerebro-spinal fluid contains one to four cells per cmm, chlorides 720–750 mg per cent, glucose 50–80 mg per cent and protein 20–40 mg per cent. Pressure is 120–150 mm of water.

In meningitis owing to the increase in cells the fluid becomes turbid and later purulent. The glucose is diminished or absent and chloride content falls. Protein is increased. Pressure rises in the early stages provided there is free circulation of cerebro-spinal fluid. There may be many variations from these conditions and the findings must be interpreted as part of the clinical picture. Organisms are now cultured from the C.S.F. only in a minority of cases of meningitis. Most patients already have received chemotherapy, so that, though conclusive, the presence of organisms is not necessary for the diagnosis of meningitis. A swab from the ear may be a useful guide to the organism and its sensitivity, and though by no means all cases of meningitis are otogenic, examination of the ear, nose and sinuses should never be overlooked in a patient with this illness.

Differential diagnosis. This concerns the various forms of meningitis, tuberculous, meningococcal and pneumococcal, and the distinctions are made chiefly by cerebrospinal fluid examination.

Prognosis. This depends to some extent on co-existent complications, but in meningitis, especially with early diagnosis and treatment, the outlook is generally good.

Treatment of meningitis. This potentially fatal disease must be controlled immediately. As soon as the patient is sufficiently recovered, as for example in chronic otitis media, surgical treatment of the primary focus can be undertaken if judged necessary.

Sulphadiazine or sulphadimidine is given because of the ease with which they enter the C.S.F. They are given in full dosage orally, unless the patient is vomiting, in which case they are given in the intravenous infusion. Penicillin in high dosage is given by injection six-hourly mainly to control the primary infection. Streptomycin is frequently used in addition.

Intrathecal penicillin is given daily by lumbar puncture after removal of C.S.F. for analysis and to relieve increased pressure and headache. It is irritating to the meninges, therefore the 10,000 units should be well diluted. Cisternal or ventricular puncture is needed only if adhesions and loculation occur. Intrathecal treatment can be abandoned when the C.S.F. is returning to normal, but systemic chemotherapy should continue for at least another two weeks after clinical recovery. This reduces the risk of formation of micro-abscesses and future recurrence of meningitis.

Lack of response to treatment usually indicates a co-existent complication rather than resistant organisms.

PETROSITIS

Though not strictly an intra-cranial complication, petrositis can be conveniently included in this chapter. It is due to the extension of infection into the body and apex of the petrous bone.

Petrositis may complicate an acute or a chronic otitis media and so occurs in acute or chronic form. It also occurs as an early or late complication of mastoid operation, during which there may have been interference with aeration or drainage of the petrous cells. Various routes are described by which the infection reaches the petrous cells, for example, through the cells around the Eustachian tube, through those posteriorly under the labyrinthine capsule, or through those behind the anterior vertical canal. The infection may show little sign for a considerable period, but gradually it softens and erodes the apex of the petrous bone. The erosion extends to the roof of the posterior surface and there produces a localized pachymeningitis, at first serous in type. This may progress and form an abscess under the dura mater. spread may take place downwards, and abscess formation in the pharynx has been recorded. Spontaneous recovery may occur by the establishment of drainage through the middle ear. On the other hand, extension of the disease may lead to a diffuse purulent meningitis.

Symptoms

Unilateral headache. The headache, which may be spasmodic in type, is usually referred to the side of the head and to the temple, and is frequently described as being behind the eye. Pain frequently radiates along the jaws into the teeth. The radiating pains in the face are due to the involvement of the fifth nerve, the ganglion of which lies immediately above the apex of the petrous bone.

Sixth nerve paralysis. Paralysis of the sixth nerve of the affected side is almost a pathognomonic sign associated with unilateral headache. Paralysis is due to oedema of the canal in which the sixth nerve runs under the sphenoidal ligament—sometimes called Dorello's canal. There may be slight elevation of temperature accompanying the onset of the characteristic headache. In post-operative cases one of the most significant symptoms is the sudden recurrence of copious discharge in an ear which hitherto has been dry or in which the discharge has been decreasing.

When these symptoms are present and fully developed, they are known as *Gradenigo's syndrome*.

Treatment. If there has been no previous surgical treatment the mastoid operation appropriate to the mastoid disease is performed, *i.e.* a simple or a radical mastoidectomy. In either operation careful search is made for any track leading medially into the petrous bone, and if found, this is opened up. With free drainage and intense chemotherapy the petrous bone has strong powers of recovery.

It is now seldom that patients require the elaborate surgical procedures designed to open the petrous apex except in those rare cases of cholesteatomatous invasion. In these patients it is necessary to utilise a mastoid approach in order to mobilise the facial nerve and enter the petrous bone through the internal ear. Only in this way can disease be cleared from the internal carotid artery and the dura of the internal auditory meatus.

38. Non-suppurative Diseases of the Middle Ear

In common with the acute and chronic suppurative disorders of the middle ear discussed in previous chapters, together with those diseases which cause obstruction of the external auditory meatus or the Eustachian tube, the following conditions also have a conductive type of hearing loss, *i.e.* bone conduction is better than air conduction and the Weber test is lateralized to the deaf ear.

ADHESIVE DEAFNESS

This type of deafness is due to fibrosis and necrosis of the mucosa, ossicles, and ligaments of the middle ear. It is essentially the end-result of healed infection which may have been either overt or such as to have passed almost unnoticed at the time. Antibiotics may have helped to mask the continuing damage. In some patients there is no history of previous ear trouble and the condition must therefore be regarded as due to chronic infection in the nasopharynx which has produced recurring tubo-tympanitis (Fig. 96).

Clinically the slowly progressive conductive deafness is often bilateral; the drum is thickened and opaque and generally reduced in mobility corresponding to the changes within the middle ear cleft. The

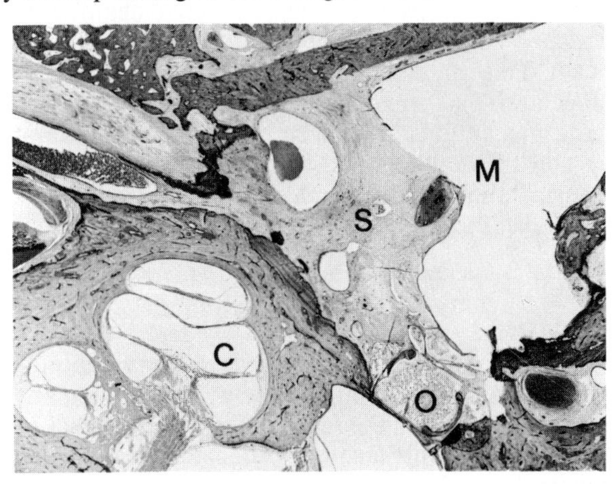

Fig. 96. Adhesive deafness. The middle ear (M) is occupied by scar tissue (S). The oval window (O) is occupied by dense scar tissue which completely envelops the stapes. The cochlea is seen at C. (by courtesy of Professor H. Schuknecht).

Eustachian tube is patent but inflation produces no improvement in hearing and the Rinne remains negative.

Tympanosclerosis is the name given to a somewhat similar disorder in which chalk-like deposits occur in the drum and middle ear mucosa with fixation of the ossicular chain. Sometimes the disorder may take the form of a fibrocystic obliteration of the middle ear cleft.

Tympanotomy can be considered if the sensori-neural reserve is adequate; limited adhesions can sometimes be divided or bypassed using techniques similar to those in tympanoplasty. Occasionally fenestration of the labyrinth is helpful, but the result of operation usually depends on the extent of the damage and is often disappointing. If the deafness is severe enough a hearing aid should be considered.

OTITIC BAROTRAUMA

This can result from any circumstances associated with increasing external pressure such as tunnelling and skin diving, but is seen most frequently after flying. To maintain an equal pressure on both sides of the intact ear drum, a normally functioning Eustachian tube is essential. The movements of swallowing allow the tube to open momentarily, but if patency is disturbed by nasopharyngeal disease (most commonly a cold) then the mechanism may fail.

Ascent, *i.e.* decompression, is generally without discomfort as air can escape readily down the Eustachian tube. On descent, however, especially if rapid, frequent and determined efforts at swallowing or performing the Valsalva manoeuvre may fail to clear the tube. This results in persistence of the low pressure in the middle ear, often with collapse of the drum and an accumulation of fluid. There may be bleeding into the ear. Severe pain and conductive deafness can occur.

The established condition can be relieved rapidly by aerating the middle ear cleft. This can be done either by Eustachian catheterization or by a paracentesis; a formal myringotomy is contraindicated. The strictest sterile precautions should be observed and antibiotic cover provided in view of the likelihood of nasopharyngeal infection. Any local predisposing abnormality should be corrected subsequently.

Exposure to noise incidental to flying can cause hearing changes. See page 318.

OTOSCLEROSIS

This is a progressive disease which as a rule causes symptoms early in adult life. Occasionally it is found in quite young children and it tends to appear more frequently in the female. There are familial tendencies which are transmitted usually through the female side of the family. The deafness may progress almost to total deafness, but in the more severe cases a sensori-neural deafness will be found to have supervened. The condition is commonly bilateral.

Symptoms. Deafness is the chief symptom, but it is frequently accompanied by tinnitus, which may be severe. Giddiness also may occur but is rarely a disability. Characteristically the patient speaks in a quiet voice in sharp contradistinction to the harsh unmodulated tones of those with sensori-neural deafness. Not infrequently patients are conscious that they hear better in a noisy environment. This is known as Paracusis Willisi, and it is marked in early cases. This is due to the fact that otosclerosis blankets ambient noise and when voices are raised to overcome noise the otosclerotic has a comparative advantage. Paracusis may be found in other kinds of conductive deafness but is characteristic of otosclerosis.

Clinical signs. Inspection of the ears usually shows the drums to be normal. Rinne's test is negative and Weber is usually lateralized to the more affected ear. In advanced cases there may be sensori-neural deafness which may be severe and masses of otosclerotic bone have been found in the cochlea. Such deafness can be assessed accurately only by audiometric testing. Its exact cause is unknown.

Pathology. The disease is caused by the laying down of spongy bone of a vascular type around the oval window. New bone may also be formed on the cochlear side of the oval window (Fig. 97). The immediate effect is fixation of the stapes. Diseased bone may also invade the otic capsule around the cochlea. Regarding the origin of otosclerosis, most authorities are agreed that there is a genetic factor. Circulatory defects, endocrine dysfunction and metabolic factors have been blamed, and the association with other bone dyscrasias has suggested the presence of osteoblastic instability, involving the necessary repair of

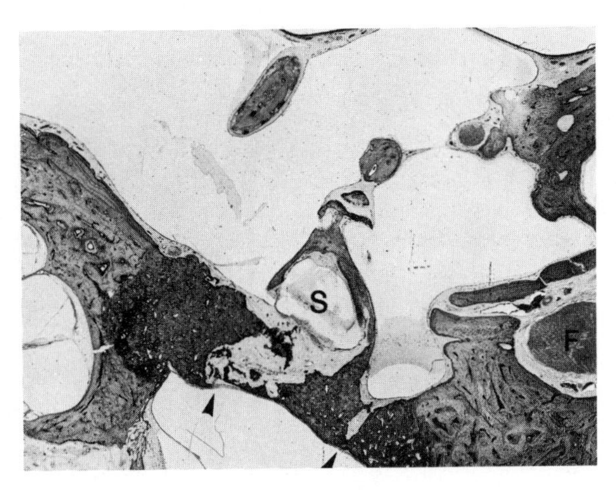

Fig. 97. Otosclerosis. Transverse section of the middle ear at the level of the oval window. The edges of the oval window are arrowed. New bone has grown over this area and entirely immobilised the stapes (S). Note the nearby presence of the facial nerve (F). (By courtesy of Professor H. Schuknecht).

unstable bone. The histological similarities between the various bone defects when undergoing repair has prompted this theory.

Treatment. The first successful surgical treatment was fenestration of the lateral semicircular canal. This operation had a number of disadvantages: it was a major procedure, and it left the patient with all the inconveniences of a mastoid cavity which was not infrequently unstable or infected. It discarded the normal middle ear mechanism and thereby caused a considerable initial loss in hearing, which rendered the operation unsuitable for patients with poor cochlear function. Its main use now is in rare cases of obliteration of the oval window by otosclerosis and some cases of congenital malformation.

The operation of stapedectomy is the modern treatment. Although this operation requires a great deal of skill and experience in microsurgical techniques it is not a serious procedure as far as the patient is concerned. It can be done under either local or general anaesthesia. The drum is elevated and folded forwards and the diagnosis of stapes fixation is confirmed by the use of a suitable probe to palpate the ossicle. There are several forms of this operation. The head neck and crura of the stapes are removed and then the diseased footplate is attacked and the whole of the footplate or a part of it is removed. A suitable prosthesis is then inserted to close the oval window and restore the continuity of the ossicular chain (Fig. 98).

Various types of prosthesis are available which may be formed from the patient's own tissues or which may be some form of piston of plastic or stainless steel. These pistons have been popular but are now suspect in that they do not provide such a safe seal around the oval

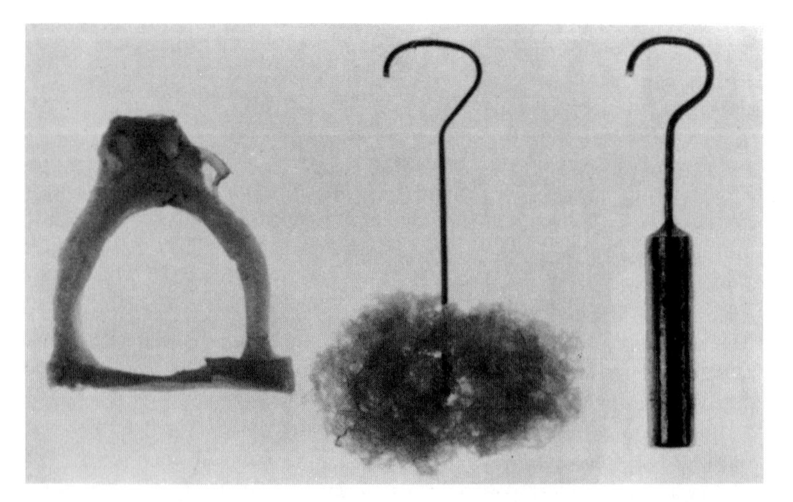

Fig. 98. Otosclerosis. The normal stapes is shown for comparison with two types of prosthesis used after stapedectomy. The hook is used to clamp the prosthesis on to the long processes of the incus.

window. There is therefore a tendency to return to the earlier method of incorporating a fragment of adipose or connective tissue in a stainless steel wire which is fastened over the long process of the incus with the plug of tissue filling the oval window. The piston techniques tend to be reserved for cases of advanced disease where the surgeon is content to drill a hole in a grossly thickened footplate (see fig. 97). These are highly specialized techniques for which the operating microscope is essential.

Perilymph fistula is a complication of stapedectomy which must be mentioned. It occasionally arises as a late complication and is characterized by a sudden fall in hearing; the hearing loss is of sensori-neural type. Some temporary recovery may occur spontaneously, but usually further episodes of sudden impairment occur until eventually a total sensori-neural deafness results. If this complication is recognized early an urgent revision operation is called for in an attempt to salvage whatever hearing remains.

Where stapedectomy is not advisable hearing aids are frequently successful and may enable the sufferer to continue to earn his or her living, or continue to enjoy public gatherings, such as churches, theatres or lectures (p. 321).

Lip reading is a valuable adjunct and should be encouraged in severely deaf patients.

INJURIES

Fractures of the temporal bone

In *longitudinal fracture*, the line runs in the axis of the external meatus. The tympanic ring is broken and the drum and the roof of the meatus torn. There is bleeding from the ear, and deafness is conductive. The laceration is frequently obscured by blood clot and swelling.

In *transverse fracture* the line is antero-posterior. The tympanic ring is spared. The inner ear is often in the line of fracture, so complete loss of function is the rule.

Examination of the tympanum shows a bluish bulging appearance owing to the presence of blood within the middle ear, but the deafness is sensori-neural. In mixed types of fracture dural laceration and C.S.F. otorrhoea may occur.

Facial paralysis can complicate fracture owing to involvement of the nerve at any level.

Treatment. This is generally conservative, the ear should be protected with a sterile dressing and systemic antibiotics given. On no account should the ear be syringed. If infection occurs it is treated on the usual lines but a special watch is maintained for intra-cranial spread, and if a chronic infection is already present it should be eliminated by the appropriate mastoid operation as soon as the patient is sufficiently recovered.

Facial palsy may require surgical treatment, although partial palsy of delayed onset generally recovers well without special attention. Head injuries not sufficiently severe to cause fracture of the temporal bone, or unconsciousness, may cause dislocation of the incus together with, in rare cases, fracture-dislocation of the stapes. Cochlear injury is frequent and its severity varies. Road accidents are responsible for the majority of these cases. Patients may also be seen in whom the dislocation dates from a previous simple mastoid operation. The tympanic membrane in these instances is intact, and the Rinne test is negative. Where the sensori-neural reserve is reasonably good a tympanotomy and examination of the ossicles should be considered.

Prognosis. Conductive deafness usually recovers as the middle ear heals, if not a tympanotomy should be done. In labyrinthine injury the sensori-neural deafness if complete is usually permanent. Less severe cochlear injury may make a partial recovery. As these fractures heal by fibrous union only, there is risk of meningitis should an ear infection occur at a later date.

TUMOURS

Glomus tumours occur but are rare. They are chemodectomas and arise from chemo-receptors in the adventitia of certain blood vessels, including the jugular bulb. They produce pulsating tinnitus owing to their great vascularity and may be seen as a red, pulsating, cherry-like swelling behind an intact drum. Although, clinically, they may be classed as benign tumours, they present serious problems in treatment, particularly if they are large, on account of their vascularity.

Carcinoma also may occur in the ear. It is usually a complication of many years of uncontrolled suppuration, either in the ear or following persistent discharge from a mastoid cavity. The onset of pain is the symptom which usually causes the patient to seek advice. Irradiation and surgery combined is the usual treatment but is often disappointing, though in certain cases radical excision of the petrous bone can cure even when previous radiotherapy and surgery have failed to control the disease.

39. Sensori-neural Deafness and Hearing Aids

As already indicated on page 225, the nomenclature is confused. The synonyms are often inaccurately applied. Sensori-neural deafness can be recognized by the fact that the patient is deaf, but on tuning-fork testing air-conduction remains better than bone conduction, and the latter may be shortened. Audiometrically, it is usually found that the loss is most severe in the high frequencies. Special tests are necessary to distinguish between a lesion of the sensory apparatus (*i.e.* the cochlea) and a neural lesion (*i.e.* a lesion of the eighth nerve, the spiral ganglion and its connections). These two types of deafness can also be accurately referred to as cochlear and retro-cochlear respectively. Other labels are best avoided.

The causes of sensori-neural deafness are many and are difficult to classify. The degenerative changes at work may arise from local or systemic, bacterial or viral infection, local injury or noise injury, toxic drugs, genetic factors, or ageing processes, as well as from other disorders affecting the internal ear and eighth nerve structures. In some patients the aetiology cannot be determined. The following types of sensori-neural hearing loss may be encountered.

TYPES OF SENSORI-NEURAL DEAFNESS

Presbyacusis

The deterioration of hearing which occurs with increasing age is so well known that it may be regarded as a normal process; beyond the age of sixty-five or seventy it does not occasion remark. There is, however, great variation in age of onset and severity. In common with other types of sensori-neural deafness the abnormality generally involves the important upper frequencies first. Histo-pathological studies of the cochlea suggest that there are various types of presbyacusis, which affect the organ of Corti, the spiral ganglion or the stria vascularis. The degenerative processes, however, probably extend all the way up to the cerebral cortex so that the anatomical and physiological defect is one of great complexity.

Toxic deafness

Deafness occasionally complicates certain virus infections such as mumps and influenza. The exact mechanism is unknown. The deafness is as a rule severe and permanent. Recent serological studies indicate that the virus disease may not be manifest clinically, but the viral labyrinthitis produces haircell damage in the organ of Corti.

Drug ototoxicity

Drugs can damage either the hair cells or the neural elements. Quinine and salicylates produce deafness which is reversible in its earlier stages. Streptomycin has been responsible for many cases of severe deafness, and careful watch must be kept for toxic effects remembering that streptomycin generally attacks the vestibular apparatus first. Kanamycin can also produce severe cochlear injury. The dosage required to cause damage is variable, but idiosyncrasy to drugs can cause injury with comparatively small dosage. The dangers are especially great if excretion is impaired as in renal disease.

Acoustic injury

This results from excessive sound stimulation. It may occur from either a sudden exposure, *e.g.* blast, or from prolonged exposure, to loud noise, as occurs in certain occupations. The disorder has long been recognized in bell-ringers and boilermakers, and is now an important hazard in many industries.

There is great individual variation in susceptibility to injury, and the lesion is essentially one of hair-cell loss in the organ of Corti; the deafness is accordingly of sensory type. Audiometric examination shows the earliest change to be at about 4,000 cycles. There is often a well-marked 'notch' at this frequency which is characteristic and disappears as the condition deteriorates and involves all the higher frequencies.

The earliest complaint may be tinnitus, and a feeling of 'cotton wool' in the ear. Only later, as the speech range is affected, does the patient complain of actual hearing loss.

There is no specific treatment, though some recovery may occur if the patient can avoid further exposure. Prophylaxis is important, though workers generally discard the special ear-muffs provided for their protection.

Concussion deafness

The labyrinth can be injured by a blow to the head insufficient to cause unconsciousness or fracture; sometimes the blow may be quite trivial. The deafness is more severe in the high frequencies and any loss persisting after six months must be regarded as permanent.

In some cases displacement of the ossicles may be found. The incus is the ossicle most frequently damaged, and replacement or other procedure may produce a dramatic relief of the associated conductive loss.

Syphilis of the ear

The *congenital* form is the result of intra-uterine disease and may result in a deaf-born child, though the deafness may not develop till the child is ten to fourteen years old. The condition is a neuro-labyrinthitis, consisting of a sensori-neural deafness with diminished vestibular function. Other stigmata such as keratitis and peg-teeth are usual.

In the *acquired* form, secondary syphilis can occasionally produce otitis media. The tertiary disease is again a neurolabyrinthitis and may be associated with attacks of vertigo and tinnitus, hearing worsening with repeated episodes.

Treatment is that of syphilis generally; it is unsatisfactory and of itself can cause an aggravation of vertigo and deafness.

Psychogenic deafness

Owing to its frequency in wartime this form of deafness has received much attention. It is due to emotional trauma and is unaccompanied by any changes in the ear.

The difficulties in diagnosis are considerable, but it is generally found that although the cochlea appears to be non-functioning, the vestibule is normal. Such a state of affairs should always arouse suspicion of psychogenic deafness. The condition must not be confused with malingering, and treatment should be given by those accustomed to dealing with psychological problems. The fact that possible compensation often confuses the situation makes diagnosis and management difficult.

TREATMENT OF SENSORI-NEURAL DEAFNESS

Any co-existing or causative condition must be sought and dealt with where possible. Unfortunately, it is rarely that any hearing improvement can be expected except in the case of psychogenic deafness and occasionally in Menière's disease. Slight fluctuation in the level of hearing is not uncommon, especially in presbyacusis, and it is tempting to attribute any improvement to vitamins, vasodilators or tonics that may have been tried. Old people are often aware that their presbyacusis is worse when they are unwell or over-tired and, accordingly, explanation and advice may be helpful. The difficulties in presbyacusis are always aggravated by upper respiratory infections, and such infections should be treated actively. In many patients a hearing aid will be necessary. Hearing therapy, lip-reading and speech therapy are also valuable in selected cases.

TINNITUS

Tinnitus means sensation of sound in the absence of a normal stimulus. Occasionally it results from a foreign body or wax impacted against the drum. Sometimes it is associated with middle ear disease, *e.g.* infection, which can be controlled. Usually the complaint is of buzzing and ringing and is associated with sensori-neural deafness; this is extremely distressing and highly resistant to treatment. Although it can occur with any type of sensori-neural deafness, tinnitus is usually at its worst in presbyacusis. Very occasionally alcohol, tobacco or aspirin are found to be aggravating the trouble. Phenobarbitone, nicotinic acid and vitamins are often prescribed but seldom help. Operative measures give no relief.

In 'objective tinnitus' a careful observer can hear the offending noise. This may occur for example with aneurysms, vascular tumours *e.g.* glomus, temporo-mandibular joint disturbance, and in myoclonus of the palatal muscles; the treatment is that of the cause if it can be found.

SENSORI-NEURAL DEAFNESS IN CHILDREN

In the examination of a deaf child it is essential to recognize and exclude such conditions as adenoids or 'glue' ear (p. 267) before coming to a diagnosis of sensori-neural hearing loss. It is also important to recognize that a child with sensori-neural hearing loss may suffer from such conditions, or may develop them at any time and require treatment. When this happens a relatively mild loss becomes severe until the middle ear condition is treated. Psychological mal-development and mental retardation may play a part. Poor eyesight may add to the problems of some deaf children.

If a child cannot hear properly then speech cannot develop normally; therefore if speech development is delayed it is of prime importance that hearing should be tested as early as possible. Normally at twelve months the child should be able to localize familiar sounds, by the age of two he should understand simple commands and begin to put words together. Children in the following 'at risk' groups should be followed up with special care.

1. Known hereditary familial defects, *e.g.* various types of cochlear malformations, atresia.
2. Pregnancy damage, *e.g.* rubella, Rh incompatibility, syphilis, drug injury.
3. Perinatal damage, *e.g.* by anoxia, traumatic labour, fits.
4. Certain illnesses can produce severe hearing damage at any age, *e.g.* measles, mumps, meningitis, otitis, mastoiditis, and if they occur early they will also interfere with speech development.
5. Finally, even when none of these factors operate but the mother is simply suspicious of a hearing defect, *e.g.* if the child seems 'inattentive', careful assessment is just as essential.

In many children with sensori-neural deafness there is no obvious cause. The hearing loss unfortunately is greatest in the important mid-

and upper-frequencies and indeed in many children the hearing loss is sub-total for the speech frequencies so that the only island of hearing that remains is in the lower part of the frequency scale. Even in these children, however, such islands of hearings can be used, especially if the diagnosis is made early.

The best results are obtained if the deafness is recognized in the first year of life; after this the difficulties are more complex and the child has lost that special readiness to listen and recognize the meaning of sound which characterizes the first two years of life. Hearing aids must therefore be fitted, and special training of the residual hearing begun as soon as the diagnosis is made. With improving methods of education of the deaf, an increasing number learn satisfactory speech, and a high proportion can now be integrated into ordinary schools, though for certain subjects special classes have to be provided for them. Lip-reading is valuable in helping these children maintain their place in the community.

Finger-spelling has less use in the ordinary community and correspondingly now receives less emphasis.

HEARING AIDS

Patients with a conductive type hearing loss can often be improved surgically, alternatively conductive type hearing loss is easily helped by means of a hearing aid. For patients with sensori-neural hearing loss operation is not possible and relief by means of a hearing aid is acoustically much more difficult.

Non-electrical aids. Auricles, trumpets and speaking tubes still have an occasional use, especially in severe sensori-neural deafness in the elderly. These instruments have the advantages of introducing little distortion, and background noise is not troublesome, but they are very conspicuous.

Electrical hearing aids. The replacement of the valve by the transistor has resulted in the progressive miniaturisation of electrical aids so that aids can now be worn around the ear itself (i.e. 'ear-level' aids) rather than at 'body-level'. Indeed, miniaturisation has advanced to such an extent that patients with a less severe hearing loss can now be given sufficient help from an instrument which is accommodated entirely in the auditory meatus.

There are two classes of instrument which can be worn at body-level or post-aurally, namely air conduction and bone conduction aids. All aids essentially consist of a microphone, an amplifier and a receiver. The microphone and amplifier are contained in one unit together with the batteries, and in body-level aids these can conveniently be concealed behind the tie, or behind a blouse or shirt with perhaps the grill of the microphone exposed. The standard type is little larger than a match box.

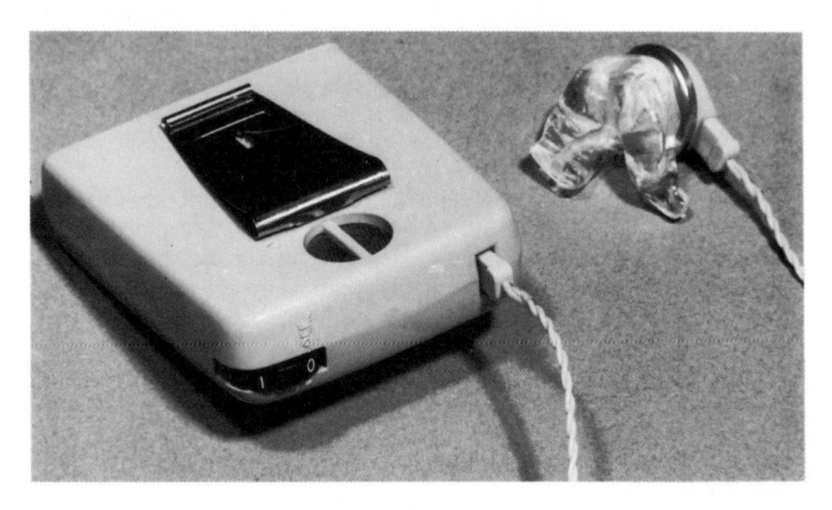

Fig. 99. Air conduction hearing aid. (The Health Service instrument).

In body-level aids a fine wire connects to a receiver which is accommodated in an 'insert' in the case of an air-conduction receiver. This insert is moulded in acrylic after taking a careful impression of the patient's concha and external ear. Whatever the kind of deafness, nearly all patients do better with an air-conduction receiver.

A substantial advance in hearing-aid technology is represented in the 'CROS' hearing aid (contra-lateral routing of signal). In this type of ear-level aid sound coming into the patient's deaf ear is routed across to the other side through fine wires which can be suitably accommodated in spectacles. These instruments are mainly intended for patients with a very great difference between the hearing levels of the two sides,

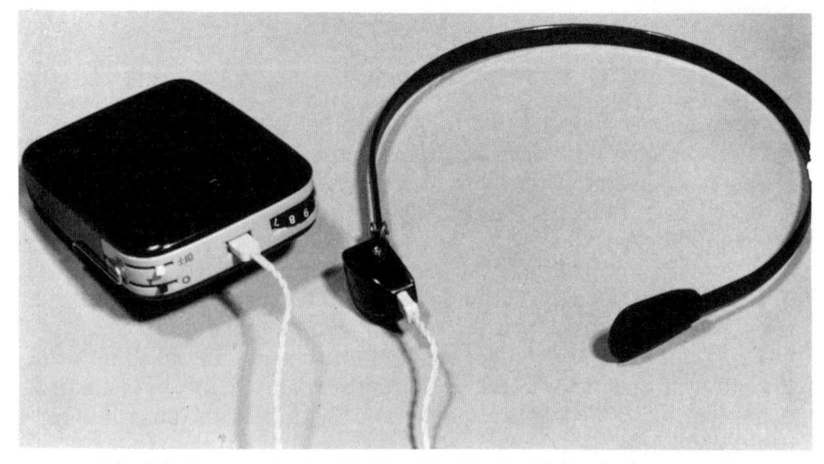

Fig. 100. Bone conduction hearing aid. (The Health Service instrument).

or even for patients with normal hearing on one side and total or sub-total hearing loss on the affected side. In the latter example these aids go a long way towards relieving the 'lop-sidedness' which is often an embarrassment to patients who have only one useful ear.

Bone-conduction is mainly used if there is an intractable external otitis or a stenosis of the meatus. The receiver presses on to the mastoid process behind the ear and is kept in position by a spring head-band.

Air and bone conduction aids are available in the British National Health Service. A complete change-over to ear-level type of instruments is envisaged during the next few years, but apart from school children many patients who wish an ear-level instrument must, at present, purchase them privately. The main advantages of ear-level aids are that they are inconspicuous, there is no interference from clothes rubbing on the microphone or the wire, and sound is received near its normal site. The main disadvantages are their limitation of power and their expense. The smaller commercially produced aids can be built into spectacles, hair slides or the entire unit (*i.e.* microphone, amplifier, receiver and batteries) concealed behind or in the ear. The sound is delivered to the meatus by a fine plastic tube which is maintained in position by a transparent skeleton mould fitting in the concha.

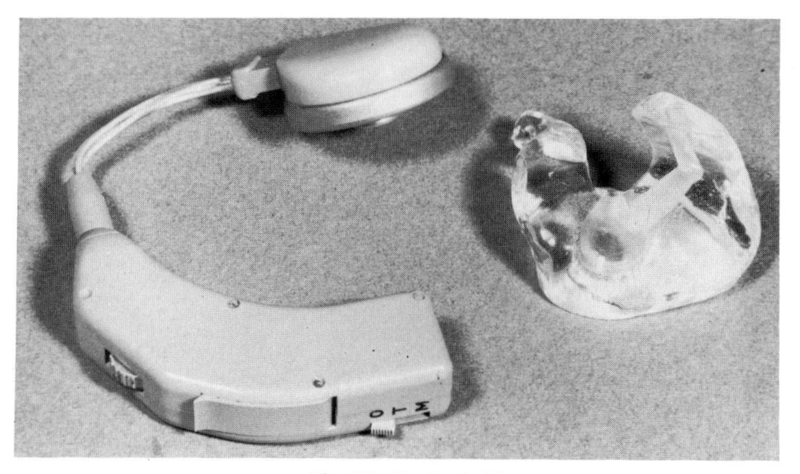

Fig. 101. Ear-level aid.

Perseverance and intelligence are needed to make the fullest use of any aid and this will require close co-operation with the hearing therapist for the very young and the very old particularly. This applies especially in sensori-neural deafness where recruitment is often troublesome and the greatest loss is for the important higher frequency components of speech. Training of residual hearing is invaluable and should whenever possible form part of the hearing aid organization.

Lip reading should always be encouraged.

The doctor recommending an electrical hearing aid must always insist that adequate trial at home, at work, or wherever the intended surroundings may be, forms part of the conditions of purchase, in the case of privately purchased instruments.

40. Vertigo

There are many causes of vertigo, for the symptoms can arise from various organs, including the ear. The ear and eighth nerve system in turn are influenced by other factors, especially circulatory. In the investigation of patients with vertigo, neurology, neuro-surgery and general medicine are involved. It is important that the patient with vertigo should be investigated by the modern methods available to the otologist. A brief account of the various audiometric and vestibular methods of examination has been given in Chapter 29.

Maintenance of satisfactory equilibrium depends upon the co-ordination of information from the various parts of the vestibular labyrinth, muscle, tendon and joint sense receptors, skin pressor receptors, as well as from visual sources. If the information received from any of these sources is at variance with signals coming from other receptors, or if there is interference with co-ordination of information because disease affects the complex connections in the brain stem and cerebellum, then vertigo is experienced. It is interesting to note that vertigo itself is strictly a cortical phenomenon.

A detailed history is of paramount importance in the attempt to reach a diagnosis. Indeed, if a diagnosis is possible the experienced clinician will often base it mainly on the history; subsequent clinical examination and special investigations may only serve to confirm his impression. For example, a somewhat ill-defined dizziness noticeable by an older patient when getting up too quickly is often vascular in origin. Severe vertigo which constantly occurs in a certain head or body position suggests a diagnosis of positional vertigo. Recurring episodes of vertigo which are associated with attacks of distorted hearing and deafness often result from Menière's disease.

Although the history is of such importance it is nevertheless essential that the ear-drums should be examined for any evidence of infection, that tuning-fork tests should be carried out to determine the presence and type of any hearing loss, or any spontaneous and positionally induced nystagmus identified. The systematic examination of the cranial nerves should form part of the routine.

Treatment of vertigo

Even for those patients in whom a precise topographical and pathological diagnosis has been possible it is seldom that specific treatment can be provided. Accordingly, before discussing the various diseases, the following plan of management for the patient suffering from vertigo may be helpful.

1. The patient seen in an acute attack.
   (*a*) Consider if there is need for urgent, surgical treatment (*e.g.* for complications of chronic otitis, or stellate ganglion block in an acute attack of Menière's disease).
   (*b*) If there is no such need suppress the symptoms by the use of prochlorperazine or a similar preparation and treat any cardiovascular or C.N.S. abnormality as appropriate.
2. Patient seen with recurring vertigo or a persistent feeling of vertigo or unsteadiness.
   (*a*) Suppress symptoms with suitable drugs, such as prochlorperazine. Correct any cardiovascular or neurological disturbance where necessary.
   (*b*) Consider if elective surgery may be indicated (*e.g.* in cerebellar tumour, or Menière's disease).

MENIÈRE'S DISEASE

This disease is characterized chiefly by acute vestibular and cochlear symptoms. The former, giddiness and vomiting, are the most disabling, but the deafness and tinnitus can be distressing. At first these attacks occur at long intervals, with increasing severity and frequency. Pathologically an endolymphatic distension occurs which can be extreme; the cause is uncertain.

The differential diagnosis of Menière's disease is often difficult. Other forms of vertigo from middle or internal ear disease, neurological and ischaemic disorders and functional states have to be considered.

Symptoms. The outstanding feature of the disease is sudden giddiness usually accompanied by vomiting, which may be of such severity as to leave the patient helpless. The attack lasts for a number of hours or days and passes off completely leaving the patient normal. Tinnitus, referred to the affected ear, precedes or accompanies the vertigo. The giddiness may have a rotatory character, but in many cases there is no definite direction of rotation. Nystagmus is observed during the attack; deafness is usual and is of sensori-neural type, and may be severe during or just after the attack. In the earlier stages it passes off completely and the hearing returns to normal, but as attacks become more frequent the deafness tends to remain and finally complete loss of hearing results. The suddenness of the attacks is one of the most characteristic features of the disease.

Another feature of the attacks is that they may occur during the night or wake the patient early in the morning. Remissions are typical of the disease and they may vary from a few weeks to several years. Sometimes remission may last so long that it seems a spontaneous cure has occurred. Usually the disease is unilateral; bilateral involvement, however, is not uncommon.

Treatment. (1) *The acute attack*. In an acute attack the patient should stay in bed and keep the head still. Injection of phenobarbitone or chlorpromazine in substantial dosage will suppress symptoms.

Stellate ganglion block can cut short an attack dramatically.

(2) *Long-term management*. The long spontaneous remissions which characterize this disorder make it difficult to assess treatment, but it seems that medical treatment, although on an empirical basis, keeps most patients well controlled.

Limitation of salt and fluid as described by Furstenberg is useful; ammonium chloride can replace common salt. Vaso-dilators are also frequently used, *e.g.* nicotinic acid at least 300 mg daily by mouth. Alternatives are buphenine and tolazine. These measures have been presumed to promote normal endolymph production; it is essential that they be combined with psychological support, strong reassurance and administration of phenobarbitone or prochlorperazine.

Antihistamine drugs are given, probably because of their association with suppression of travel sickness, and partly because of their sedative effect. Ergot preparations can be tried if migrainous symptoms are present.

If medical treatment has failed surgery should be considered.

If hearing in the ear is poor and the opposite side is healthy, the labyrinth can be destroyed. This can be done by disrupting the membranous labyrinth and injecting alcohol, either by a mastoid approach with fenestration of the lateral semicircular canal or by elevating the drum permeatally and working through the oval and round windows. These operations are followed by acute labyrinthine vertigo; remedial exercises are helpful until compensation occurs.

If hearing is still at a useful level in the ear, or if there is any question of the other ear being abnormal, then a selective destruction of the vestibular labyrinth by ultrasound should be considered. The ultrasound is delivered by direct application of the special probe to the lateral semicircular canal utilizing a Schwartze approach. Hearing is usually retained at its pre-operative level and disturbance is minimal.

The operation of vestibular neurectomy may save the hearing. In this procedure a middle fossa approach is used to provide access to the internal auditory meatus by drilling away the overlying part of the petrous bone. Alternatively, hearing may also be preserved by decompression of the saccus endolymphaticus as it lies on the posterior surface of the petrous bone. Good results are claimed for both types of operation.

Mention should also be made of cervical sympathectomy, which is mainly of use in the earlier stages of the disease, and of streptomycin therapy. In the latter, the bilateral vestibulotoxic effect of the drug is utilized. This method is not without danger to the cochlea.

BENIGN POSITIONAL VERTIGO

In this disorder vertigo occurs in a particular head position. It may follow a head injury or there may be no evident cause. The characteristic fatigueable nystagmus can be elicited by the postural tests described in Chapter 29. The symptoms result from a lesion of the crista of the posterior semicircular canal. This must be differentiated from the important central type of the disorder. Hearing and caloric tests are normal.

The symptoms generally abate within about three months during which wearing a felt collar will help to prevent the patient turning the head into the critical position.

Treatment is otherwise symptomatic.

VESTIBULAR NEURONITIS

This disease is thought to be of virus origin, possibly following a vague upper respiratory infection, and sometimes occurs in small epidemics. The symptoms and signs are those of acute vestibular failure, cochlear involvement being notably absent.

Treatment is entirely symptomatic while waiting for recovery to occur by compensation. Subsequent caloric testing will frequently fail to elicit a response from the affected ear, though true recovery of function may occur.

LATERAL MEDULLARY SYNDROME

Severe paroxysmal vertigo with vomiting occurs. The diagnosis is usually clarified early by the appearance of other neurological signs resulting from medullary infarction. Deafness will occur if infarction extends beyond the point of entry of the eighth nerve into the brain stem.

DRUG TOXICITY

Streptomycin and its derivatives can destroy vestibular function and produce severe disability. A non-specific effect on the vestibular system can arise from a wide variety of drugs, but generally does not produce a well-defined dizziness. Drugs which are usually to blame are those given for epilepsy, mental depression and hypertension.

PSYCHOGENIC VERTIGO

The neurotic patient usually describes his dizziness in such a vague manner, but in such flowery terms that the diagnosis may be self-evident. The absence of any abnormality on repeated audiometric, vestibular and neurological examination helps towards the diagnosis in doubtful cases. It must be borne in mind, however, that even the best methods of investigation available in modern vertigo clinics may well be too insensitive to detect some abnormalities. Electro-nystagmography will minimize error and avoid labelling as 'neurotic' patients who have an abnormality, even though it cannot be identified precisely. If more sensitive tests were available it is possible that fewer patients would be regarded as neurotic.

EPIDEMIC VERTIGO

The precise nature of this disorder is not known. It usually occurs in otherwise healthy young adults, it may follow an upper respiratory infection and, as the name indicates, it is not unusual to see a number of cases together. The patients may be incapacitated with vertigo and vomiting. Hearing is unaffected; nystagmus is usually present on gazing to either side. If other disorders can be excluded the symptoms may be suppressed by suitable drugs in the expectation of recovery within a few days.

VERTEBRO-BASILAR ISCHAEMIA

The patient is usually elderly and complains of a mild vertigo of varying duration, generally described as a 'swimming' sensation. Frequently it is known that the patient has cardiovascular disease. Although the vertigo can occur at any time it is most troublesome when rising suddenly from a sitting position or on getting out of bed. Bilateral sensori-neural deafness and tinnitus usually co-exist in these elderly patients. Treatment of the underlying cause is often unsatisfactory and suppression of the symptoms by suitable drugs is uncertain. Occasionally a cervical collar is helpful if the symptoms are aggravated by turning the head.

NUCHAL VERTIGO

An ill-defined giddiness occasionally complicates 'whiplash', *i.e.* flexion-extension injuries of the neck. Where matters of legal compensation arise, it can be difficult to exclude functional causes. Dizziness, associated with neck pain, stiff neck or a sub-occipital headache, is sometimes produced by disturbances of the neck and proprioceptive mechanisms. This usually responds to short-wave diathermy and the wearing of a surgical collar.

41. Neural Affections of the Ear

EIGHTH NERVE TUMOUR

This arises in the Schwann cell of the neurilemma sheath of the vestibular nerve. Similar symptoms occur from other tumours in the cerebello-pontine angle. The lesion may be bilateral, especially in neurofibromatosis.

The first symptom is usually a slowly progressive, unilateral deafness which is of sensori-neural type. Recruitment is absent and speech discrimination is severely impaired, indicating a neural rather than a sensory type of lesion. The deafness is generally accompanied by tinnitus which may develop over two or three years or even decades. The slow destruction of the vestibular nerve permits excellent compensation to take place. Accordingly, dizziness is seldom severe, and acute attacks of vertigo are usually absent. Most patients complain merely of a vague unsteadiness or clumsiness in walking. Vertigo of any severity occurs only in a minority of cases although it can occasionally be sufficiently severe to cause confusion with Menière's disease. Only at a later stage do facial nerve involvement and loss of the corneal reflex occur. Symptoms arising from involvement of other cranial nerves or brain-stem pressure are found only in advanced disease.

Improved methods of diagnosis are now rendering recognition possible during the earlier otological stage, rather than in the neurological stage when interference with brain stem and cerebellar function has begun. A raised C.S.F. protein in a patient with a unilateral neural type of deafness is highly significant though again is a very late finding. Studies with contrast media are essential for early diagnosis; enlargement of the internal auditory meatus on plain X-ray films or on tomograms is found only with large tumours.

Treatment is surgical. The optimum time for operation is no longer debated. These tumours should be operated on as soon as diagnosed. It is futile to expect good results from a 'wait and see' policy and to delay operation until major symptoms and massive tumours are present. It is also accepted that the average time interval between the occurrence of comparatively minor symptoms and the development of major neurological disability is only in the order of about three years.

Intra-capsular nucleation of these tumours invites recurrence. Therefore the only justifiable operation is total removal of the tumour using micro-surgical techniques. This is best accomplished through a trans-labyrinthine approach in which the Otologist clears the tumour from the internal auditory meatus and exposes very wide areas of middle fossa and posterior fossa dura. The neuro-surgeon proceeds to remove that part of the tumour lying in the posterior fossa. This may be done at the same operation, or at a second stage a day or two later.

Operations of this kind, although requiring a high degree of surgical skill, are associated with very small mortality and morbidity in comparison with the classical posterior fossa approach; the patient recovers far more quickly, the facial nerve can often be preserved and the operation offers a cure.

FACIAL PARALYSIS

Facial paralysis may be caused by intra-cranial, intra-temporal, or extra-temporal lesions.

Upper motor neurone paralysis is recognised by (*a*) the upper part of the face being spared, (*b*) emotional movements and muscle tone being preserved. These cases belong to the field of the neurologist and so need not be further discussed here.

Intra-cranial lower motor neurone lesions are mostly within the region of the cerebello-pontine angle.

Intra-temporal lesions may occur as a complication of acute or chronic ear disease. Paralysis may be caused also through fracture or operative accident. Other causes are virus diseases, which include herpes zoster oticus (Ramsay Hunt syndrome). Extra temporal causes include trauma, either direct or operative and tumours such as parotid, carcinoma.

The most common kind of lower motor neurone paralysis, however, is Bell's palsy. It is important that the eponym should be used purely for lower motor neurone lesions of idiopathic type and that it should not be used loosely for any other kind of facial paralysis.

The site of the lesion in Bell's palsy is not known, but the evidence suggests that it may be in the internal auditory meatus. The condition must only be diagnosed when all other types of facial palsy have been excluded.

Diagnosis. It is essential that all patients with a facial palsy are seen by a competent otologist. Otherwise Bell's palsy may be diagnosed when in fact the paralysis is secondary to disease in or around the temporal bone which requires treatment. Tumours and cholesteatomata sometimes present with this symptom.

Having made a routine examination of the ear it is necessary to decide upon the level of the lesion. The effects on the chorda tympani, stapedius muscle and tear secretion give useful clues.

It is also necessary to decide whether the paralysis is a non-degenerative (*i.e.* a neuropraxia) or a degenerative one. For this, various electrical tests of conductivity and excitability are necessary.

Treatment. If paralysis occurs in the course of a chronic otitis or follows operation for this, immediate exposure and examination are necessary.

On the other hand the surgeon will save himself a great deal of anxiety if he makes a practice of examining the facial movement at the end of every ear operation. Should paralysis occur within a short period after conclusion of the operation, provided alar or other facial movement has been verified nothing more need be done unless the surgeon has some suspicion that he was working in dangerous proximity to the nerve, when perfect control was difficult. Any tight packs in the ear should be loosened and nerve conductivity tests should be repeated daily and if degeneration threatens the nerve should be explored.

In the case of Bell's palsy no special treatment is required as long as the weakness is only partial, but if it becomes complete (and certainly if degeneration threatens) prednisolone should be given without delay. The evidence indicates that the risk of denervation with consequent delayed and incomplete recovery can be significantly reduced by such treatment.

The chief problem in Bell's palsy is to decide when to decompress the swollen nerve in its bony canal and when to refrain. It can be said with certainty that in a non-degenerative lesion this is not necessary. Excellent recovery can be expected early, with or without massage, electrical therapy, etc.

The selection of patients with degenerative lesions, suitable for decompression is difficult. All cases of nerve degeneration recover slowly and often incompletely. Because of this incomplete or unsatisfactory recovery, urgent decompression is recommended by some otologists as soon as degeneration is diagnosed by daily conductivity tests. In skilled hands this may produce some benefit and cannot do harm. Decompression of the nerve may allow some fibres to survive which otherwise would not have done so, and more satisfactory conditions are provided to encourage normal re-generation. Comparative series of cases are few and there is as yet no definite statistical evidence to show that decompression produces any better results than inactivity.

HERPES ZOSTER OTICUS

Herpes oticus, or Ramsey Hunt syndrome, is probably due to the chickenpox virus. It affects the geniculate and other cranial nerve ganglia.

As is usual in inflammation of posterior root ganglia, one of the chief symptoms is herpes, which involves the external auditory meatus and the auricle. The seventh and eighth nerves are those most frequently involved, but other nerves may be affected.

Symptoms of herpes and facial paralysis are referable to the seventh nerve involvement and vomiting, giddiness, nystagmus and deafness are referable to the eighth nerve.

Treatment is palliative, the herpetic pain should be relieved with the usual remedies and the condition allowed to settle spontaneously. The value of surgical decompression of the nerve in those patients whose conductivity tests indicate impending degeneration is still a matter of argument.

42. Chemotherapy

ANTIBIOTICS

The penicillins are virtually non-toxic, though dangerous allergic reactions can result from sensitization. They are chiefly effective against cocci and gram-positive organisms. Penicillins diffuse readily into tissue fluids except for the cerebro-spinal fluid (but will cross the inflamed meninges). The majority of acute ear, nose and throat infections remain responsive to penicillin in proper dosage. If a satisfactory response is obtained therapy generally continues for about six days, but if the response is poor after two or three days, or if an unsatisfactory bacteriological report is received, a change of antibiotic is indicated.

Benzyl-penicillin must be given by injection. The usual dose is 500,000 units (300 mg) six-hourly. In less severe infections a daily injection of procaine penicillin can follow the loading dose or, alternatively, an oral preparation such as Phenoxymethylpenicillin can be used.

Cloxacillin and methicillin should be used only for staphylococcal infections which have been shown to be resistant to other penicillins. In severe illness they can be given by injections, although cloxacillin is also effective by mouth.

Ampicillin is similarly acid-resistant and so can be given orally; although covering a broad spectrum of organisms it is destroyed by staphylococcal penicillinase. It is a useful antibiotic in those infections which are suspected to be due to haemophilus influenzae. The usual adult dose is 1 to 4 g daily in divided doses given by mouth for five to six days.

Streptomycin has limited use in otolaryngology but is sometimes useful against penicillin-resistant or gram-negative organisms. Given with penicillin, the drugs are synergie. Except in tuberculosis the course should not exceed 1 g daily for five days, and its ototoxicity is a hazard.

Tetracycline and oxytetracycline are mainly used for infections which do not respond to sulphonamides or penicillin. 250 mg q.i.d. is the standard adult dose, and is given orally for five days. The effect of these antibiotics on the intestinal flora can produce severe bowel complications.

Erythromycin has a range similar to penicillin and is useful against penicillin-resistant organisms or for patients with penicillin sensitivity. It is given orally.

Nystatin is valuable in the local treatment of fungus infections of the ear and upper alimentary tract. This drug is poorly absorbed from the intestinal tract and is too toxic for parenteral use. Other fungicides can be used such as amphetericin B.

Neomycin, Polymycin, Bacitracin and Gramicidin applied locally in external otitis are valuable, and as their systemic use is limited by their toxicity they are the antibiotics of choice for topical application. They should nevertheless be applied in combination with a steroid.

It will be appreciated that this account of individual drugs is far from exhaustive but is intended only to emphasize the most important points as they apply to E.N.T. practice. For further information on new developments reference should be made to the current literature.

CHEMOTHERAPY OF CANCER

Reference has already been made (p. 91) to the use of cytotoxic drugs in the treatment of cancer of the upper jaw and nasopharynx, and it is recognized that the place of this form of treatment is not yet fully evaluated in malignant disease of the head and neck. Up to the present it has been used most often as a palliative, especially for the relief of pain. It seems possible that in the future, with increasing knowledge and the development of new agents, the main use of these drugs may be in association with radiotherapy as an initial form of treatment in preparation for planned surgery. Progress, however, remains disappointingly slow.

The drugs fall into various groups, the most frequently used at present being the anti-metabolites and the radiomimetic drugs, the action of which is indicated by their names. Certain antibiotics also have an anti-mitotic action. Other drugs arrest cell-division in the stage of metaphase and are known as metaphase-inhibitors.

The majority of these drugs are highly toxic to all dividing cells and can produce dangerous suppression of the bone marrow. In order to obtain the maximum local effect, therefore, these agents are often given by intra-arterial perfusion. The anatomical arrangement of the external carotid system makes head and neck cancers particularly suited to continuous perfusion by means of an indwelling catheter in the external carotid artery through its superior thyroid or superficial temporal branches. The position of the catheter is adjusted as necessary after injecting a dye such as methylene blue until the desired area is shown to be satisfactorily perfused. Infusion of the selected agent is then begun.

The best methods of administration and dosage are not yet agreed. In the case of antimetabolites such as methotraxate, a continuous intra-arterial infusion is probably the best method. With radiomimetic drugs, many of which have half-lives of a few minutes only, intermittent intra-arterial injection is preferable. These drugs are highly reactive and it is important that the injection should be confined to those branches of the carotid which supply the tumour. In other programmes of treatment drugs may be given by a series of intravenous injections, or they may be given by mouth, especially when the patient is on a maintenance dose.

It is essential to examine the blood count each day whatever type of drug is chosen and to adjust treatment according to the white blood count. In spite of continuing pharmacological research, marrow suppression continues to be a problem which is inseparable from the use of many cytotoxic agents. Bleomycin is an important exception to this statement and is particularly valuable in producing regression of squamous cell carcinomas. Toxic side-effects continue to be a very serious problem in this type of treatment and the patient's condition can very easily be worsened.

Appendix

INSTRUCTIONS FOR THE PREPARATION OF PATIENTS FOR OPERATION

The same precaution should be observed in the preparation of ear, nose and throat patients as in the preparation of any surgical case.

Nasal Cases. Wherever possible the patients should be clean shaved or clipped closely. In the event of patients being unwilling to lose their moustaches, these must be washed and rendered aseptic. Mouthwashes should be given before preparing the nose. Many nasal operations can be done satisfactorily with suitable pre-medication combined with local anaesthesia, but even when general anaesthesia is used the nose should still be prepared with cocaine and adrenalin in order to reduce vascularity and shrink down the mucosa.

The nose is first sprayed with 1 to 2 ml of 5 per cent cocaine. If the nose is to be packed it must be done by someone accustomed to working within the nose using a good headlight. Packing must be carried out 30 minutes before the patient is required in the operating theatre. A long strip of gauze is used in each side of the nose, the gauze having been soaked and wrung out in a mixture of 4 ml each of 10 per cent cocaine and 1 in 1,000 adrenalin.

As an alternative, 25 per cent cocaine paste can be used. This is smeared on the mucous membrane with cotton-tipped applicators. There are various other methods, but the packing method can be relied upon for satisfactory results and when properly carried out has no permanent ill effects upon the nasal mucous membrane.

Block anaesthesia can be achieved by placing dressed probes moistened with a strong solution of cocaine, one over the spheno-palatine foramen and one over the point of emergence of the anterior ethmoidal nerve in the roof of the nose. It is important to remember that this method must not be used after shrinking the nasal mucous membrane by weaker solutions as described, otherwise cocained intoxication may result, with grave danger to the patient.

Accessory sinus cases should be prepared in the same way.

Aural cases. A gauze strip soaked in adrenalin and cocaine reduces vascularity prior to removing polyps or granulations.

Endoscopy cases. The patient is given an injection of atropine and pethedine an hour before operation. Endoscopic examination is usually done under general anaesthesia, but for examination under local anaesthesia the throat is sprayed with 1 to 2 ml of 10% cocaine. The mouth should be cleaned with mouthwash before spraying.

The tongue is first sprayed, then held down, while the epiglottis and pharynx are sprayed.

As an alternative to spraying, the patient can be given an anaesthetic lozenge to suck twenty minutes before the examination.

A Jackson cross-action forceps is then used to hold a small swab soaked in 20 per cent cocaine in the pyriform fossa. This gives block anaesthesia of both superior laryngeal nerves and so causes complete anaesthesia of the larynx. Where possible, the larynx should also be sprayed with cocaine.

NOTES ON LOCAL ANAESTHESIA

Cocaine is an excellent topical anaesthetic for mucous membranes but produces very dangerous toxic effects if absorbed or injected. The use of cocaine is governed by rules regarding concentration and amount. The duration of application is also of importance and these points are dealt with above. Cocaine is especially valuable in nasal surgery, for in addition to its anaesthetic action is produces profound local vasoconstriction and retraction of the soft tissues. These effects are assisted by adding adrenalin.

The symptoms of cocaine poisoning or sensitivity are confusing. Excitation and depression can occur, so that any abnormal sign in a patient being anaesthetized with cocaine must be heeded. Initial excitation may be followed by pallor, sweating and faintness. Unconsciousness and convulsions may precede respiratory arrest and death. Cocaine can be highly dangerous by injection; it is therefore a good rule never to allow cocaine into a syringe.

If a cocaine reaction occurs, the patient should be laid flat and kept warm, and a stimulant such as caffein may be needed. Convulsions may occur and should be treated with barbiturates.

Lignocaine hydrochloride in a concentration of 2 to 4 per cent is useful as a topical anaesthetic but lacks the vascoconstrictor and tissue-retracting effects of cocaine; addition of adrenalin or ephedrine is therefore essential. Lignocaine can be used by injection.

Procaine hydrochloride has no effect as a surface application but is valuable for infiltration on account of its low toxicity. Up to 200 ml of $\frac{1}{2}$ per cent solution can be used. If adrenalin is added its final concentration must not exceed 1 in 200,000.

FORMULAE

OINTMENTS—

Mercuric oxide ointment

℞ Yellow mercuric oxide ... 1 per cent.
Liquid paraffin ... ... q.s.
Soft paraffin ... ... to 100 per cent.

Ichthammol ointment

℞	Ichthammol	10 per cent.
	Wool fat	45 per cent.
	Soft paraffin	45 per cent.

These ointments are useful in dermatitis or eczema occurring round the nasal vestibule or the ear.

Also useful are:

℞	Neomycin	0.5 per cent.
	Fluociniline ointment (0.025 per cent B.P.C.) ...	to 100 per cent.

Beta-methasone valerate ointment B.N.F.

℞ (0.1 per cent in a bland base)

These can be supplied after bathing the area in Cetamide solution B.P.C. (Cetavlon).

LOTIONS –

Solution of ichthyol in water, 30 per cent, is useful in cases of streptococcal dermatitis of the nasal vestibule.

The nose

INHALATIONS –

℞ Menthol. Two crystals are placed in a jug half-filled with hot water just off the boil, and the steam is inhaled. The strength of the solution is maintained by addition of crystals as required. The patient must be warned not to expose himself to cold air for one to two hours after inhalation.

℞	Menthol	2 per cent.
	Benzoin inhalation B.P.C. ...	to 100 per cent.

Fifteen to twenty drops are placed in hot water and used as an inhalation. This inhalation is useful in rhinitis and Eustachian catarrh.

℞ *Compound tincture of benzoin*

Thirty drops of the tincture are placed in hot water and used as an inhalation. This inhalation is useful in laryngitis and bronchitis.

Ephedrin nasal drops

℞	Ephedrin hydrochloride ...	1 per cent.
	Sodium chloride	0.5 per cent.
	Chlorbutol	0.5 per cent.
	Water	to 100 per cent.

SPRAYS –

℞		
℞	Menthol	0.5 per cent.
	Camphor	2 per cent.
	Liquid paraffin	to 100 per cent.

This is useful in rhinitis.

DOUCHES –

℞		
℞	Sodium bicarbonate ...	25 per cent.
	Sodium biborate	25 per cent.
	Sodium chloride	50 per cent.

Half a teaspoonful of the powder is dissolved in a cup of warm water.

The ear

EAR DROPS –

℞		
℞	Phenol glycerin	37 per cent.
	Glycerin	100 per cent.

N.B. – These drops are caustic if diluted with water.

Four to five drops are poured into the ear.

℞		
℞	Phenol glycerin	37 per cent.
	Cocaine hydrochloride ...	37 per cent.
	Glycerin	to 100 per cent.

N.B. – These drops are caustic if diluted with water.
Four to five drops are poured into the ear.
These drops are useful for the relief of pain in acute otitis media.

℞		
℞	Boric acid	2 per cent.
	Industrial methylated spirit	20 per cent.
	Water	to 100 per cent.

Six to ten drops are instilled into the ear once or twice daily to aid drying up of the discharge in chronic otitis media.

℞		
℞	Sodium bicarbonate ...	5 per cent.
	Glycerin	35 per cent.
	Water	to 100 per cent.

This is used to soften wax in the ear. Warm olive oil is also effective.

Bonain's drops –

℞		
℞	Menthol. ...	equal parts
	Acid. carbol. ...	
	Cocaine. hydrochlor.	

Blegvad's drops—

℞	Cocaine. hydrochlor.	
	Acid. salicyl.	*aa* 4 g.
	Spirit. rect.	4 ml.

Used to obtain anaesthesia of the ear-drum by the placing of pledgets of wool soaked in the solution against the drum.

PACKINGS—

℞	Solution of aluminium acetate	8 per cent.
℞	Ichthammol in glycerin ...	10 per cent.

INSUFFLATIONS—

℞	Iodine	0.75 per cent.
	Boric acid	to 100 per cent.

The throat

PAINTS—

Mandl's paint—

℞	Iodine	1 per cent.
	Potassium iodide	5 per cent.
	Peppermint oil	1 per cent.
	Glycerin	to 100 per cent.

Used as a paint in chronic pharyngitis.

℞	Tannic acid	5.5 per cent.
	Glycerin	to 100 per cent.

An astringent paint, useful in chronic pharyngitis.

GARGLES—

Potassium chlorate and phenol gargle

℞	Potassium chlorate ...	3.5 per cent.
	Liquified phenol	1.5 per cent.
	Sulphan blue solution ...	1.5 per cent.
	Water	to 100 per cent.

To be diluted to one tablespoonful in half a glass of warm water.

℞	Hydrogen peroxide ...	10 vols.

Dilute with an equal quantity of water.

℞	Mist A.P.C.	
	Acetyl-salicyl.	300 mg
	Phenacetin	300 mg
	Caffein Citrate	150 mg
	Pulv. Trag. Co	200 mg
	Syrup	2 ml.
	Chloroform water to 10 ml.	

Disguise in Blackcurrant juice or similar e.g. 'Ribena'.

Index

U

V

W

X

APPENDIX